ADVANCES IN EQUINE NUTRITION IV

Advances in Equine Nutrition IV

Edited by Joe D. Pagan Ph.D.
Kentucky Equine Research, Versailles, Kentucky, USA

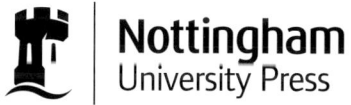

Nottingham University Press
Manor Farm, Main Street, Thrumpton
Nottingham, NG11 0AX, United Kingdom
www.nup.com

NOTTINGHAM

First published 2009
© Kentucky Equine Research Inc. 2009

All rights reserved. No part of this publication
may be reproduced in any material form
(including photocopying or storing in any
medium by electronic means and whether or not
transiently or incidentally to some other use of
this publication) without the written permission
of the copyright holder except in accordance with
the provisions of the Copyright, Designs and
Patents Act 1988. Applications for the copyright
holder's written permission to reproduce any part
of this publication should be addressed to the publishers.

British Library Cataloguing in Publication Data
Advances in Equine Nutrition IV
Pagan, J.D.

ISBN 978-1-904761-87-7

Disclaimer

Every reasonable effort has been made to ensure that the material in this book is true, correct, complete and appropriate at the time of writing. Nevertheless, the publishers and authors do not accept responsibility for any omission or error, or for any injury, damage, loss or financial consequences arising from the use of the book.

Typeset by Nottingham University Press, Nottingham
Printed and bound by the Charlesworth Group, Wakefield

CONTENTS

General Nutrition

Nutrient Requirements: Applying the Science 1
   J.D. Pagan

Making Nutrient Composition Tables Relevant 7
   P.K. Sirois

Forages: The Foundation for Equine Gastrointestinal Health 17
   J.D. Pagan

Grazing Preferences of Horses for Different Cool-Season Grasses 25
   J. Ringler, B. Cassill, S. Hayes, J. Stine, and L. Lawrence

Carbohydrates in Forage: What is a Safe Grass? 29
   K.A. Watts

Assessing Energy Balance 43
   L. Lawrence

Beta-Carotene: An Essential Nutrient for Horses? 51
   E. Kane

Vitamin E: An Essential Nutrient for Horses? 61
   E. Kane

Equine Behavior: A Nutritional Link? 77
   C. McCall

Nutrition and Management of the Performance Horse

The Efficiency of Utilization of Digestible Energy During Submaximal Exercise 89
   J.D. Pagan, G. Cowley, D. Nash, A. Fitzgerald, L. White, and M. Mohr

Efficacy of an Herbal Feed Supplement in Reducing Exercise-Related
   Stress in Horses 97
   V.E. Wilkins, H.M. Greene, and S.J. Wickler

Update on Bone Disease: The Impact of Skeletal Disease on Athletic Performance ... 101
   C.W. McIlwraith

Nutrition and Management of the Broodmare

The New NRC: Updated Requirements for Pregnancy and Growth 123
  L. Lawrence

Oral Water-Soluble Vitamin E Supplementation of the Mare in Late Gestation,
  Its Effects on Serum Vitamin E Levels in the Pre- and Postpartum Mare
  and the Neonate: A Preliminary Investigation.. 133
  E Drury, T. Whitaker, and L. Palmer

Body Weight and Condition of Kentucky Thoroughbred Mares and Their Foals
  as Influenced by Month of Foaling, Season, and Gender...................................... 137
  J.D. Pagan, C.G. Brown-Douglas, and S. Caddel

The Effect of Dietary Calcium on Indicators of Bone Turnover in Broodmares....... 147
  B. Cassill, S. Hayes, J. Ringler, K. Janicki, and L. Lawrence

Nutrition of the Dam Influences Growth and Development of the Foal.................... 151
  L.A. Lawrence

Nutrition and Management of the Growing Horse

Nutrition of the Young Equine Athlete.. 161
  J.D. Pagan and D. Nash

Development of the Equine Gastrointestinal Tract 173
  L.A. Lawrence and T.J. Lawrence

Skeletal Adaptation During Growth and Development: A Global Research Alliance.. 185
  C.E. Kawcak

Muscle Adaptations During Growth and Early Training 193
  S.J. Valberg and L. Borgia

The Balancing Act of Growing a Sound, Athletic Horse.. 203
  C.G. Brown-Douglas

Body Weight, Wither Height and Growth Rates in Thoroughbreds Raised in
  America, England, Australia, New Zealand and India.. 213
  C.G. Brown-Douglas and J.D. Pagan

Size Matters at the Sales 221
  J.D. Pagan, A. Koch, and S. Caddel

Thoroughbred Growth and Future Racing Performance.. 231
  C.G. Brown-Douglas, J.D. Pagan and A.J. Stromberg

Managing Growth to Produce a Sound, Athletic Horse... 247
  J.D. Pagan and D. Nash

Pathological Conditions

Feeding the Atypical Horse 259
    L. Lawrence and T. Weddington

Nutritional Management of Metabolic Disorders 269
    J.D. Pagan

Pathology of Metabolic-Related Conditions 277
    F.M. Andrews and N. Frank

Recent Research into Laminitis 293
    P. Huntington, C. Pollitt, and C. McGown

Colic Prevalence, Risk Factors and Prevention 313
    N.A. White

Colic Treatment and Post-Colic Nutrition 327
    N. A. White

Overview of Gastric and Colonic Ulcers 347
    F.M. Andrews

Insulin Resistance – What Is It and How Do We Measure It? 355
    S. Valberg and A. Firshman

Exercise-Induced Pulmonary Hemorrhage 367
    K.W. Hinchcliff

Food Allergy in the Horse: A Dermatologist's View 379
    Dawn Logas   379

Beyond the X-Ray: The Latest Methods to Detect and Predict Skeletal Damage 385
    C.W. McIlwraith

Managing the Sick Foal to Produce a Sound Athlete 403
    W. Bernard

Rational Approaches to Equine Parasite Control 411
    C.R. Reinemeyer

Index 421

GENERAL NUTRITION

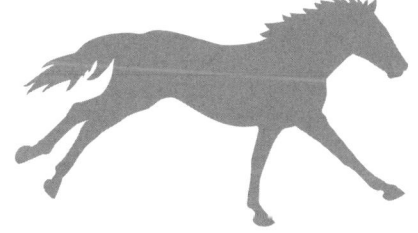

NUTRIENT REQUIREMENTS: APPLYING THE SCIENCE

JOE D. PAGAN
Kentucky Equine Research, Versailles, Kentucky

Introduction

Because the recommendations outlined in the current NRC *Nutrient Requirements of Horses* are based mostly on small controlled studies conducted with horses, ponies, and other species of livestock, it remains unclear how they should be applied to feeding horses under a range of management conditions. How should a feed manufacturer use NRC requirements to formulate horse feed and evaluate nutrient adequacy in rations? This paper will explore how well the NRC requirements fit the real world of horse feeding and will make suggestions about how they can best be utilized by the feed manufacturer.

Requirements or Recommendations?

The most fundamental question that we should ask about the NRC is what do the requirements represent? Are they the levels of nutrients that should be included in a horse's ration or are they the bare minimums required to prevent clinical disease? The 1989 NRC states that its nutrient requirements represent the minimum amounts needed to sustain normal health, production, and performance of horses. It cautions, however, that horses should be fed as individuals and that, when applying the recommendations, consideration should be given to factors such as: 1) digestive and metabolic differences between horses; 2) variation in production and performance capabilities of the animal and expectations of the owner; 3) health status of the animal; 4) variations in the nutrient availability in feed ingredients; 5) interrelationships among nutrients; 6) previous nutritional status of the horse; and 7) climatic and environmental conditions. In other words, the requirements probably shouldn't be strictly followed in real-life feeding situations where any or all of these factors come into play. Unfortunately, the 1989 NRC doesn't provide recommendations to adjust for any of these factors.

It is crucial that we differentiate between nutrient *requirements* and *recommendations* when evaluating the nutrient adequacy of a specific equine ration. Kronfeld (2001) stated that NRC nutrient *requirements* for companion animals are levels that are sufficient to prevent lesions or growth retardation in 50% of animals. Recognizing that the nutrient requirements for dogs and cats have little practical value,

2 Nutrient Requirements: Applying the Science

the Association of American Feed Control Officials (AAFCO) created nutrient profiles for dogs and cats that were about 1.3 to 2 times the corresponding NRC values. In human nutrition, nutrient recommendations are expressed as RDAs (recommended daily allowances) that are two standard deviations above mean minimum requirements, thereby being sufficient for 98% of the population.

Kentucky Equine Research (KER) created its own set of nutrient "requirements" for horses shortly after the publication of the last NRC. These values should more correctly be termed recommendations rather than requirements because they are intended to account for many of the variables that affect nutrient adequacy, which were noted in the current NRC. They do not use a set multiplier of NRC requirements since many of the NRC values are already appropriate as practical recommendations under most management situations. Other KER recommendations are considerably higher than NRC values, while some are lower than the NRC requirement (Table 1). Even though KER's recommendations account for many variables encountered in feeding horses, they are too general to be used in every situation. Therefore, more specific recommendations are under development by KER for different breeds, disciplines, geographic regions, and pathological conditions.

Table 1. KER recommendations as multiples of NRC requirements.

Nutrient	Class of Horse				
	Maintenance	Pregnancy	Lactation	Performance	Growth
Protein	1.1	1.1	1.0	0.75-0.9	1.0
Energy	1.0	1.1	1.0	1.0	1.0
Macrominerals	1.3-2.1	1.1-1.9	1.1-2.3	0.8-1.9	1.3-3.1
Microminerals	1.0-2.3	1.4-2.6	1.4-2.7	1.0-2.4	1.4-2.6
Vitamins	0.9-2.3	0.9-1.8	0.9-2.3	1.0-2.4	0.9-3.6

The NRC provides equations to calculate only eight nutrient requirements (DE, CP, lysine, Ca, P, Mg, K, and vitamin A) using information about the horse's age, body weight, and average daily gain. Requirements for 13 other nutrients (nine minerals and four vitamins) are given as adequate concentrations in total rations for horses. No requirements are listed for seven additional B-complex vitamins or vitamin C, and surprisingly, no requirement is given for chloride except to say "chloride requirements are presumed to be adequate when the sodium requirements are met with sodium chloride." Many of these nutrients are important for different classes of horses and recommendations should be given for them even if concrete experimental data are not available to quantify a requirement. Additionally, there are several other feed constituents that affect the health and well-being of the horse. The 1989 NRC does not provide recommendations about the level of fiber required in the horse's ration other than to offer the rule of thumb that horses should be fed at least 1% of their body weight per day of good-quality roughage or be given access to pasture for sufficient time to consume at least 1% of body weight as dry matter per day. The 1989 NRC discusses different sources of energy for the horse but does not provide recommendations for either safe or optimal levels of each source in the horse's ration. This is an area of prime importance for all classes of horses and should be a major focus of research in the future.

Acceptable Ranges

Only under very artificial experimental conditions will the intake of every nutrient exactly match the recommendation. Some nutrients will exceed recommendations by a large margin, while others might be slightly below. In truth, horses can tolerate and thrive on a range of nutrient intakes. That range, however, can vary tremendously depending on the nutrient and class of horse being fed. For example, potassium intakes are often much higher than required because forages are rich sources of potassium and high forage intakes are desirable for most horses. Energy intakes, on the other hand, must closely match the horse's requirement or the horse will gain or lose weight.

Kronfeld (2001) endorsed setting goals for intakes of energy and nutrients. These goals were not specified as single numbers or requirements, but rather as optimal or target ranges, with upper and lower limits as well as middle values (Figure 1).

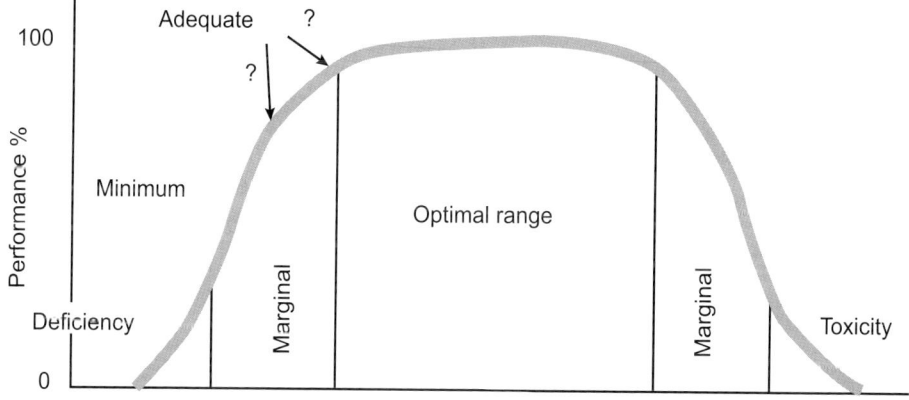

Figure 1. Optimal ranges for nutrient intakes.

KER has adopted this philosophy of assessing nutrient adequacy and has divided levels of nutrient intake into seven ranges as follows:

- *Deficient*: Nutrient intakes in this range will likely result in either the clinical expression of disease or a marked reduction in performance. Additional fortification is absolutely necessary.

- *Underfortified*: Nutrient intakes are marginal and may lead to deficiency symptoms or a drop in performance if the animal is stressed or if inhibitory substances are present in the ration. If practically feasible, the ration should be fortified with this nutrient.
- *Adequate (low range)*: The nutrient intake is below the target range, but under most circumstances should be adequate.
- *Target Range*: This range is very near the RDA for the nutrient, with slight variation to allow for uncertainties related to intake and ingredient composition.
- *Adequate (high range)*: Higher than recommended, but no undesirable effects other than possibly expense.
- *Overfortified*: Higher than required and may lead to problems related to interactions with other nutrients in the ration. If practical, nutrient intake should be reduced.
- *Excessive*: A level of intake that will likely result in toxicity symptoms or a drop in performance. Every effort should be made to reduce the level of intake of this nutrient.

Evaluating Rations

Table 2 and Figures 2 and 3 illustrate how KER recommendations and acceptable ranges can be used to evaluate a ration for a mare in the third trimester of pregnancy. This mare is in a desirable body condition and is gaining weight at an acceptable rate for late pregnancy. She is eating 5 kg of mixed orchard grass/alfalfa hay, 1.5 kg of oats, and 500 g of All-Phase balancer pellet per day. She is also allowed to graze a high-quality pasture during the day. Based on the caloric intake from hay, grain, and supplement, it is estimated that she is consuming 4 kg of pasture dry matter per day.

In Figure 2, daily intakes for each nutrient evaluated are expressed as a percentage of the KER recommendation. These nutrient intakes range from 90% of recommended for zinc (Zn) to 210% of the recommended intake for potassium (K). Are these nutrient intakes acceptable for a late pregnant mare? Figure 3 shows that all of the nutrients evaluated are well within either the target or acceptable ranges for pregnancy. Additionally, Ca:P ratio, % forage, and % dry matter fall within acceptable ranges. In conclusion, NRC requirements for horses are of little practical value for evaluating rations unless they are expressed as recommended daily allowances with acceptable ranges of nutrient intake. The next revision of the NRC will hopefully include more of this type of information.

Table 2. Nutrient intakes of a Thoroughbred mare during the third trimester of pregnancy.

Daily Nutrient Intake	Fall Pasture	Mix Hay 20A:80G	Oats	All-Phase	Salt	RDA* (KER)	Total Nutrients
Intake (kg/day)	4.0	5.0	1.5	0.5	0.03		11.03
DM (kg/day)	4.0	4.5	1.338	0.45	0.029	9.977	10.317
Protein (g/day)	640.0	500.0	177.0	125.0		1058.4	1442.0
Lysine (g/day)	22.4	19.0	5.9	7.5		37.0	54.8
DE (Mcal/day)	8.8	9.4	4.5	1.4		24.1	24.1
Ca (g/day)	22.0	26.3	1.2	15.0		53.8	64.5
P (g/day)	12.0	11.0	5.1	9.0		35.8	37.1
Mg (g/day)	8.0	10.0	2.1	2.0		13.4	22.1
Na (g/day)	0.4	0.5	0.8	3.4	12.0	15.0	17.0
Cl (g/day)	10.0	5.0	1.4	5.0	18.0	22.4	39.4
K (g/day)	68.0	66.2	6.0	6.5		69.8	146.7
Cu (mg/day)	48.0	45.0	9.0	75.0		171.0	177.0
Se (mg/day)	0.40	0.5	0.32	1.05		2.49	2.27
Zn (mg/day)	140.0	88.0	52.5	182.5		513.1	719.0
I (mg/day)	0.20	0.55	0.17	1.00		2.00	1.92
Mn (mg/day)	280.0	265.0	54.0	120.0		513.1	719.0
Vit. A (IU/day)	20000.0	30000.0	66.0	10000.0		49884.0	60066.0
Vit. D (IU/day)	2000.0	2750.0		1000.0		4988.0	5750.0
Vit. E (IU/day)	480.0	220.0	23.0	75.0		798.0	798.0

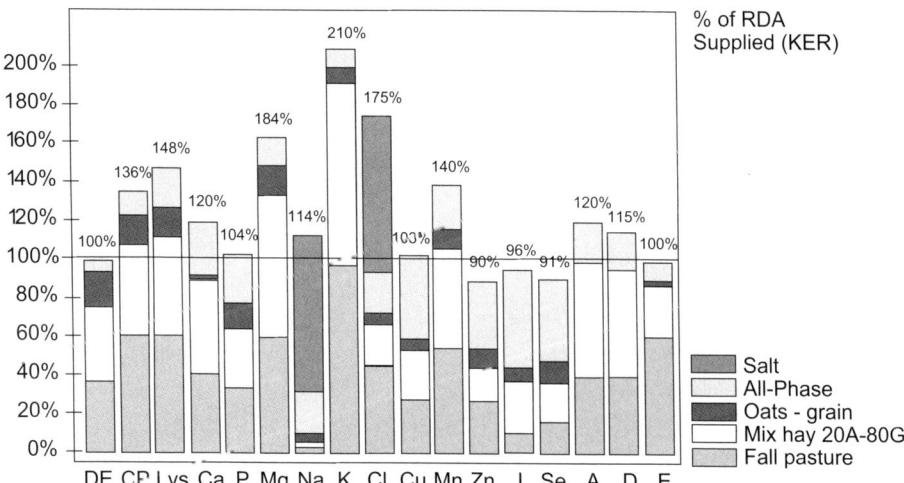

Figure 2. Daily intakes as a percentage of KER recommendations.

6 Nutrient Requirements: Applying the Science

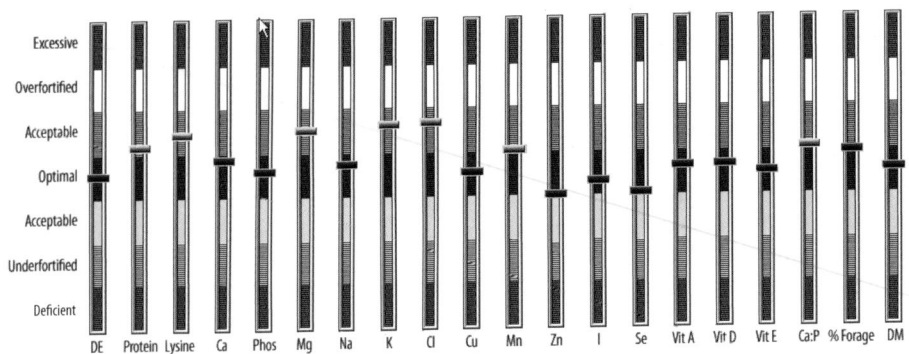

Figure 3. Daily intakes as they compare to acceptable ranges.

References

Kronfeld, D. 2001. A practical method for ration evaluation and diet formulation: An introduction to sensitivity analysis. In: Pagan, J.D., and R.J. Geor (Eds.). *Advances in Equine Nutrition II*. p. 153-160. Nottingham University Press, Nottingham, U.K.

NRC. 1989. Nutrient Requirements of Horses. (5th Ed.). National Academy Press. Washington, DC.

MAKING NUTRIENT COMPOSITION TABLES RELEVANT

PAUL K. SIROIS
Dairy One Forage Lab, Ithaca, New York

Nutrient requirements, feed intake, and feed composition form the trifecta of ration balancing. Requirements are determined using published tables or computer programs. Intake is reasonably established with stable-fed animals but more difficult to estimate for horses on pasture. Feed composition is based on actual analyses or from nutrient composition tables. The best rations are based on feed analyses. Nutrient composition tables should be used only as a secondary source in the absence of analytical data. To provide the best information, tables should incorporate data from a variety of contemporary sources.

Source of Data

The *United States-Canadian Tables of Feed Composition* (NRC, 1982) was the last comprehensive set of nutrient values published by the National Research Council (NRC). The data are reported to be from "individuals in both industry and public institutions." In order to complete the table, missing values were estimated using regression equations or estimated from similar feeds. No information is given regarding the number of samples or the standard deviation for each nutrient. Individual forages can vary widely in nutrient composition. Table 1 illustrates the variation in legume hays analyzed by our lab. Reporting the standard deviation improves the usefulness of the tables. For example, if an individual forage is recognized as being better than average in quality, the crude protein plus one standard deviation and the ADF minus one standard deviation can be used to better estimate the quality of the feed.

No overt reference is made to the origins of the data in *Nutrient Requirements of Horses* (NRC, 1989), heretofore referred to as the 1989 Horse NRC. Presumably, the information comes from other NRC sources. A big improvement in this table was the inclusion of the number of observations used in the statistics along with the standard deviation. Disappointingly, many feed types are based on few observations. For example, commonly fed timothy hay listed an average of four observations per nutrient.

The challenge for the next NRC equine committee will be to construct tables using current, relevant information. Securing data based on large numbers of observations will enhance the meaningfulness of the tabular values and provide measures of variation for individual feeds.

8 Making Nutrient Composition Tables Relevant

Table 1. Composition of legume hays (DM basis) from 5/01/00 to 4/30/04.

	n	Mean	sd
CP, %	51389	21.1	2.8
ADF, %	51032	30.0	4.1
NDF, %	51055	38.6	5.5
DE, Mcal/kg		2.63	
Fat, %	23856	2.5	0.5
Ash, %	24048	10.8	1.8
Ca, %	44327	1.56	0.28
P, %	44336	0.28	0.05
Mg, %	43663	0.31	0.07
K, %	43773	2.44	0.54
Na, %	14082	0.14	0.13
Fe, ppm	14025	353	320
Zn, ppm	14012	36	
Cu, ppm	14008	9	7
Mn, ppm	14011	35	17
S, %	26023	0.28	0.17

Commercial Analyses

Commercial forage analysis began to grow in the latter part of the 1960s. Initially targeted at the dairy industry, the number of labs and nutrient analyses available continue to grow. The National Forage Testing Association (NFTA) started with 25 labs in the late 1980s and enlists over 150 labs today. Forage analysis was seen as a way to optimize feed costs by providing the nutrients required and avoiding the costs incurred with over- and underfeeding. Commercial forage analysis is now a virtual requirement for doing business with today's dairies. This is evidenced by the growth of Dairy One services. In 1975, just over 5,000 samples were analyzed, primarily from New York and New England. In 2003, analyses were performed on over 120,000 samples from all across the world.

Commercial labs typically perform a greater number of nutrient analyses per sample than would be found in research trials, where the focus tends to be on specific or few components. In 1975 Dairy One provided 20 nutrients compared to 63 values in 2003. These more complete profiles would serve to greatly enhance aggregate tabular values.

Labs also receive samples from a greater number of different sources. This enables the lab to produce a more robust database and truer indication of variation within a feed type. Table 2 compares summarized data for commonly fed grains from Dairy One compared with data from the 1989 Horse NRC. The corn data were relatively consistent across the two sources. Compare this to the oats and barley data. Calculated

Table 2. Comparison of small grains (DM basis) from Dairy One (5/01/00-4/30/04) and the NRC (NRC, 1989).

	Dairy One Oats			NRC Oats			Dairy One Corn			NRC Corn			Dairy One Barley			NRC Barley		
	n	mean	sd	n	mean	sd	n	mean	sd	n	mean	sd	n	mean	sd	n	mean	sd
CF, %	270	12.9	2.4	110	13.3	1.3	1699	9.4	1.8	527	10.4	1.4	439	12.9	2.2	304	13.2	1.9
ADF, %	206	13.2	5.3	2	15.9	1.6	1361	3.6	1.3	5	4.1	0.8	416	7.7	4.1	13	7.0	5.2
NDF, %	208	27.2	9.8	14	27.3	4.5	1376	10.0	3.1	3	10.8	2.1	427	19.6	7.1	25	19.0	3.3
DE, Mcal/kg		3.34			3.20			3.87			3.84			3.65			3.69	
Fat, %	184	7.2	2.0	108	5.2	1.	1090	4.4	1.6	89	4.1	0.6	231	2.7	1.3	208	2.0	0.5
Ash, %	155	2.7	1.3	91	3.4	0.5	789	1.5	0.5	64	1.5	0.3	181	3.1	1.2	217	2.7	0.3
Starch, %	92	44.4	10.5				737	70.4	4.4				141	53.7	9.7			
Ca, %	189	0.15	0.15	64	0.09	0.03	1147	0.05	0.16	48	0.05	0.07	336	0.10	0.12	117	0.05	0.02
P, %	189	0.42	0.08	71	0.38	0.05	1137	0.33	0.12	47	0.31	0.04	336	0.44	0.11	134	0.38	0.07
Mg, %	185	0.15	0.03	48	0.16	0.03	1129	0.13	0.13	41	0.12	0.03	335	0.15	0.04	73	0.15	0.02
K, %	185	0.58	0.20	47	0.45	0.12	1130	0.41	0.10	35	0.37	0.03	335	0.59	0.17	71	0.50	0.13
Na, %	122	0.03	0.10	15	0.06	0.03	745	0.04	0.20	26	0.03	0.01	255	0.04	0.13	19	0.03	0.02
Fe, ppm	122	108	80.2	38	73	25.2	712	63	104	29	35	12.6	255	99	131	59	83	30
Zn, ppm	122	36	28.6	40	39	10.9	712	24	18	33	22	5.5	255	32	15.2	65	19	18
Cu, ppm	122	8	4.6	27	7	1.8	712	3	3.2	33	4	1.3	255	6	2.6	45	9	4.1
Mn, ppm	122	51	21	37	40	10	712	9	15.2	31	6	1.5	255	20	10.5	60	18	3.7
S, %	97	0.14	0.04	13	0.23	0.01	756	0.1	0.02	7	0.13	0.02	203	0.13	0.03	14	0.17	0.01

coefficients of variation (cv) for NDF (36.0%, 36.2%) and starch (23.6%, 18.0%) in the Dairy One data for oats and barley, respectively, are greater than the NRC (NDF: 16.4%, 17.3%; no starch figures available). The wide variation in starch is extremely important as the management of carbohydrates in equine diets continues to receive increasing emphasis. Table users need to be aware of the diversity in nutrient composition of commodities.

The area of mineral composition values needs an infusion of fresh data. Table 3 compares the mineral values of common grasses from the 1989 Horse NRC to Dairy One. There is a large disparity in the number of observations (NRC <4, Dairy One >6000). Of particular interest is the difference in copper values. The NRC values are 2.0 to 2.9 times the Dairy One values and inconsistent with values from other NRC publications. Table 4 compares the Horse NRC values for grasses with other NRC publications.

As a result, some commercial labs have created large databases of nutrient values. Dairy One published an annual summary of analytical results until 1996 when it became cost-prohibitive. This information was of great value to the feed industry and was sorely missed. The advent of the Internet allowed us to establish a platform for storing and updating information and making it available in a readily accessible form. Nutrient composition data are available to the public on both our dairy (dairyone.com) and equine (equi-analytical.com) Web sites. Data are summarized on annual and cumulative bases and serve as valuable references for industry professionals and laymen alike. The large numbers of observations provide the industry with confidence in the published values. For example, the crude protein values for legume hay reported in Table 1 are from 51,389 observations compared to 63 observations in the 1989 Horse NRC.

Building Tables

Feed composition tables are a necessary component of the nutrient requirement series to provide users with baseline values for different feed types. To be useful, the tables should be built on large numbers of observations to accurately represent feed and forages commonly fed to today's livestock. Future NRC committees should seek out as many sources as possible to ensure the robustness of the data presented in the tables. Commercial labs perform the bulk of nutrient analyses in the U.S. and hopefully would be willing to share information for the betterment of the industry. A precedent was set when the committee writing Nutrient Requirements of Dairy Cattle (NRC, 2001) sought and extensively used commercial analyses in the development of its published tables. This greatly increased the number of observations and the value of the information therein. Table 5 compares the 1989 Horse NRC to the 2001 Dairy NRC. The large difference in the number of observations inspires greater confidence in the use of these values.

Table 3. Comparison of grass hay mineral values (DM basis) between the *Nutrient Requirements of Horses* (NRC, 1989) and Dairy One (5/C1/00 - 04/30/04).

	NRC Bermuda 56d growth		NRC Brome mid bloom		NRC Fescue mature		NRC Orchard late bloom		NRC Timothy full bloom		Dairy One Grass		
	n	mean	n	mean	n	mean	n	mean	n	mean	n	mean	sd
Ca, %	1	0.26	1	0.29	2	0.41	1	0.26	3	0.43	14309	0.54	0.22
P, %	1	.018	1	0.28	2	0.30	1	0.30	4	0.20	14311	0.25	0.08
Mg, %	1	0.13	1	0.10	2	0.16	1	0.11	3	0.09	14246	0.21	0.08
K, %	1	1.30	1	1.99	2	1.96	1	2.67	4	1.99	14324	1.89	0.57
Na, %		x	1	0.01	1	0.02	1	0.01	3	0.07	6374	0.05	0.11
Fe, ppm		x	1	91	2	132	1	84	2	140	6359	177	220
Zn, ppm		x	1	30	2	35	1	38	1	54	6362	23	14
Cu, ppm		x	1	25	2	22	1	20	2	29	6360	10	5
Mn, ppm		x	1	40	2	97	1	167	2	93	6361	66	57
S, %		x		x		x		x	3	0.14	8291	0.18	0.07

x = no values reported

Table 4. Comparison of grass hay mineral composition (DM basis) between NRC publications (NRC, 1982, 1989, 2001).

	NRC* Horse 1989	NRC* US-Can 1982	NRC** Dairy 2001
Ca, %	0.43	0.43	0.58
P, %	0.20	0.20	0.23
Mg, %	0.09	0.14	0.20
K, %	1.99	1.64	2.01
Na, %	0.07		0.04
Fe, ppm	140	157	156
Zn ppm	54		31
Cu, ppm	29	5	9
Mn, ppm	93		72
S, %	0.14		0.21

*Values for full bloom timothy hay
**Values for all grass hays

Table 5. Comparison of grass hays (DM basis) from the dairy (NRC, 2001) and horse (NRC, 1989) nutrient requirement series.

	Dairy NRC 2001*		Horse NRC 1989**	
	n	mean	n	mean
CP, %	4702	10.6	15	8.1
ADF, %	4695	39.5	8	37.5
NDF, %	4695	64.4	8	64.2
DE, Mcal/kg		1.97		1.94
Fat, %	542	2.6	7	2.9
Ash, %	1791	7.6	8	5.2
Ca, %	4653	0.58	3	0.43
P, %	4653	0.23	4	0.20
Mg, %	4653	0.20	3	0.09
K, %	4653	2.01	4	1.99
Na, %	1321	0.04	3	0.07
Fe, ppm	1321	156	2	140
Zn, ppm	1321	31	1	54
Cu, ppm	1321	9	2	29
Mn, ppm	1321	72	2	93
S, %	1448	0.21	3	0.14

*Values for all grass hays
**Values for full bloom timothy hay

Classifying Feeds

Previous editions of NRC publications have attempted to characterize forages by species and stage of maturity. No one can argue the impact of these two factors on forage quality, but assembling data of this nature is difficult. From a commercial lab standpoint, consider the following:

1. True sample identification is often missing.
2. Stage of maturity is rarely reported.
3. More often than not, samples are mixtures rather than pure forages.
4. Ability of the person submitting the sample to accurately identify the species and stage of maturity is unknown.

All attempts are made to properly identify feeds at the lab. Dairy One uses 471 different codes to categorize feeds. No feeds are classified by stage of maturity. There are some individual forage codes, but to simplify matters for our customers, hay crop forages are divided into four broad categories: legume, mixed mostly legume (MML), mixed mostly grass (MMG), and grass forages. Customers can usually place forages correctly into one of these groups. Evidence of this can be seen in Table 6. Note the expected decline in CP and rise in ADF and NDF as samples move across the continuum from legumes to grasses.

Table 6. Comparison of major nutrients (DM basis) for broad categories of hays as classified by Dairy One (5/01/03-4/30/04).

	Legume	*MML**	*MMG**	*Grass*
CP, %	21.1	17.0	12.1	10.6
ADF, %	30.0	35.3	38.7	39.1
NDF, %	38.6	49.7	60.6	63.7

*Mixed mostly legume and mixed mostly grass hays

Cherney et al. (1993) reported similarity in nutrient composition across grass species and stage of maturity. Table 7 is a comparison of late bloom orchardgrass, full bloom timothy, and mid bloom timothy from the 1989 Horse NRC and grass data from Dairy One. Based on the lack of observations in the NRC data, it is clear that the broad grass category used by Dairy One would provide sufficient values to be used for any of these.

The 2001 Dairy NRC committee recognized this fact. Species and maturity data were eliminated from the nutrient composition tables and were replaced by broader forage categories. This enabled them to:

14 *Making Nutrient Composition Tables Relevant*

1. Increase the numbers of observations.
2. Report better standard deviations.
3. Provide current, robust data for industry use.

Table 7. Comparison of several grass hays (DM basis) across species and maturities (NRC, 1989) with Dairy One grass hays (5/01/03-4/30-04).

	Late bloom orchard (NRC)		Full bloom timothy (NRC)		Mid bloom timothy (NRC)		Mean of hays (NRC)		Grass (Dairy One)	
	n	mean	n	mean	n	mean	n	mean	n	mean
CP, %	1	8.4	15	8.1	20	9.7	36	8.7	15097	10.6
ADF, %	3	37.8	8	37.5	13	36.4	24	37.2	14815	39.1
NDF, %	3	65.0	8	64.2	13	63.7	24	64.3	15030	63.7
DE, Mcal/kg		1.94		1.94		2.02		1.97		1.98
Fat, %	1	3.4	7	2.9	11	2.6	19	3.0	8074	2.5
Ash, %	3	10.1	8	5.2	8	6.1	19	7.1	8170	7.6
Ca, %	1	0.26	3	0.43	2	0.48	6	0.39	14309	0.54
P, %	1	0.30	4	0.20	2	0.23	7	0.24	14311	0.25
Mg, %	1	0.11	3	0.09	3	0.13	7	0.11	14246	0.21
K, %	1	2.67	4	1.99	3	1.82	8	2.16	14324	1.89
Na, %	1	0.01	3	0.07	1	0.01	5	0.03	6374	0.05
Fe, ppm	1	84	2	140	3	149	6	124	6359	177
Zn, ppm	1	38	1	54	1	43	3	45	6362	23
Cu, ppm	1	20	2	29	2	16	5	22	6360	10
Mn, ppm	1	167	2	93	2	56	5	105	6361	66
S, %			3	0.14	1	0.13	4	0.14	8291	0.18

Summary

Feed composition tables are an essential component of the nutrient requirement publication series created by the NRC. It is the charge of the committees to locate and assimilate data to provide the industry with meaningful reference/baseline values. Confidence in values improves when represented by larger numbers of samples. Measures of variation must be included to reflect the variation inherent in the population. Commercial forage/feed laboratories conduct the majority of analyses in today's market. Many have large nutrient databases. Commercial labs should be sought out to see if they are willing to share this information with the committee. The previous NRC dairy committee recognized this fact and included extensive commercial data in its tables. The large number of observations and inclusion of standard deviations has improved the robustness and usefulness of the nutrient composition tables. A good goal would be to create a single Web-based nutrient composition table for all species that would be routinely updated and upgraded.

References

Cherney, D.J., J.H. Cherney, and R.F. Lucey. 1993. In vitro digestion kinetics and quality of perennial grasses as influenced by forage maturity. J. Dairy Science 76:790-797.

NRC. 1982. United States-Canadian Tables of Feed Composition. (3rd Ed.). National Academy Press, Washington, DC.

NRC. 1989. Nutrient Requirements of Horses. (5th Ed.). National Academy Press, Washington, DC.

NRC. 2001. Nutrient Requirements of Dairy Cattle. (7th Ed.). National Academy Press, Washington, DC.

FORAGES: THE FOUNDATION FOR EQUINE GASTROINTESTINAL HEALTH

JOE D. PAGAN
Kentucky Equine Research, Versailles, Kentucky

Introduction

Horses have evolved over millions of years as grazers, with specialized digestive tracts adapted to digest and utilize diets containing high levels of plant fiber. They are capable of processing large quantities of forage to meet their nutrient demands. In an attempt to maximize growth or productivity, horses are often fed diets that also contain high levels of grains and supplements. Unfortunately, this type of grain supplementation often overshadows the significant contribution that forages make in satisfying the horse's nutrient demands and can lead to serious gastrointestinal disturbances.

Digestive Function

Horses are classified anatomically as nonruminant herbivores or hindgut fermenters. The large intestine of the horse holds about 21 to 24 gallons (80-90 liters) of liquid and houses billions of bacteria and protozoa that produce enzymes which break down (ferment) plant fiber. These microbes are absolutely essential to the horse, because the horse cannot produce these enzymes without them. The by-products of this microbial fermentation provide the horse with a source of energy and micronutrients.

The equine digestive tract is designed in this fashion to allow the horse to ingest large quantities of forage in a continuous fashion. The small capacity of the upper part of the tract is not well-suited for large single meals, a fact that is often ignored by horsemen. Large single meals of grain overwhelm the digestive capacity of the stomach and small intestine, resulting in rapid fermentation of the grain carbohydrates by the microflora in the hindgut. This fermentation may result in a wide range of problems including colic and laminitis.

The fact that horses are hindgut fermenters has several implications for the person feeding the horse. First, since horses are designed to live on forages, any feeding program that neglects fiber will result in undesirable physical and mental consequences. Horses have a psychological need for the full feeling that fiber provides.

Horses fed fiber-deficient diets will in extreme cases become chronic woodchewers, 1000-pound termites that can destroy a good deal of fencing or stall front. It is also important to maintain a constant food source for the beneficial bacteria in the hindgut. Not only does the fermentation of fiber provide a great deal of energy for the horse, but the presence of beneficial bacteria prevents the proliferation of other, potentially pathogenic bacteria. Horses, like humans, need a certain amount of bulk to sustain normal digestive function. Horses have an immense digestive system designed to process a large volume of feed at all times. Deprived of that bulk, the many loops of the bowel are more likely to kink or twist, and serious colic can result.

Forage should remain the foundation of a horse's feeding program, regardless of where it is raised or how it is used. Additional grains or protein and mineral supplements should be used only to supply essential nutrients not contained in the forage. This is the most logical and economical way to approach feeding horses, because it eliminates the needless duplication or dangerous excess of fortification. The problem with this method of ration balancing is that the quantity and quality of forage eaten by most horses is not precisely known. Horsemen pay close attention to a difference of a few percentage points of protein in a grain mix, but rarely assay hay or pasture for nutrient content. To compound the problem, intakes of hay and pasture are difficult to measure. This does not mean, however, that reasonable estimates of forage intake cannot be made.

Forage Composition

Forages are composed of two components, cell contents and cell walls. Cell contents contain most of the protein and all of the starch, sugars, lipids, organic acids, and soluble ash found in the plant. These components are degraded by enzymes produced by the horse and are highly digestible. The cell wall contains the fibrous portion of the plant, which is resistant to digestive enzymes produced by the horse. The primary components of the cell wall are cellulose, hemicellulose and lignin. The nutritive value of forages is determined by two factors:

1)   Fiber content (the proportion of the plant that is composed of cell wall).
2)   Fiber quality (the degree of lignification).

These factors are important because the horse can digest practically all of the cell contents contained in forages, but bacterial fermentation can digest only 50% or less of most plant cell wall. The degree to which plant cell wall is digestible is largely dependent on the amount of lignin that it contains.

Factors Affecting Forage Quality

Many factors affect the quality of forage. Most important of these are the species of plant, stage of maturity, location where the plant was grown, and content of inhibitory substances. All of these factors should be considered when assessing the suitability of a particular forage for horses.

Species. Most plants that serve as forages for horses can be divided into two different categories, grasses and legumes. Grasses contain much structural matter in their leaves and leaf sheaths, and this can be as important as or more important than the stem in holding the plant erect. Examples of grass forages used for horses include temperate species such as timothy, orchard grass, brome grass, and fescue and tropical species like pangola, guinea, Bermuda, and kikuyu. Legumes, on the other hand, tend to be treelike on a miniature scale. Their leaves have very little structural function and tend to be on the ends of woody stems. The primary legumes used as horse forage are alfalfa and clover.

At a similar stage of maturity, legumes tend to be higher in protein, energy, and calcium than grasses. ADF (acid detergent fiber; lignin + cellulose) does not vary that much between grasses and legumes at the same stage of maturity. NDF (neutral detergent fiber; lignin + cellulose + hemicellulose), however, is much higher in grasses than legumes. This is because grasses contain a great deal more hemicellulose than legumes. Therefore, evaluating the fiber content of forages based on ADF alone underestimates the total cell wall content and overestimates the total energy content of a grass. Remember, hemicellulose is typically only 50% digested in the horse, and cell solubles are almost completely digested. By only considering ADF, the assumption is that the rest of the forage (besides protein, fat, and ash) is soluble sugar. This is truer in legumes, which contain only around 10% hemicellulose, than in grasses, which can have hemicellulose contents of 30% or more. The fiber that is in legumes tends to be less digestible than the fiber in grasses, largely because legumes tend to have higher lignin content per unit of total fiber. This means that the digestible fiber content of grasses is much higher than it is in legumes of similar maturity.

Because of the factors mentioned above, legumes contain 20-25% more digestible energy than grasses at the same maturity. In certain instances, the amount of legume hay fed may be limited so that the horse doesn't get too fat. This can result in intakes of digestible fiber that are below optimal levels, particularly in extremely high-quality hays.

Stage of maturity. Generally, as plants mature they become less digestible. This is because a greater proportion of their mass becomes structural and less metabolic. Legumes tend to mature by decreasing leafiness and increasing the stem-to-leaf ratio.

Alfalfa leaves maintain the same level of digestibility throughout their growth. Their stems, however, decrease dramatically in digestibility as they mature. This is because they become highly lignified to support the extra weight of the plant. The ultimate example of lignification for support is the oak tree. The wood of the oak tree is highly lignified and practically indigestible. When pulp wood is processed to make paper, the lignin is removed using harsh chemicals such as sulfuric acid (hence the sulfur smell around paper mills).

The leaves of grasses serve more of a structural function than in legumes. As they mature, these leaves become more lignified and less digestible. Since the stems of certain grasses serve a reserve function, they may actually be more digestible than the leaves of these grasses at a later stage of maturity. When forage is grazed as pasture, its nutrient quality is almost always higher than when it is harvested as hay unless the pasture is the dead aftermath left over from the previous growing season. New spring pasture can be quite low in fiber content and high in soluble carbohydrates. In spring, it is often a good management practice to continue to offer horses on pasture additional hay even if the pasture appears thick and lush. If the horses are getting adequate fiber from the pasture, then they will ignore the hay.

Latitudinal effects. The digestibility of tropical forages averages on the order of 15 units of digestibility lower than temperate forages (Van Soest, 1994). Plants that grow in the tropics have been genetically selected for a larger proportion of protective structures such as lignin to avoid predation. At the other extreme are the perennial plants in the far northern regions of the world. These plants have very short growing seasons and need to store energy in reserves as sugars and fructans rather than in irretrievable substances such as lignin and cellulose. Care should be taken when feeding high-fructan forages to horses since these compounds are poorly digested in the small intestine and may lead to colic or laminitis due to excess lactic acid fermentation in the hindgut.

Inhibitory substances. Besides lignin, a number of other substances in forages can reduce digestibility of fiber and minerals. Silica is used as a structural element complementing lignin to strengthen and add rigidity to cell walls. Alfalfa and other temperate legumes restrict absorption of silica and never contain more than a few hundred ppm in their tissues (Van Soest, 1994). Cereal straws are quite high in silica. This gives the straw a clean, glassy appearance and it also reduces its digestibility. Rice hulls are extremely high in silica and indigestible by horses. There are also substances contained in forages that can inhibit mineral digestibility. Two that are particularly important are phytate and oxalate. Phytates contain phosphorus in a bound form that is unavailable to the horse. Phytate may also inhibit the digestibility of other minerals such as calcium, zinc, and iodine.

Oxalates can reduce the digestibility of calcium in forages if the calcium-to-oxalate ratio in the forage is 0.5 or less on a weight-to-weight basis (Hintz, 1990). This is a common problem in tropical forages which tend to be high in oxalates and low in calcium. Low calcium availability in tropical forages can lead to nutritional secondary hyperparathyroidism or "big head" disease. Therefore, when tropical forages are fed to horses, supplemental sources of calcium should be available.

There is a common misconception that oxalates reduce calcium digestibility in alfalfa hay. This is not true because the calcium:oxalate ratio is much higher than 0.5, even in alfalfa hays that contain high levels of oxalates. Hintz et al. (1984) demonstrated this in an experiment in which no difference was found in the absorption of calcium from alfalfa containing 0.5% and 0.9% oxalic acid in which the calcium:oxalate ratios were 3 and 1.7, respectively. The true digestibility of the calcium from both hays was estimated to be >75%.

Buffering Capacity of Forage

Gastric ulcers are very common in performance horses, affecting over 90% of racehorses and 60% of show horses and most commonly occurring in the upper portion of the horse's stomach, which is composed of nonglandular squamous epithelium. These ulcers are primarily the result of prolonged exposure of this tissue to gastric acid. Unlike the glandular portion of the stomach, the upper half of the equine stomach does not have a mucous layer and does not secrete bicarbonate onto its luminal surface. The only protection that this portion of the stomach has from gastric acid and pepsin comes from saliva production and the buffering capacity of feed.

The high incidence of ulcers seen in performance horses is a man-made problem resulting from the way that we feed and manage these horses, as ulcers are extremely rare in nonexercised horses maintained solely on pasture. Meals of grain or extended periods of fasting lead to excess gastric acid output without adequate saliva production. Additionally, production of VFAs (particularly butyric acid) from the fermentation of grain in the stomach makes the nonglandular epithelium more susceptible to acid damage. Horses secrete acid continually whether they are fed or not. The pH of gastric fluid in horses withheld from feed for several hours has consistently been measured to be 2.0 or less (Murray, 1992). Horses that received free-choice timothy hay for 24 hours had mean gastric pH readings that were significantly higher than fasted horses (Murray and Schusser, 1989). Higher pH readings in hay-fed horses should be expected since forage consumption stimulates saliva production. German researchers measured the amount of saliva produced when horses ate either hay, pasture, or a grain feed (Meyer et al., 1985). When fed hay and fresh grass, they produced twice as much saliva compared to when a grain-based feed was offered.

There is growing evidence that the type of hay fed to horses has a significant impact on acid neutralization and the incidence of gastric ulcers. Tennessee researchers reported a study where 6 horses with gastric cannulae were fed either alfalfa hay and concentrate or brome grass hay without grain supplementation (Nadeau et al., 2000). It was predicted that the alfalfa hay and concentrate diet would produce more ulcers due to greater gastric VFA production and less saliva production compared to when the horses were fed only grass hay. Surprisingly, they found that feeding alfalfa hay and concentrate increased the pH of gastric fluid and reduced the number and severity of squamous mucosal ulceration compared to feeding the diet of brome grass hay. Saliva production was not measured in this study, but it was suggested that the buffering capacity of the alfalfa and/or concentrate was greater than grass hay.

A more recent study at Texas A&M University suggests that the differences seen in the Tennessee study were related to the type of hay fed. In this study, the incidence of ulceration was compared in horses fed a pelleted concentrate along with either Bermuda grass hay or alfalfa hay (Lybbert et al., 2007). Twenty-four Quarter Horse yearlings, 12-16 months of age, were included in a crossover design conducted over a 77-day period consisting of two 28-day periods separated by a 21-day wash-out period. Gastric endoscopy was performed at the beginning of the study, and each horse was assigned an ulcer severity score, using a grading system ranging from 0 (intact gastric epithelium with no hyperemia or hyperkeratosis) to 4 (submucosal penetration). The horses were assigned to one of two treatment groups, using a randomized block method to ensure equivalent ulcer severity scores in the two treatment groups. Group 1 horses were fed a diet consisting of coastal Bermuda grass hay and a pelleted concentrate (15% protein) in a weight:weight ratio of 1:1, and group 2 horses were fed a diet consisting of alfalfa hay and the same concentrate in a weight:weight ratio of 1:1. The horses were housed in small dry lots and subjected to an exercise regimen 3 days/week using a mechanical horse-exerciser. After the end of the first 28-day period, gastroscopy was repeated, and horses were turned out to pasture with no forced exercise and fed a diet comprised of grazing and 1.8 kg/horse of the same pellet. After 21 days in pasture, gastric endoscopy was repeated and diet regimens were switched (i.e., group 1 horses were switched to group 2 and vice versa).

The ulcer severity scores were significantly ($p < 0.001$) lower for horses in the alfalfa hay group than horses fed coastal Bermuda grass hay. Among horses fed alfalfa, 12 had no ulcers at baseline and 11 had ulcer scores of 2 ($N = 6$) or 3 ($N = 5$). Of the 11 horses with ulcer scores >0, all improved by at least two ulcer grades while on the alfalfa diet; 1 of the 12 horses without ulceration developed gastric ulceration during the time it was fed alfalfa. In contrast, of the 12 horses fed coastal Bermuda grass hay that had ulcer scores >0, 5 horses had scores were improved, and only 2 were improved by at least 2 grades; of the 12 horses with initial ulcer scores of 0 fed coastal Bermuda, only 3 remained free of ulcers and 7 developed ulcer scores ≥2. Among horses fed coastal Bermuda grass during period 1, ulcer scores did not change significantly between the end of period 1 and the end of the wash-out period; however, the ulcer severity scores of horses fed alfalfa during period 1 were significantly ($p<0.007$) higher after the wash-out period ended than at the end of period 1.

Relative to feeding coastal Bermuda grass hay, feeding alfalfa hay reduced ulcer severity scores in horses with gastric ulceration and prevented ulcer development in 11 of 12 (92%) horses fed alfalfa hay that did not have ulcers, whereas only 25% (3/12) of the horses without evidence of ulceration fed coastal Bermuda grass hay did not appear to develop ulcerations. Moreover, horses that were initially fed alfalfa hay had a significant worsening of ulcer severity scores during the wash-out period.

Alfalfa hay provides greater buffering capacity compared to Bermuda grass hay for several reasons. First, alfalfa contains higher levels of protein and calcium, both of which buffer gastric acid. Also, alfalfa fiber has a higher cation exchange capacity compared to graminaceous plants, due largely to its higher content of lignin and other polyphenolics (Van Soest, 1994). McBurney et al. (1983) showed that alfalfa cell wall has a much higher buffering capacity than either timothy or oat cell wall when titrated with HCl acid.

Jasaitis et al. (1987) measured the in vitro buffering capacity of 52 feeds to determine the buffering capacity range within and among feed types. Buffering capacity was lowest for energy feeds, intermediate for low-protein feeds (15 to 35% crude protein) and grass forages, and highest for high-protein feeds (>35% crude protein) and legume forages.

The buffering capacity of feed and forage plays an important role in the prevention of gastric ulcers in horses. Alfalfa hay has been shown to be effective in reducing the severity of ulcers in horses by providing superior buffering capacity compared to grass hay. Unfortunately, high levels of alfalfa hay may not be desirable for performance horses because of the detrimental effects of excess protein intake (Pagan, 1998). More research is needed to identify other feeds and forages that also possess high buffering capacities while containing more desirable nutrient compositions.

References

Hintz, H.F. 1990. Factors affecting nutrient availability in the horse. In: Proceed. Georgia Nutrition Conference. p. 182-193.

Hintz, H.F., H.F. Schryver, J. Doty, C. Lakin, and R.A. Zimmerman. 1984. Oxalic acid content of alfalfa hays and its influence on the availability of calcium, phosphorus and magnesium to ponies. J. Anim. Sci. 58:939-942.

Jasaitis, D.K., J.E. Wohlt, and J.L. Evans. 1987. Influence of feed ion content on buffering capacity of ruminant feedstuffs in vitro. J. Dairy Sci. 70:1391-1403.

Lybbert, T., P. Gibbs, N. Cohen, B. Scott, and D. Sigler. 2007. Feeding alfalfa hay to exercising horses reduces the severity of gastric squamous mucosal ulceration. In: Proc. Amer. Assoc. Equine Practnr. 53:525-526.

McBurney, M. I., P. J. Van Soest, and L. E. Chase. 1983. Cation exchange capacity and buffering capacity of neutral detergent fibers. J. Sci. Food Agric. 34:910–916.

Meyer, H., M. Coenen, and C. Gurer. 1985. Investigations of saliva production and chewing in horses fed various feeds. In: Proc. Equine Nutri. Physiol. Soc. p. 38-41.

Murray, M.J. 1992. Aetiopathogenesis and treatment of peptic ulcer in the horse: A comparative review. Equine Vet J. Suppl. 13:63-74.

Murray, M.J., and G. Schusser. 1989. Application of gastric pH-metry in horses: Measurement of 24 hour gastric pH in horses fed, fasted, and treated with ranitidine. J. Vet. Intern. Med. 6:133.

Nadeau, J.A., F.M. Andrews, and A.G. Matthew. 2000. Evaluation of diet as a cause of gastric ulcers in horses. Amer. J. Vet. Res. 61:784-790.

Pagan, J.D. 1998. Energy and the performance horse. In: J.D. Pagan and R.J. Geor (Eds.) Advances in Equine Nutrition, Vol. II. Nottingham University Press, United Kingdom.

Van Soest, P.J. 1994. Nutritional Ecology of the Ruminant. Cornell University Press.

GRAZING PREFERENCES OF HORSES FOR DIFFERENT COOL-SEASON GRASSES

JENNIFER RINGLER, BRYAN CASSILL, SUSAN HAYES, JEFF STINE, AND LAURIE LAWRENCE
University of Kentucky, Lexington, Kentucky

Cool-season grasses are the predominant plants used in central Kentucky horse pastures. Within a species there may be varieties that differ in agronomic characteristics. Previous studies at the University of Kentucky have evaluated the tolerance of cool-season grass varieties to intense grazing by horses (Spitileri et al., 2004). This study was conducted to determine whether horses demonstrate preferences for certain cool-season grasses. Cool-season grasses in the study included timothy (two varieties), orchardgrass (one variety), Kentucky bluegrass (two varieties), bromegrass (one variety), and tall fescue or tall fescue-cross (nine varieties).

Fifteen varieties of cool-season grasses were seeded in a 0.5-acre paddock in fall of 2003. The fifteen varieties were distributed among 90 individual plots (1.5 m x 4.6 m each) so that each variety was seeded into six plots in the paddock. In the spring of 2004, plots were scored for plant density and mean forage height was measured before horses were allowed to graze in the paddock. These observations were repeated 2 d, 5 d, 7 d, and 14 d after the horses were given access to the paddock. In addition, plots were scored for grazing intensity 2 d, 5 d, 7 d, and 14 d after the horses were given access to the paddock. On each day, observations were made in the following order: grazing intensity, plant density, and forage height. Observers completed all scores for grazing intensity before scoring the plots for plant density, and all plant density scores were completed before forage height was measured. Ratings were made by four trained observers; however, each plot was rated by only two individuals. Two observers rated plots 1-45 and the other two observers rated plots 46-90. Each observer worked independently. The two independent observations were averaged for each plot to yield one grazing intensity score, one plant density score, and one forage height measurement per plot. The average of the six plots for each variety was then determined for grazing intensity, plant density, and forage height for each measurement day. Measurements were made during the spring growing season (mid-May) when plants were in a vegetative state. All observations were made between 8 a.m. and 10 a.m.

Plant density was scored from 0 to 10, where 0 was a plot with none of the seeded variety present, and 10 was a plot with complete coverage by the seeded variety. Intermediate scores represented the percentage of the plot that was covered so that a score of 5 indicated a plot with 50% coverage. Grazing activity was also scored from

0 to 10, where 0 was a plot with no grazing activity and a 10 was a plot where 100% of the plants had been grazed. Intermediate scores represented a percentage of the plants in the plot that had been grazed so that 5 represented a plot where 50% of the plants had been grazed. Each observer measured forage height at five locations across a diagonal of each plot. For each plot, the one observer measured across the right to left diagonal and the other observer measured across the left to right diagonal. The five measurements made by each observer were averaged to produce one measurement per observer per plot.

Prior to being given access to the test paddock, four horses were kept in a holding pasture that was adjacent to the test paddock for 2 wk. Once the pre-grazing observations were made, the gate between the test pasture and the holding pasture was opened. Horses were able to enter the test paddock area at will and were not confined in the test paddock at any time. Water was available in the adjacent pasture.

Initial height of forage available for grazing in the test paddock was higher ($P < 0.05$) for the tall fescue/fescue-cross varieties than for the non-fescue varieties (34.6 +/- 1.8 cm vs 32.0 +/- 2.2 cm, respectively, mean +/- SE). The difference in initial height could be attributed to the two bluegrass varieties that had an average initial height of 28.0 +/- 2.2 cm. By day 2, forage height was reduced for some varieties. The greatest mean reduction in forage height on day 2 was observed for a variety of timothy (9.3 +/- 1.0). The mean reduction in forage height was not different for tall fescue/fescue-cross varieties compared to non-fescue varieties on day 2. By day 5, however, the mean reduction in forage height for non-fescue varieties was greater ($P<0.05$) than for tall fescue/fescue-cross varieties (10.6 +/- 2.9 cm vs 6.9 +/- 2.0 cm, respectively). This difference persisted through 14 d with forage height reductions of 17.8 +/- 2.5 cm for the non-tall fescue varieties and 12.5 +/- 2.4 cm for the tall fescue/fescue-cross varieties.

Initial plant density scores were 7 or above for all varieties, with scores above 8 for all tall fescue/fescue-cross varieties, the orchardgrass, and one timothy variety. Density scores decreased with grazing time, but at 2 wk, several tall fescue/fescue-cross varieties still had density scores above 8. By comparison, the bromegrass variety sustained the greatest change in density from an initial score of 7.4 to a 2 wk score of 4. In general, greater reductions in density were observed for the non-fescue varieties than for the tall fescue/fescue-cross varieties. As expected, grazing scores increased during the grazing period. On day 2, several varieties had minimal evidence of grazing (mean score < 1.0) but one variety had grazing scores above 5. Interestingly, the two varieties with the lowest grazing score on day 2 also had low reductions in forage height, and the variety with the greatest reduction in forage height had the highest grazing score. By 2 wk, grazing scores were above 6 for all varieties except for two tall fescue/fescue-cross varieties. The variety with the lowest grazing score at 2 wk was also the variety with the lowest reduction in forage height.

Observations in this study suggest that horses select among cool-season grass forages. The reasons horses select one grass over another are unknown but may relate

Carbohydrate Source-Sink Dynamics

An important concept to the understanding of carbohydrate concentration and distribution in grass is the dynamic nature of its production and utilization. A brief overview is presented by Nelson (1995). Plant scientists use the term "source" to indicate where carbohydrate is produced and "sink" to explain where carbohydrate is utilized. Plant organs can be either source or sink depending on stage of growth and environmental conditions. In early spring, carbohydrates stored in seed, crown, stem base, root, or rhizome tissues are the source for carbon and energy utilized in the formation of the first new leaves, which in this case are the sink. When enough leaf area has formed, such that the surface area has sufficient photosynthetic capacity to produce more carbohydrate than that required for growth, that leaf then becomes a source of sugar. Once the leaf is fully extended, the sink for growth is removed. Thereafter, sugars produced in excess of respiratory needs are available for translocation to sinks in other parts of the plant. Meristematic tissues, which are undifferentiated growth points throughout a plant, have priority for allocation of NSC. The sink for excess NSC might be new leaf, tiller, root, stem, or seed production. During the stem-elongation phase, the developing reproductive organs inside the stem are the sink. During seed filling, the stem is then the source and the seed is the sink. If adverse conditions limit seed filling, excess sugars may be left over in the stem. During germination, the seed is once again the source for NSC. High respiratory rates in cool-season grasses during hot weather may become a sink, burning up sugars that might otherwise go towards growth or seed production. In some winter-hardy types of perennial grass, onset of freezing temperatures may trigger translocation of sugars back to stem bases or underground storage organs. Leaf tissue in this case is the source; the storage organs are the sink. The source-sink relationship between various plant organs is dynamic, and can change hourly as environmental conditions affect photosynthetic capacity, respiration, and growth. Polysaccharides are too large for transport, so they are hydrolyzed to sugars for translocation. Much of the translocation of sugars from source to sink occurs in stem tissue. This is why stems are often higher in sugar concentration than leaves.

When growth slows or stops due to cold temperatures or a lack of water or other nutrients, the sink is removed. As long as there is still green leaf tissue and adequate sunlight to allow production of photosynthates, accumulation may occur whenever carbohydrate production exceeds utilization.

Concentration of Various Forms of Carbohydrate in Grass

SUGAR

All types of grass contain sugar. Under simulated conditions of 10° C days/5° C nights, some selections of both C3 and C4 grasses had sucrose concentrations ranging from

CARBOHYDRATES IN FORAGE: WHAT IS A SAFE GRASS?

KATHRYN A. WATTS
Rocky Mountain Research & Consulting, Inc., Center, Colorado

Introduction

The ability to accumulate high levels of nonstructural carbohydrates (NSC) confers superior agronomic characteristics to grass. Grass species that accumulate NSC are more persistent under drought stress than species that do not (Boschma et al., 2003). Drought tolerance (Volaire and Lelievre, 1997; Volaire et al., 1998) and the ability to grow under cool temperatures (Brocklebank and Hendry, 1989) are linked to high fructan levels. Grasses that retain higher levels of NSC after grazing or hay production have faster regrowth and better persistence (Donaghy and Fulkerson, 1997). Grasses with larger seeds containing more starch are faster to germinate and establish after planting. Animal preference and better performance of meat- and milk-producing animals are also associated with higher levels of NSC in forage. High sugar concentration in grass allows more efficient utilization of nitrogen in the rumen, preventing excess from being excreted and contaminating the environment (Miller et al., 2001; Lovett et al., 2004). For all of these reasons, high concentration of NSC in grass is a major focus for grass breeders (Humphreys et al., 2006).

While the ruminant livestock enterprises benefit from higher levels of NSC in grass, various forms of carbohydrate intolerance are being recognized in horses. Obesity, laminitis, insulin resistance (Treiber et al., 2006), developmental orthopedic disease (Hoffman et al., 1999), and polysaccharide storage myopathy (Firshman et al., 2003) all involve excess dietary NSC in their etiology. Traditionally, these conditions were attributed to consumption of excess starch from grain; however, recent studies now include NSC in forage as a potential trigger factor (Longland and Byrd, 2006). Hyperinsulinemia may cause laminitis in ponies (Asplin et al., 2007), which implicates carbohydrates that elicit a glycemic response as triggers. Inulin, a form of short-chain fructans found in some broad-leaf plants, may trigger laminitis in horses via mechanisms involving microbial population dynamics (van Eps et al., 2006) and hyperinsulinemia (Bailey et al., 2007). Laminitis may also be induced with inulin in cows (Thoefner et al., 2004). A better understanding of the NSC concentration of various grass species and variation throughout the growing season would be valuable to those managing horses at risk for illness associated with excess carbohydrates.

to forage chemical composition or forage morphology. Similarly, the impact of forage preferences of horses is unknown, but further research is needed to determine whether total intake of preferred varieties is greater than intake of less preferred varieties.

References

Spitaleri, R.F., M. Collins, L.M. Lawrence, G.D. Lacefield, T.D. Phillips, B. Coleman, and D. Powell. (2004). 2003 Cool-season Grass Grazing Variety Report: Tolerance to Horses. PR-496 UK Agricultural Experiment Station, University of Kentucky, Lexington.

12-15% DM (Chatterton et al., 1989). Drought stress may increase sugar concentration. The ratio of sugars to starch in a drought-stressed plant can be different depending on whether the drought came on suddenly or developed slowly. In setaria (*Setaria sphacelata*), a C4 tropical grass, the relationship between sucrose, hexoses (glucose and fructose), and starch was studied after dramatic short-term drought of exposed leaf discs, and a long-term drought of 45-day duration. While short-term water loss caused a reduction of sucrose and starch, presumably due to increased respiration, a long-term gradual drought caused sucrose to increase twofold to almost 50% of the dry matter; glucose and fructose increased significantly; and starch decreased (da Silva and Arrabaca, 2004). When sugar concentration reaches a threshold, formation of storage polysaccharides commences.

FRUCTANS

C3 cool-season grasses generally, but not always, store fructans. Chatterton et al. (1989) suggested that accumulation of fructan in most cool-season grasses did not occur before a threshold value of 15% NSC. Other studies showed that tall fescue may accumulate fructan when NSC level is lower than that. Highest mean level of fructan across the growing season in Idaho for eight varieties of tall fescue over the growing season was 119 g NSC kg^{-1} DM (equivalent to 11% total dry matter) (Shewmaker et al., 2006). Tall fescue and perennial ryegrass tend to have the highest levels of fructans when compared to other grasses under the same conditions. Fructan is stored in vacuoles inside cells throughout the plant where it is readily available as needed. In some species of grass, the lower part of the stem is a carbohydrate-storage organ.

Extrapolation of dosage of inulin, given as a bolus, necessary to induce laminitis in a clinical setting would require 28% DM fructan in grass and high intake rates over the course of a full day (Longland and Byrd, 2006). While this level has been documented in stem tissue and whole plants or excised leaves grown under artificial, controlled conditions, this concentration of fructan in whole-plant grass samples grown under field conditions is not supported in existing published literature. As per Chatterton (personal communication), maximum concentration of fructan in grass under field conditions is around 20% (DM), although dandelions may have more fructan than grass.

STARCH

C4 warm-season grasses store starch in chloroplasts in leaf tissue. While they do not contain fructans, they may contain small amounts of short-chain fructooligosaccharides (FOS) (Chatterton et al., 1991). C4 grasses have different respiratory mechanisms than C3 grasses, allowing them to conserve energy under hot conditions when C3 grasses may burn off carbohydrates. Under high heat in growth chambers (32.2° C days/26.7° C nights), vegetative growth from two tropical grasses accumulated high levels of starch (16-19% DM), while the NSC of perennial ryegrass stayed fairly low (Wilson and Ford, 1971). C4 grasses such as Bermuda, paspalum, and Rhodes grass grown under heat stress may contain considerable starch content in leafy tissue. When hays made from C4 grasses are fed to carbohydrate-intolerant horses, analysis for starch is recommended even if no seed heads are present.

Environmental Factors Trigger Genetic Potential

Appropriate environmental conditions are necessary to trigger the genetic potential for higher NSC concentration. Cool temperatures, short day length, intense sunlight, drought, and limited nutrients may cause NSC to accumulate. If a required stimulus is lacking, the mechanisms that produce excess carbohydrate are not initiated. Varieties of ryegrass considered "high sugar" in the United Kingdom did not express this characteristic when grown under field conditions in New Zealand. Further investigations in controlled environment chambers found that sugar production was triggered by temperatures below 10° C for 14 days, especially if followed by 10 weeks at 5° C, and accompanied by short day length (Parsons et al., 2004). These same ryegrass varieties were higher in sugar than local commercial standard varieties when grown in Oregon (Downing, 2007). Sometimes, varieties developed in the United Kingdom and considered high in sugar do not express the trait when grown there (Lovett et al., 2004). In orchard grass grown in a Mediterranean climate, drought stress triggered accumulation of WSC in leaf bases and increased as the drought progressed through the summer (Volaire and Lelievre, 1997). Crested wheatgrass is known as a fructan accumulator but fructans were not detected when grown at temperatures optimum for growth (20° C days/15° C nights). Only at cool temperatures (10/5° C) did fructan accumulation occur (Chatterton et al., 1986). In the intermountain region of the United States, where winters are subfreezing and grass becomes dormant, fructan concentrations in crested wheatgrass were least in midwinter when daily maximum temperatures were near 0° C, and greatest in spring and fall. When temperatures increased above freezing, fructan accumulation increased, reaching maximum concentrations when the ambient temperatures reached 15° C and then declining during the summer when optimum growth allowed full utilization of the NSC produced (Chatterton et al., 1988). The total concentration and ratio of NSC components may vary even in the same species depending on slow or rapid onset of cold temperatures, which affects enzymatic activity for first- and second-stage cold hardening (Livingston and Henson, 1998). First-stage cold hardening in cool-season perennial grasses triggers fructan accumulation when temperatures dip below 5° C. Second-stage hardening occurs with onset of prolonged hard freezing, generally causing fructans to hydrolyze to simple sugars. Rapid freezing without a long enough first-stage hardening period to accumulate fructan to use as a substrate for energy through a long winter may affect winter hardiness, even in species that have the genetic potential to accumulate high levels of fructan under optimum conditions.

Photosynthetic rate response to temperature and the resulting carbohydrate levels may vary by grass species within the same genus (Borland and Farrar, 1987). NSC concentration of cultivars within the same species can vary significantly (Shewmaker et al., 2006). In a study conducted in the Netherlands during summer, perennial ryegrass cultivars differed up to 37% in WSC concentration under the same field conditions (Smit et al., 2005). In a growth chamber study, a new, improved cultivar of Italian ryegrass had 16% higher NSC under warm conditions and 22% higher NSC under cool growing conditions when compared to a standard commercial cultivar (Hopkins et al., 2002).

Because of confounding factors, many studies comparing NSC content of various grass species have been conducted in growth chambers or greenhouses where factors can be controlled. While these studies are valuable to assess genetic potential to accumulate NSC under controlled conditions, they do not provide information about the NSC content of individual grass species and how it may vary under fluctuating field conditions.

Seasonal Variation

The temperatures and day length that trigger accumulation of NSC are specific for each genus, species, and variety of grass. Generally, when night temperatures are below 5-10° C, NSC will begin to accumulate. Care must be taken to avoid extrapolating data on seasonal variation of NSC to areas with different climatic conditions. The United Kingdom has mild winters with temperatures frequently just above freezing, so grass stays mostly green, although growth may slow or stop during a cold spell. These conditions are similar to spring in the northern half of the United States, and midwinter conditions in the southern regions. Yet, it is common worldwide to associate "spring grass" with laminitis. Since the theory that fructan may be involved in grass-associated laminitis has received so much attention, it is often assumed that fructan is highest in spring. Seasonal patterns of fructans concentration in four major species of C3 pasture grasses grown in England had greatest fructan concentrations in midwinter (Pollack and Jones, 1978). Fescue in Idaho had highest fructan levels in July (Shewmaker et al., 2006). Periods corresponding to times when NSC fluctuates are about weather, not season, especially in a global perspective. Recommendations for low-NSC forage must be qualified with information about specific growing conditions.

Growth Rate

It is often incorrectly assumed that fast-growing grass or a "new flush" of grass is high in NSC concentration. The first two to three leaves of new growth are generally low in NSC concentration as reserves are depleted to accomplish the growth. New growth is a carbohydrate sink. The first new shoots do not have enough surface area for the photosynthetic capacity to function as a source of carbohydrate. When grass is growing the fastest in midsummer warmth, NSC is at the lowest concentration of the year. Accumulation of sugars occurs when growth is slowed such that the products of photosynthesis exceed demand for growth.

In Tasmania, warm temperatures cause rapid growth and increased respiratory rate while cloudy conditions decrease photosynthetic rate. These conditions necessitate intensive management of grazing land based on cool-season grasses. Dairymen must hold off grazing until the critical stage when grass starts accumulating carbohydrates to replenish reserves. If the sink (new growth) is continually removed, the carbohydrate source will be exhausted and grass will die. New growth of perennial ryegrass switched from sink to source at the three-leaf stage (Fulkerson and Donaghy, 2001), and orchard grass at the four-leaf stage under these growing conditions (Rawnsley et al., 2002). It is likely that these critical stages to maintain sustainable grazing would differ in regions with different environmental conditions.

So why is it recommended that horses prone to laminitis avoid rapidly growing grass? While concentration of NSC per mouthful of grass is lower when growth rate is high, the amount of NSC per acre is increasing. Rainfall or application of fertilizer increases carbohydrate per acre (Belesky et al., 1991). Limitations to intake may be removed by the sheer abundance of grass available when growth rate is high. The horse suddenly has the opportunity to overeat. If laminitis is associated with a new "flush" of green grass that grows rapidly and steadily during warm weather, factors other than high NSC concentration should be considered.

Maturity

Sometimes it is incorrectly assumed that very mature forage is safer for horses with metabolic problems. Stage of growth is but one factor in the NSC concentration of grass. Generally, later stages of maturity are considered less nutritious, but care should be taken when interpreting such general terms in the context of NSC. Nutritionists generally quantify fractions as a percentage of total dry matter, which might lead to thinking that an increase of one fraction leads to a decrease of the others. While this may be true of ground feedstuffs, it is not true of carbohydrate fractions found in separate parts of a plant cell.

Cellulose, hemicellulose, and lignin concentrations increase with increasing maturity and are found in cell walls. NSC concentration is more a function of environmental conditions. NSC is found in storage organs inside plant cells. Apoplastic sugars are found between plant cells. Since fiber and NSC are found in different parts of a plant cell, they are not mutually exclusive. High levels of NSC may be found in very mature, high-fiber forage when grown under environmental conditions conducive to its accumulation.

Plant scientists generally quantify nonstructural dry matter as a ratio of structural dry matter (mg gSDM^{-1}), fully acknowledging that they vary independently (Chatterton et al., 1989). Sometimes this is referred to as adjusted dry weight (ADW) (Shewmaker et al., 2006). The following example shows how to convert ADW to % total dry matter:

333 mg gSDM^{-1} = 333 mg nonstructural dry matter + 1000 mg structural dry matter = 1333 mg total dry matter. 333 mg/1333 mg = 25% NSC (total DM).

When NSC are expressed as ratio to ADW, plant scientists show that NSC vary significantly independently from structural dry matter (fiber), even over the course of a single day. In Idaho, daily carbohydrate accumulation in tall fescue was studied. Rates of daily NSC gain varied over the season, with the highest rate of increase from dawn to dusk in September at 30.8 g kg^{-1} ADW, or nearly 3% of total dry matter in one day (Shewmaker et al., 2006).

Stage of Growth vs. Environmental Conditions

To investigate whether environmental conditions were more important than stage of growth as a factor of NSC concentration, a study was conducted comparing early- and late-planted oat hay. The spring planting was subjected to freezing temperatures at early stages of growth, and the adjacent summer-planted oats were subjected to freezing temperatures as they matured in late fall. The study was conducted at Rocky Mountain Research & Consulting, Inc. in Center, Colorado. The site is a high alpine desert at 7700 ft altitude with usually cloudless skies, a relatively short growing season, and wide diurnal temperature fluctuations. Samples were cut at seven different stages of growth and air-dried, with four replications. The spring-planted oat hay had peak NSC concentration at boot stage, with 29% NSC (total DM) and 36% NDF, averaged over two growing years. The summer-planted oat hay had peak NSC concentration at soft dough stage, with an average of 27% NSC and 49% NDF. Maximum fructan concentration was near 12% and occurred at boot stage in the second year of spring planting following a period of near-freezing night temperatures. Peak NSC concentration followed trends in temperature more closely than stage of growth (Chatterton et al., 2006). Maturity is a factor in the NSC concentration of forage, but environmental conditions may override stage of growth, producing very mature forage with high NSC concentration.

At the same Colorado site, thirteen perennial grass varieties from a randomized block with four replications were cut in late July, a full month after the optimum time for hay production. All were headed out. Samples were frozen immediately and shipped frozen to Dairy One (Ithaca, New York) for analysis. Correlation (r) between WSC and NDF was -0.61 (P< 0.0001) and between NSC and NDF was -0.66 (P< 0.0001). A scatter plot of the data (Figure 1) for means presented in Table 1 illustrates

Table 1. Overmature fresh grass NSC vs. NDF (DM).

Variety	NSC	WSC	NDF
Roadcrest crested wheatgrass	20.2	19.2	61.6
Garrison meadow foxtail	19.9	19.2	57.3
Climax timothy	17.2	15.9	59.6
Potomac orchardgrass	15.5	14.4	61.9
NewHy Crested wheatgrass	15.1	14.1	64.0
Cache meadow brome	13.8	12.2	66.5
Sherman big bluegrass	13.4	12.6	67.5
Regar meadow brome	13.0	12.1	64.7
Ginger Kentucky bluegrass	12.8	11.5	63.8
Fawn tall fescue	12.8	9.5	62.3
Wideleaf orchardgrass	12.4	11.3	61.9
Manchar smooth brome	12.0	8.3	63.3
Redtop	10.7	9.5	64.5
LSD (P=0.05)	3.6	3.5	3.4

Mean of 4 reps, Analysis by Dairy One, Ithaca, NY

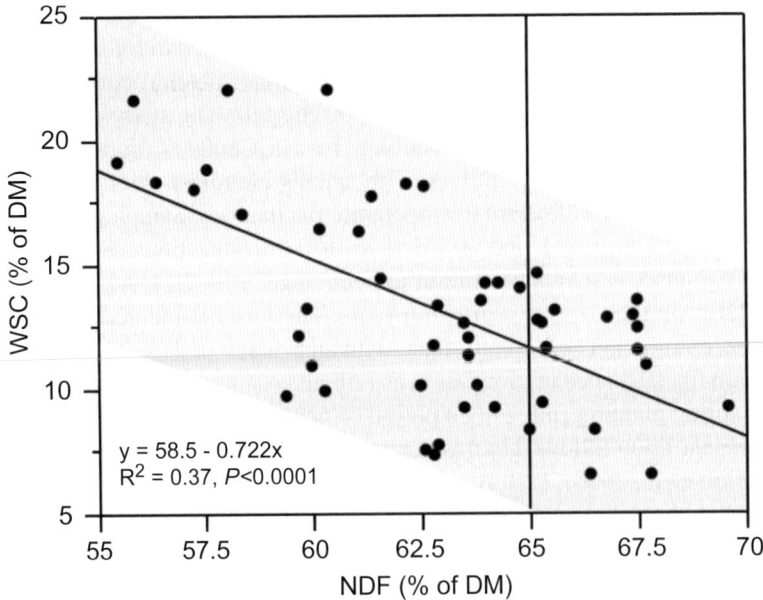

Figure 1. Even when NDF was as high as 65%, WSC concentration was up to 15%.

that even when NDF was as high as 65%, WSC concentration was up to 15%. For a forage entry similar to the sample population evaluated, one would expect that 95%

of the time an entry with 65% NDF would have a WSC value that would fall within a range of about 5 to 17.5% WSC. Fresh grass forage samples (n=3500) submitted to Dairy One (online database through April, 2007) have a mean of 10.4% WSC (DM), and 13.1% NSC (DM). High-fiber grass can still have a considerable amount of WSC under certain conditions.

Purposely allowing grass to become overmature does not necessarily result in low NSC content. Photosynthetic capacity diminishes in mature leaf tissue, but as growth ceases, sugar production may still exceed utilization, especially under cloudless skies and cool night temperatures. While protein and mineral concentrations decrease consistently with increasing maturity, sugar and fructan contents are more closely linked to environmental conditions. Until appropriate studies on availability of NSC in various fiber matrices are conducted in horses, it may be prudent to avoid assuming NSC are unavailable for fermentation or absorption even when fiber content is considered high.

Inverse Relationship Between NSC Concentration and Yield

When breeders select for more productive varieties of grass, management practices for maximum production are implemented. This may inadvertently select for those varieties that require higher management inputs, such as higher amounts of fertilizer or water. If these are not supplied as needed, the grass will be under stress. Stressed grass is higher in NSC. Far too frequently, horse owners overgraze and neglect pastures. When grass is perceived as the enemy, it seems intuitive to many owners of carbohydrate-intolerant horses to discourage its growth or vigor. Benign neglect becomes the prevailing pasture management practice. If "lush" grass to be avoided, they believe that dry, sparse grass is safer. This may be counterproductive. While NSC per acre may be less, the NSC per mouthful of grass can be greater with nutrient stress. Nitrogen has an inverse relationship with NSC (Lovett et al., 2004). An irrigated paddock of Paddock meadow brome (*Bromus riparius*) and Garrison meadow foxtail (*Alopecurus arundinaceus*) in Center, Colorado was divided into a randomized complete block with four replications. A moderate rate of ammonia nitrate decreased NSC concentration significantly compared to the unfertilized grass (Table 2). Dry matter production increased threefold on the fertilized plots, resulting in a large increase in NSC per acre (Watts, 2005a). In a study conducted in Georgia, fescue fertilized with nitrogen was also lower in carbohydrate concentration, with carbohydrate yield per acre higher on fertilized grass. Higher carbohydrate yield per acre tended to correspond to lower carbohydrate concentration, especially after high rainfall. In the same study, ungrazed fescue had higher carbohydrate yield per acre than fescue after grazing (Belesky et al., 1991). In fescue grown under simulated short-term drought conditions, sucrose levels in leaf bases increased 258% (Spollen and Nelson, 1994). While rapidly growing grass is lower in NSC concentration, sheer volume may remove limitations to intake imposed by overgrazing, drought, or neglect. Weeds that thrive when grass is stressed may be higher in sugar than grass (Watts, 2005b). While we cannot control the weather, we can do a better job correcting nutrient deficiency and controlling high-sugar weeds to decrease carbohydrate concentration per mouthful. Limiting intake when grass is in abundance seems a more useful approach than purposely stressing grass by ignoring good agronomic practices.

Table 2. NSC content of fertilized vs. nonfertilized pasture.

	NSC* % dry matter	Yield tons DM/acre	NSC lb/acre
35 lb N/acre nitrogen as AmNO$_3$	17.88	0.6	631
No nitrogen	23.10	1.8	285
LSD (P=0.05)	2.33	0.8	274

Mean of 4 reps
Analysis by Dairy One, Ithaca, NY. *NSC=WSC + starch.

Growing Low-NSC Grass May Be Difficult

It will be easier to grow low-NSC grass in warm, cloudy climates, and more difficult in sunny, cool climates. The most commonly used grasses in horse pasture in regions with hard winters must have a genetic potential for high levels of NSC in order to be productive throughout a long grazing season and to withstand the stress of intensive grazing, cold, and perhaps drought. High-NSC grasses grow in spite of the abuse and neglect that is too often the case in horse pastures. Warm-season C4 grasses tend to be lower in NSC concentration than C3 cool-season grasses, especially under cool growing conditions (Chatterton et al., 1989). When subjected to frost that dramatically raises NSC concentration in C3 cool-season grasses, C4 warm-season grasses go dormant. While these may be a viable lower NSC alternative in subtropical regions, in temperate regions their growth season is very short. They will not break dormancy until the soil temperature is above around 10° C, and are productive only during summer months with adequate rainfall or irrigation. As they tend not to store as much NSC reserves as cool-season grasses, they would not be sustainable under yearlong intensive grazing by horses outside of their region of adaptation. A possible strategy for utilizing some of the more winter-hardy, warm-season grasses in temperate regions might be to set aside a paddock that is grazed only in spring or fall as standing hay, when many cool-season grasses are peaking in NSC content. Keeping invasive indigenous cool-season grasses from taking over the less competitive low-sugar grasses will be a challenge. Many of the low-sugar grasses native to the intermountain region spring up quickly after snowmelt or summer rains. They remain dormant during times of drought, so they don't have to hoard NSC to stay alive. They will not be competitive when grown where sod-forming grasses thrive. Even in their preferred habitat, they are not sustainable without intensive management that includes rotational grazing and destocking when conditions are suboptimal. Horse owners are generally not willing to withhold access to grazing for the sake of the grass. These low-NSC native grasses comprise a large part of the diet of free-ranging feral horses and wildlife in the intermountain region of the United States. Assessments of the condition of rangelands are done continuously by range managers to determine carrying capacity and assure sustainability. It is unlikely these native grasses will provide a viable alternative for grazing horses confined on small parcels of land, even in areas where they are well-adapted.

A more successful approach to growing low-sugar forage may be to choose a grass species that is well-adapted to the growing area, and apply best management practices for minimizing stress and optimizing growth. Stress causes accumulation of NSC, and growth utilizes NSC. Management systems for individual grass species in specific regions have been developed to facilitate utilization of grass when carbohydrate concentrations are maximized without depleting carbohydrate reserves beyond that which is necessary for optimum regrowth and sustainability of the sward (Fulkerson, 2001). Cutting or grazing grass when NSC are lowest depletes energy reserves (Nelson, 1995). It will be more difficult to manage grass for low NSC content sustainably. Field studies to develop grazing management strategies when NSC are lowest need to be conducted. Studies will be necessary for each type of grass in each bioregion. A rotational grazing plan that allows grass to replenish carbohydrate reserves after grazing will be necessary to sustain the grass sward.

Summary

The NSC content of a grass species at any given time is dependent upon a complex array of interacting factors. Clearly we cannot consider the concentration or ratio of various NSC fractions in any given grass species without considering the environmental conditions under which it was grown. Horses that cannot tolerate any grass when weather is sunny and cool may be at less risk during warm or cloudy weather. Unstressed regrowth after mowing or intensive grazing when weather is warm will have far less NSC content than grass that is heading or is subjected to cold, drought, or nutrient stress. Overmature grass is not always lower in NSC. While some native grasses are lower in NSC than those adaptable to continuous grazing, a very large acreage per animal, a climate suitable to each species of grass, and intensive management utilizing sophisticated agronomic science will be required to graze such grasses sustainably. Lower productivity will likely be associated with grass species that have relatively lower NSC content than currently popular species. If lower sugar alternatives to the types of grass traditionally recommended for horse pasture are deemed necessary, appropriate studies to determine suitable varieties and to develop sustainable management systems should be conducted in each bioregion. All the most commonly recommended varieties of grass have the potential to have high levels of NSC under certain conditions. Rather than recommending a different grass, my best current advice for safer grass is to manage existing stands for lower NSC concentration and limit access, or restrict access when this is not possible.

Acknowledgements

Thanks to Charles MacKown, USDA-ARS Grazing Lands Research Lab, for producing Figure 1.

References

Asplin, K.E., M.N. Sillence, C.C. Pollitt, and C.M. McGowan. 2007. Induction of laminitis by prolonged hyperinsulinaemia in clinically normal ponies. Vet. J. 174:530-535.

Bailey, S.R., N.J. Menzies-Gow, P.A. Harris, J.L. Habershon-Butcher, C. Crawford, Y. Berhane, R.C. Boston, and J. Elliot. 2007. Effect of dietary fructans and dexamethasone administration on the insulin response of ponies predisposed to laminitis. J. Amer. Vet. Med. Assoc. 231:1365-1373.

Belesky, D.P., S.R. Wilkinson, and J. A. Stuedemann. 1991. The influence of nitrogen fertilizer and *Acremonium coenophialum* on the soluble carbohydrate content of grazed and non-grazed *Festuca arundinacea*. Grass and Forage Sci. 46:159-166.

Borland, A.M., and J.F. Farrar. 1987. The influence of low temperature on diel patterns of carbohydrate metabolism in leaves of *Poa annua* L. and *Poa X jemtlandica* (ALMQ) Richt. New Phytol. 105:255-263.

Boschma, S.P., M.J. Hill, J.M. Scott, and G.G. Rapp. 2003. The response to moisture and defoliation stresses, and traits for resilience of perennial grasses on the northern tablelands of New South Wales, Australia. Aus. J. Ag Res. 54:903-916.

Brocklebank, K. J., and G.A.E. Hendry. 1989. Characteristics of plant species which store different types of reserve carbohydrates. New Phytol. 112:255-260.

Chatterton, N.J., P.A. Harrison, and J.H. Bennett. 1986. Environmental effects on sucrose and fructan concentration in leaves of *Agropyron* spp. In: Phloem Transport p. 471- 476, Alan R. Liss, Inc.

Chatterton, N. J., P. A. Harrison, J.H. Bennett, and K. H. Assay. 1989. Carbohydrate partitioning from 185 accessions of gramineae grown under warm and cool temperatures. J. Plant Physiol. 134:169-179.

Chatterton, N.J., W.R. Thornley, P.A. Harrison, and J.H. Bennett. 1988. Dynamics of fructan and sucrose biosynthesis in crested wheatgrass. Plant Cell Physiol. 29:1103-1108.

Chatterton, N.J., W.R. Thornley, P.A. Harrison, and J.H. Bennett. 1991. DP-3 and DP-4 oligosaccharides in temperate and tropical grass foliage grown under cool temperatures. Plant Physiol. and Biochem. 29:367-372.

Chatterton, N.J., K.A. Watts, K.B. Jensen, P.A. Harrison, and W.H. Horton. 2006. Nonstructural carbohydrates in oat forage. J. Nutr. 136:2111S-2113S.

da Silva, J.M., and M.C. Arrabaca. 2004. Contributions of soluble carbohydrates to the osmotic adjustment in the C4 grass *Setaria sphacelate*: A comparison between rapidly and slowly imposed water stress. J. Plant Physiol. 161:551-555.

Donaghy D.J., and W.J. Fulkerson. 1997. The importance of water-soluble carbohydrate reserves on regrowth and root growth of *Lolium perenne* (L.). Grass Forage Sci. 52:401-407.

Downing, T. 2007. Nonstructural carbohydrates in cool-season grasses. Oregon State University. Ext Serv. Spec. Report 1079-E.

Firshman A.M., S.J. Valberg, J.B. Bender, and C.J. Finno. 2003. Epidemiologic characteristics and management of polysaccharide storage myopathy in Quarter Horses. Amer. J. Vet. Res. 64:1319-1327.

Fulkerson, W.J., and D.J. Donaghy. 2001. Plant-soluble carbohydrate reserves and senescence- key criteria for developing an effective grazing management system for ryegrass-based pasture: A review. Austral. J. Exper. Agric. 41:261-275.

Hoffman, R.M., L.A. Lawrence, D.S. Kronfeld, W.L. Cooper, D.J. Sklan, J.J. Dascanio, and P.A. Harris. 1999. Dietary carbohydrates and fat influence radiographic bone mineral content of growing foal. J. Anim. Sci. 77:3330-3338.

Hopkins, C., J.P. Marais, and D.C.V. Goodenough. 2002. A comparison, under controlled environmental conditions, of a *Lolium multiflorum* selection bred for high dry matter content and nonstructural carbohydrate concentration with a commercial cultivar. Grass Forage Sci. 57:367-372.

Humphreys M.W., R.S. Yadav, A.J. Cairns, L.B. Turner, J. Humphreys, and L. Skøt. 2006. A changing climate for grassland research. New Phytol. 169:9–26.

Livingston, D.P., and C.A. Henson. 1998. Apoplastic sugars, fructans, fructan exohydrolase, and invertase in winter oat: Responses to second-phase cold hardening. Plant Physiol. 116:403-408.

Longland A.C., and B.M. Byrd. 2006. Pasture nonstructural carbohydrates and equine laminitis. J. Nutr. 136:2099S-2102S.

Lovett, D.K., A.P. Bortolozzo, P. Conaghan, P. O'Kiely and F.P. O'Mara. 2004. In vitro total and methane gas production as influenced by rate of nitrogen application, season of harvest and perennial ryegrass cultivar. Grass Forage Sci. 59:227–232.

Miller, L.A., J.M. Moorby, D.R. Davies, M.O. Humphreys, N.D. Scollan, J.C. MacRae, and M.K. Theodorou. 2001. Increased concentration of water-soluble carbohydrate in perennial ryegrass (*Lolium perenne* L.): Milk production from late-lactation dairy cows. Grass Forage Sci. 56: 383-394.

Nelson, J.C., 1995. Photosynthesis and carbon metabolism. Page 40 in Forages: An Introduction to Grassland Agriculture. Iowa State University Press, Ames, Vol. 1.

Parsons, A.J., S. Rasmussen, H. Xue, J.A. Newman, C.B. Anderson, and G.P. Cosgrove. 2004. Some "high sugar grasses" don't like it hot. In: Proc. New Zeal. Grassland Assoc. Conf. 6:265-271.

Pollock, C.J., and T. Jones. 1978. Seasonal patterns of fructan metabolism in forage grasses. New Phytol. 83:9-15.

Rawnsley, R. P., D.J. Donaghy, W.J. Fulkerson, and P.A. Lane. 2002. Changes in the physiology and feed quality of cocksfoot (*Dactylis glomerata* L.) during regrowth. Grass Forage Sci. 57:203-211.

Shewmaker, G.E., H.F. Mayland, C.A. Roberts, P.A. Harrison, N.J. Chatterton, and D.A. Sleper. 2006. Daily carbohydrate accumulation in eight tall fescue cultivars. Grass Forage Sci. 61:413-421.

Smit, H.J., B.M. Tas, H.Z. Taweel, S. Tamminga, and A. Elersma. 2005. Effects of perennial ryegrass (*Lolium perenne* L.) cultivars on herbage production, nutritional quality and herbage intake of grazing dairy cows. Grass Forage Sci. 60:297-309.

Spollen, W.G., and C.J. Nelson. 1994. Response of fructan to water deficit in growing leaves of tall fescue. Plant Physiol. 106:329-336.

Thoefner, M.B., C.C. Pollitt, A.W. van Eps, G.J. Milinovich, D.J. Trott, O. Wattle, and P.H. Andersen. 2004. Acute bovine laminitis: A new induction model using alimentary oligofructose overload. J. Dairy Sci. 87:2932–2940.

Treiber, K.H., D. S. Kronfeld, and R.J. Geor. 2006. Insulin resistance in equids: Possible role in laminitis. J. Nutr. 136:2094S-2098S.

van Eps, A.W., and C.C. Pollitt. 2006. Equine laminitis induced with oligofructose. Equine Vet J. 38(3):203-208.

Volaire F., and F. Lelievre. 1997. Production, persistence and water-soluble carbohydrate accumulation in 21 contrasting populations of *Dactylis glomerata* L. subjected to severe drought in the south of France. Aust. J. Agric. Res. 48:933-944.

Volaire, F., H. Thomas, and F. Lelievre. 1998. Survival and recovery of perennial forage grasses under prolonged Mediterranean drought. New Phytol. 140:439-449.

Watts, K. 2005a. Nitrogen-deficient grass is higher in nonstructural carbohydrates than grass fertilized with ammonium nitrate. In: Proc. Equine Nutr. Physiol. Soc. Symp.

Watts, K. 2005b. A review of unlikely sources of excess carbohydrates in equine diets. JEVS. 25:338-344.

Wilson, J.R., and C.W. Ford. 1971. Temperature influences on the growth, digestibility, and carbohydrate composition of two tropical grasses, *Panicum maximum* Var. Trichoglume and Setariasphacelata, and two cultivars of the temperate grass *Lolium perenne*. Aust. J. Agric. Res. 22:563-571.

ASSESSING ENERGY BALANCE

LAURIE LAWRENCE
University of Kentucky, Lexington, Kentucky

Introduction

"The eye of the master fattens the ox." Anyone who has heard this adage may have wondered how the master knew how much to fatten the ox. Many horse owners have a similar question about their horses. How fat is too fat? How thin is too thin?

In the last 25 years, the use of portable scales has allowed us to gain a lot of information on body weights in horses. But, knowing a horse's body weight doesn't tell us if that is the best body weight for that horse. Henneke and coworkers (1983) developed a body condition scoring system that has been widely used in the horse industry. Their system applies a score of 1 to an emaciated horse and a score of 9 to an extremely obese horse. A score of 5 is given to a horse with "moderate" condition. A horse in moderate condition has enough fat cover to make the withers feel rounded and to make the back appear flat. The ribs are easily felt but cannot be visually distinguished. The neck and shoulders blend smoothly into the body. Henneke et al. (1984) reported that broodmares had higher reproductive efficiency if they entered the breeding season with a condition score of at least 5. There was no benefit to much higher condition scores, but there was also no negative effect on reproductive performance. Because it is a subjective system, there is always some variation from one user to another. However, researchers have reported that performance horses usually have condition scores between 4 and 6.

Few feeding guidelines for mature horses give recommendations on how to manipulate the diet to alter condition score. However, there are many horses that are deemed to be either too thin or too fat. Mares entering the broodmare herd from a performance career may have a condition score that is too low for optimum reproductive efficiency. Conversely, horses going back to work after a period of rest may have a condition score that is too high. These horses must be fed diets that permit a change in body condition through weight gain or weight loss. The most recent NRC (2007) provides a small amount of information on feeding mature horses for weight gain, but there is little information on feeding horses for weight loss.

My Horse is Too Skinny!

When a horse is in less-than-desirable body condition, it will need to gain weight to improve condition. There seems to be a lot of variation in how much weight gain is needed to produce a noticeable change in condition. The NRC (2007) suggests that weight gain of 16 to 20 kg will increase the body condition of a 500-kg horse from a 4 to a 5. However, Quinn et al. (2007) have reported that the condition score of Thoroughbred geldings that gained 93 kg increased from 4.3 to 7.0. Their results suggest that about 34 kg of gain were associated with each unit increase in condition score. The NRC (2007) has suggested that each kilogram of gain in a mature horse will require about 20 to 25 Mcal of digestible energy(above maintenance). The results of Quinn and coworkers (2007) suggest that this value may be too low, so the exact value is not known. The amount of digestible energy needed to achieve a kilogram of gain may be affected by the composition of the gain. Weight gain will consist of some protein, some fat, and some water. A pound of gain in a fat individual will probably contain less protein and water and more fat than a pound of gain in a lean individual. Therefore, the calories stored in a kilogram of weight gained by a lean horse will be less than in a kilogram gained by a fat horse. The percentage of protein in the whole body is relatively constant at about 18-21%, but the percentages of body fat and body water are more variable. In a study conducted at the University of Illinois, carcass fat ranged from 8 to 21%, and body water ranged from 56 to 64% (Lawrence, unpublished data). Ultrasound measurement of rump fat thickness has been used to estimate total body fat in horses. Cavinder et al. (2005) reported that broodmares with a condition score of 5 had about 12% body fat, whereas mares with a condition score of 7 had about 15% body fat. Other researchers have reported that horses with a condition score of about 4 had approximately 7 to 11% body fat (Henneke et al., 1984; Lawrence et al., 1992). If the calories stored in each kilogram of gain are approximated from the change in body weight and the change in body composition, a kilogram of gain should contain 5 to 6 Mcal. The NRC (2007) estimates that 20 to 25 Mcal of digestible energy are needed for a kilogram of gain, so the efficiency of digestible energy use for gain would be about 20-30%. Pagan et al. (2005) suggested that the efficiency of digestible energy use for gain was at least 28% in horses.

Daily energy balance is the first factor to consider when developing a dietary plan for a thin horse. It will be important to provide additional amounts of other nutrients (weight gain is not just fat) but energy intake will be the focus of this discussion. The first step is to determine the animal's current energy intake. In true energy balance (sometimes called "zero energy balance"), an individual consumes enough energy to exactly replace the energy that is expended. If a horse is in thin condition but has a stable weight, then the current diet is meeting the horse's current energy expenditures and the horse is in zero energy balance. However, if a horse is in thin condition and is progressively losing weight, then energy expenditure exceeds energy intake and the horse is in negative energy balance. So, before this horse can start to gain weight, it must be fed enough to attain a daily energy balance of zero. The NRC (2007) provides three levels of maintenance for adult horses. The elevated level is suggested for horses with above average voluntary activity, but it could be a starting point for horses that are in negative energy balance as well. On a body weight basis, maintenance requirements are higher for lean animals than for fat animals, and therefore it is suggested that the elevated maintenance level be used for horses on a weight-gaining diet. Actual daily maintenance requirements of horses may be much higher than levels proposed by the NRC (2007). The NRC values apply to maintenance in nonstressful, thermoneutral environments. Horses kept outside in challenging climates may have maintenance needs as much as 50% above the NRC levels.

If evaluation of the diet and the horse's environment suggests that the horse is being fed a diet that should provide adequate energy and the horse is still losing weight, then the possibility of underlying disease should be considered and a veterinarian consulted. A veterinarian should also be consulted if the horse's feed intake is unusually low, if weight loss is severe, or if there are any other indications of poor health. If the diet evaluation indicates that the horse is receiving inadequate amounts of dietary energy, then a new diet should be formulated. Inadequate energy intakes may result from low feed intake, poor-quality feed (particularly the forage component), or both.

Using the information above, it is possible to develop diets that will result in weight gain for most clinically normal horses. The first step is to determine how much digestible energy the horse should receive each day to meet its maintenance requirements. The second step is to estimate the amount of weight the horse should gain to achieve the desired condition score. The third step is to determine the number of days available to accomplish this weight gain. For example, if you would like a mare to gain enough weight to increase her condition score from a 4 to a 5 before the onset of the breeding season (February 1), you will have 120 days if you start on October 1, but only 60 days if you wait until December 1. Finally you will have to calculate the amount of digestible energy needed to achieve the desired daily weight gain. The estimated daily digestible energy intakes that would be needed to change the condition score of a 500-kg mare from a 4 to a 5 are shown in Table 1. The shorter the available time to change body weight, the higher the amount of digestible energy that must be fed. Some horses in poor body condition may already have suboptimal gastrointestinal health (racehorses on layup), so diets that promote normal gastrointestinal function should be used. The higher the quality of the forage, the higher the expected forage intakes and the lower the amount of concentrate that will be needed. When 90 days are available, the diet could consist of about 10 kg of good-quality forage and 2 to 3 kg of concentrate. When only 30 days are available, a very high level of concentrate (6 to 8 kg) will be needed even if high-quality forage is available. This level of concentrate may not be ideal for gastrointestinal health. Management programs should allow for longer periods of time to adjust body weights so that it is not necessary to feed extremely high levels of concentrate.

Assessing Energy Balance

Table 1. Daily digestible energy (Mcal) intakes needed for weight gain in a mature idle mare with an initial body condition score of 4.

Initial Condition Score = 4   Target Condition Score = 5
Initial Weight = 500 kg   Target Weight = 525 kg

Days to target weight	ADG (kg/d)	DE to maintain current wt (Mcal)*	DE for gain (Mcal)	Total daily DE (Mcal)
120 d	0.2	18.6	5.0	23.6
90 d	0.3	18.6	7.5	6.1
60 d	0.4	18.6	10.0	28.6
30 d	0.8	18.6	20.0	38.6**

*Based on an average BW of 512.5 kg
**Not recommended

The estimates in Table 1 are based on a horse that is not receiving regular exercise. If a horse is being exercised, then additional energy must be fed to meet the needs for exercise. The 500-kg mare in Table 1 would have to consume about 26 Mcal of digestible energy a day just to maintain her body weight if she is being exercised at a moderate level. She would need an additional 10 Mcal/d to gain 25 kg in a 60-day period, so her total digestible energy intake would have to be about 36 Mcal/d. It is almost impossible to achieve this digestible energy intake without feeding very high levels of concentrate. An alternative is to reduce daily energy expenditure (exercise) to make it easier to achieve a positive energy balance.

Although increases in weight gain and condition score are positively correlated, many people observe that a change in body weight can occur without a change in body condition. It is likely that this occurs because of changes in gut fill and/or gastrointestinal tissue mass. A relatively small increase in dry matter intake of 2 kg/d could increase body weight by 6-8 kg due to the water that is associated with the food. As feed intake increases there may also be an increase in gastrointestinal tissue mass. Ironically, as gastrointestinal weight increases, so does an animal's maintenance requirement. Therefore, as an animal is adapted to a diet with increased feed intake, there may be a fairly immediate increase in body weight due to changes in the gastrointestinal tract, followed by a period of slower body weight change. The change in condition score will frequently lag behind a change in body weight.

My Horse is Too Fat!

It seems that every month there is an article about obesity in horses. However, there is hardly any good scientific information that allows us to define "obese" in terms of

BETA-CAROTENE: AN ESSENTIAL NUTRIENT FOR HORSES?

ED KANE
Stuart Products, Bedford, Texas

Introduction

Beta-carotene (ß-carotene) is one of many carotenoids found in nature. In the human nutrition field, evidence suggests that higher blood levels of ß-carotene as well as other carotenoids such as alpha-carotene, lycopene, lutein, zeaxanthin, and ß-cryptoxanthin may be associated with lower risk of several chronic diseases. ß-carotene, α-carotene, and ß-cryptoxanthin have pro-vitamin A activity, while the other carotenoids have no pro-vitamin A activity (DRI, 2000).

Earlier publications on nutrient requirements of horses (NRC, 1961) suggested that horses had both a carotene and vitamin A requirement; however the latest edition (NRC, 1989) has published only a vitamin A requirement and not a carotene requirement for all horse classes. Thus, nutritionists typically do not consider the intake of carotenoids when formulating rations for horses.

Do all horse classes only need pre-formed vitamin A and not ß-carotene, or is there also a need to supplement some classes of horses with ß-carotene as well as vitamin A?

What Are Carotenoids?

Carotenoids occur in almost all plants and animals. Carotenoids are essential to green plants for photosynthesis, acting in light harvesting, and protecting against destructive photooxidation. Without carotenoids photosynthesis in an oxygen-containing atmosphere would be impossible. In addition to those in green plants, carotenoids are also compounds easily recognized as the orange-red colors of foods like oranges, tomatoes, and carrots. Some animals use carotenoids for coloration, especially birds (yellow and red feathers; e.g., flamingos), fish (e.g., goldfish and salmon), and a wide variety of invertebrate animals (shrimp, lobster, and other crustaceans), where binding with protein may modify their colors to blue, green, or purple.

Straub (1987) described 563 different carotenoids, not counting their various cis- and trans-isomers. A few of the main carotenoids and polyenes found in foodstuffs and feeds are α- and ß-carotene, zeaxanthin, lutein, ß-Apo-8;-carotenoids, ß-cryptoxanthin, astaxanthin, canthaxanthin, citranaxanthin, lycopene, neoxanthin, phytoene and phytofluene, and violaxanthin. The naturally occurring carotenoids are fat-soluble and are completely insoluble in water. They are often associated with lipids, to which they impart their color (e.g., milk fat, egg yolks, and animal fat). In fish and shrimp, however, carotenoids are typically protein-bound.

Of the major carotenoids, ß-carotene has the highest pro-vitamin A activity, thus it has received most attention by scientists. More recently, protective effects against serious disorders such as cancer, heart disease, and degenerative eye disease have been recognized for ß-carotene and the other carotenoids lutein, lycopene, and zeaxanthin. Roles other than pro-vitamin A activity have stimulated intensive research into various effects of carotenoids in humans and animals. Of the commercially available carotenoids, ß-carotene is the least expensive.

ß-carotene Absorption, Transport, and Tissue Retention

Like other fat-soluble nutrients, ß-carotene must be emulsified prior to metabolism and/or absorption via the action of bile acids. ß-carotene can either be converted in the mucosa to retinal by the action of a specific enzyme—15,15´-dioxygenase—and subsequently reduced to retinol or absorbed intact and incorporated in the chylomicrons. The ß-carotene is then transported via the lymph into the blood. In either case, ß-carotene or vitamin A must then be incorporated into chylomicrons and passed into the lymphatics. There are no data in horses, but in humans 60-75% of the ß-carotene is absorbed as vitamin A, while 15% is absorbed intact (Goodman et al., 1966). ß-carotene is transported in the blood exclusively via lipoproteins, predominantly by low-density ones (LDL). ß-carotene is excreted in the urine and bile.

Yang and Tume (1993) suggested that differences in the selective absorption process in the small intestine are responsible for the various concentrations of carotenoids observed in different species of animals. It is generally thought that carotenoids move into the enterocytes by passive diffusion (Furr and Clark, 1997). If this is the case, species differences in intestinal pH, gut motility, liposome and micelle formation, as well as the variation in the type and amount of dietary fat consumed, may influence carotene absorption. In addition, little is known concerning how carotenoids are incorporated into lipoprotein fractions and enter the circulation (Furr and Clark, 1997). Species variations in lipoprotein handling are also likely to be large contributors to differences in the accumulation of carotenoids (Slifka et al., 1999).

Horses and certain breeds of cattle have the ability to absorb ß-carotene intact as well as be converted to vitamin A (Parrish et al., 1947; Van der Noot et al., 1964; Bondi and Sklan, 1984). This conversion appears not to be very efficient in horses, and differences in utilization of carotenes from various forages may occur (NRC, 1989).

The utilization of ß-carotene is dependent on the animal species and on the carotene and vitamin A supply status. In ruminants, with a vitamin A supply approximately covering the requirement, a conversion rate of ß-carotene to vitamin A of 6:1 (1.8 µg of ß-carotene provides 0.3 µg of vitamin A alcohol = 1 IU of vitamin A) can be assumed. For horses the conversion is similar, 1mg ß-carotene provides 333 IU vitamin A activity (Fonnesbeck and Symons, 1967).

Measuring tissue concentration, horse-related species (Perissodactyla) had carotenoids ranging from not detectable in the black rhinoceros to 13 µg/dl in the Grant's zebra (Slifka et al., 1999). The serum concentration of ß-carotene in the Grant's zebra was similar to the 14.6 µg/dl reported in horses by Baker et al. (1986), but considerably lower than the 52.46 µg/dl value reported for horses by Van der Noot et al. (1964).

Functions and Actions

For the horse, the main recognized function of ß-carotene is as a precursor to vitamin A. Through other actions, it may provide benefits other than a source of vitamin A, especially to those horses not consuming adequate ß-carotene from green, lush pasture. ß-carotene, like vitamin E, can serve as an antioxidant and enhance the immune system. It has been shown to enable immune cells to act more efficiently by increasing lymphocyte response to mitogens, and to assist helper T cells and natural killer cells (Santos et al., 1996; Hughes et al., 1997; Kramer and Burri, 1997). Disease resistance has also been observed in animals with high circulating ß-carotene levels (DRI, 2000). Whether the action is due to the ß-carotene-moiety or its conversion to vitamin A is still being debated.

Benefit to Reproduction and Lactation

In the horse and other species, ß-carotene supplementation has been shown to enhance reproduction (Van der Holst, 1984; Brief and Chew, 1985; Michal et al., 1994; Chew et al., 1994). Fertility, especially of females, can be improved through the consumption of adequate ß-carotene. Reduced ß-carotene intake occurs mainly when horses do not have access to feedstuffs containing high levels of ß-carotene, such as lush, green grass. Confinement feeding and/or feeding ß-carotene-low diets has been shown to reduce circulating levels of ß-carotene in animals. ß-carotene supplementation was found to have a positive effect on fertility in cattle. Its deficiency resulted in higher incidence of silent estrus, decreased conception rates, increased embryonic death, early abortion, and poor-quality colostrum (Simpson and Chichester, 1981).

Pres et al. (1993) found that sows fed supplemental ß-carotene had more piglets per litter, and that synthetic ß-carotene in addition to vitamin A supplementation increased the number of viable embryos and corpus lutei in sows slaughtered on the 28th day of gestation. Moreover ß-carotene subsequently improved the fertility of sows in the next reproductive cycle. Coffey and Britt (1993) reported that sows injected with various levels of ß-carotene had decreased embryonic mortality and higher plasma ß-carotene levels for up to 13 days post-injection. By day 18, there were no differences in plasma levels.

Iwanska and Strusinska (1997) suggested that ß-carotene specifically, not as a precursor of vitamin A, was an important factor in bovine reproduction. They found that the number of inseminations per cow was reduced and the conception rate was significantly higher in cows supplemented with 300 mg of synthetic ß-carotene with or without vitamins A, D_3 and E.

Weng et al. (2000) found that ß-carotene was taken up by canine blood and luteal and endometrial tissues in a dose-dependent manner, as had been shown in sows (Chew et al., 1994), and cows (O'Fallon and Chew, 1994). They suggested that ß-carotene may be beneficial in optimizing the functional integrity of these tissues and, as an antioxidant, protecting ovarian and endometrial tissues from oxidative stress. As the endometrium undergoes dramatic changes to ensure successful implantation and survival of the conceptus, ß-carotene may act to decrease embryonic mortality. They stated that "uptake of ß-carotene by the uterine endometrium could protect the highly active uterine environment against oxidative damage, thereby ensuring a more optimal uterine environment for embryo development."

For horses, Van der Holst (1984) reported that ß-carotene supplementation produced stronger heats, improved conception rates, and tended to reduce embryonic mortality. Ferraro and Cote (1984) suggested that feeding 100 mg ß-carotene/day induced earlier and stronger heats, improved conception rates, and aided in maintenance of pregnancy. Ralston et al. (1985) found that 17-19 mg ß-carotene /kg DM in grass hay was adequate for semen production and libido in stallions.

Schweigert and Gottwald (1999) found that ß-carotene concentrations in colostrum were positively correlated with corresponding plasma levels in mares during the period 12 weeks around parturition. They suggested the possible reasons for the increase in plasma ß-carotene around parturition may be an improved absorption of carotene and/or reduced conversion to vitamin A, as well as mobilization from tissue storages or a reduced uptake in tissues other than the mammary gland. Increased ß-carotene in the colostrum would be favorable to enhanced immune status in the newborn foal. Mares readily pass significant amounts of ß-carotene to their offspring via the colostrum.

Intake and Supplementation

What is the daily vitamin A intake of horses grazing green pasture? The answer is zero! Unlike carnivores, grazing horses do not consume vitamin A per se. They consume ß-carotene, which is converted to vitamin A (retinol) in the intestine. *Nutrient Requirement for Horses* (NRC, 1961) noted a specific requirement for carotene and that those horses on grain and forage diets consume approximately 360 mg natural ß-carotene per day. It stated that a horse at maintenance required 1.5 mg/100 lb body weight; thus a 1200-lb mare would require 18 mg ß-carotene daily. A lactating mare required 7 mg ß-carotene per 100 lb body weight; thus a 1200-lb lactating mare would have a daily requirement of 84 mg ß-carotene.

Horses on fresh green pasture typically consume ß-carotene at much higher levels than horses consuming stored roughages. ß-carotene is also found in yellow corn at much lower levels. It is rapidly oxidized by light and heat, and therefore cured and storage forages readily lose ß-carotene content over time. After two years of storage, ß-carotene content of hay declined to less than 10% of its original concentration (Waite and Sastry, 1949). If hay is rained on during curing and drying time is extended, further losses will occur. ß-carotene content of fresh growing grass and alfalfa is 400-600 mg/kg DM, whereas content in alfalfa and timothy hay (US 1) is 40 and 20 mg/kg DM, respectively (NRC, 1989).

ß-carotene intake also varies seasonally from a high level during early spring and summer, and in some climes during the fall, to a decline during winter that lasts until new plant growth begins. Garton et al. (1964) noted that plasma ß-carotene concentration of mares was 7.9 µg/dl during the winter on hay and 114.1 µg/dl on early spring pasture, with a subsequent decrease to 15.6 µg/dl during the following winter. They reported a mean concentration of summer and fall pastures of 204 mg/kg DM. Fonnesbeck and Symons (1967) found that Standardbreds consuming hay (bromegrass, canarygrass, fescue, red clover, and alfalfa) supplying 198 mg ß-carotene/day did not maintain initial plasma vitamin A concentrations, which declined from 14.6 to 8.5 µg retinol/dl over a 24-week feeding period. Plasma ß-carotene was very low and ranged from 1.9 to 8.5 µg/dl during the same time period. Ahlswede and Konermann (1980) reported that horses on pasture had plasma carotene concentrations 8 to 13 times higher than horses kept in stables, and that ß-carotene supplementation of stabled mares tended to improve ovarian activity. Other researchers (Mäenpää et al., 1988) found seasonal variation in vitamin A status, an indicator of seasonal ß-carotene intake. In a survey of pastured horses, Barton (1997) found that serum ß-carotene levels ranged from a low of 3.3 µg/dl to a high value of 293 µg/dl with an average of 55 µg/dl. In stabled horses, the range was 1.8 to 16 with an average of 8.4 µg/dl.

Griewe-Crandell et al. (1997) fed vitamin A- and ß-carotene-depleted mares either 72,000 IU vitamin A palmitate or 216 mg ß-carotene /d utilizing a 10% water-dispersible beadlet equivalent to 72,000 IU vitamin A. They found that the beadlet form of ß-carotene was poorly absorbed and did not improve vitamin A status of depleted mares. ß-carotene concentrations in serum were found to be undetectable. Watson et al. (1996) also found poor availability from a water-dispersible beadlet when fed to Thoroughbreds and ponies. They found approximately 40% of the supplemental beta-carotene in the feces. Kienzle et al. (2002) fed approximately 225 mg ß-carotene from either grass meal (natural-source) or a water-dispersible beadlet for 4 weeks. Plasma ß-carotene levels increased from approximately 2.5 µg/dl to 30 µg/dl when oil was added to the diet. When oil was not added, the magnitude of response was not as high (Figure 1).

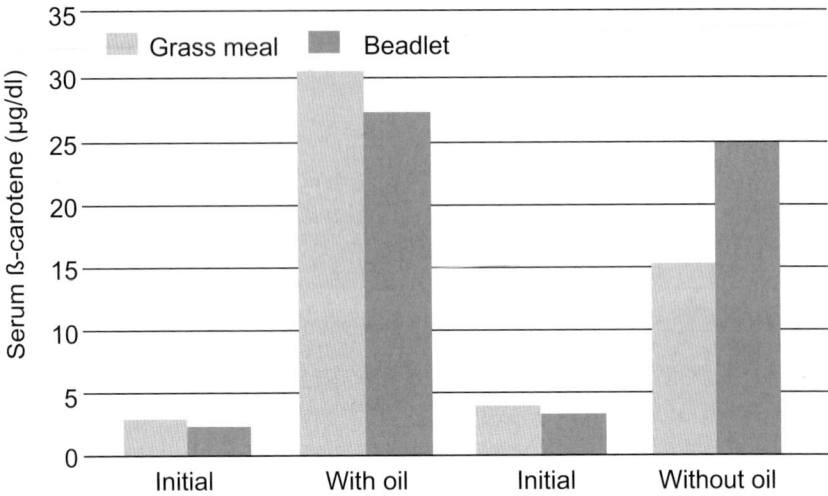

Figure 1. Effects of natural or synthetic ß-carotene sources on ß-carotene status in ponies (Kienzle et al., 2002).

These studies demonstrate the variation in the bioavailability of ß-carotene products supplemented to horses. Some appeared to improve ß-carotene status, while others did not. More research is needed to determine what commercial sources are effective in enhancing ß-carotene status of horses. A product containing ß-carotene does not necessarily mean that the form and source is biologically available to the horse.

Recommended Intakes

It should be kept in mind that ß-carotene has pro-vitamin A activity to meet a horse's vitamin A needs; however, if beta-carotene is needed for other metabolic purposes, vitamin A cannot meet those needs. The 1989 NRC's vitamin A requirement ranges from 30 to 60 IU /kg BW. Guilbert et al. (1940) suggested that the minimal requirement of ß-carotene for horses could be defined as that level to prevent nyctalopia (night blindness) to be 20-30 µg/kg BW; that would be equivalent to 6.6-10 IU vitamin A/kg BW. This level supported normal growth and freedom from signs of deficiency. The minimal carotene requirement for significant tissue storage and reproduction was raised to 125 µg/kg BW, but that level was based on research with other species besides horses.

In general, the supply of ß-carotene appears to be adequate when horses are grazing lush pasture. Due to higher cost compared to vitamin A, ß-carotene is not typically supplemented in horse diets. From review of the literature, breeding horses and foals in confinement or on poor winter pasture and fed stored forages could benefit from ß-carotene supplementation.

From various horse studies, ß-carotene has been fed at levels of 100 mg/day (Ferraro and Cote, 1984); 400 mg/day (Van der Holst, 1984); and 500 mg/day (Ahlswede and Konermann,1980; Eitzer and Rapp, 1985). While the NRC (1989) suggests that ß-carotene supplementation is not beneficial to mares on pasture or fed forages containing high levels, it does suggest that the daily dietary requirement for ß-carotene to supply vitamin A activity is 72-144 µg/kg BW.

Horses grazing lush pasture appear not to require additional ß-carotene supplementation, no matter what their life stage or physical condition. However, young foals, yearlings, and breeding animals not on pasture should be supplemented with 1000 mg ß-carotene per horse daily. Working performance horses and breeding stallions should be supplemented daily with 500 mg ß-carotene (Table 1). Since excess ß-carotene supplementation has not caused any reported toxicities in horses, these recommended supplemental levels are well within safe levels (NRC, 1989).

Table 1. Supplemental ß-carotene recommendations for horses.

Class	Forage source	Supplemental ß-carotene (mg/day)
Foals and yearlings	Stored roughages	1,000
	Lush grass	Not needed
Working horses	Stored roughages	500
	Lush grass	Not needed
Pregnant and Lactating mares	Stored roughages	1,000
	Lush grass	500-1,000
Stallions	Stored roughages	500
	Lush grass	Not needed

Summary

ß-carotene is a naturally occurring plant pigment readily obtained by horses grazing lush pasture. A 500-kg horse on pasture consuming 1.5-2% of its body weight as forage would consume approximately 3000 mg natural ß-carotene daily. Due to ß-carotene losses during processing and storage, a confined horse would consume approximately 300 mg. Though its primary functions are as the major pro-vitamin A source and as an antioxidant, ß-carotene has been shown to enhance immunity and be beneficial to reproduction. It is found in abundance in the mare's colostrum and corpus luteum. There is also evidence it is beneficial for stallion fertility. Because all commercial sources of supplemental ß-carotene are not equally bioavailable, it is important to supplement a horse with the most biologically absorbed source of ß-carotene.

ß-carotene is naturally absorbed with the aid of bile acids and micelle formation, so therefore micellized sources of ß-carotene allow for more efficient absorption and uptake. ß-carotene should be supplemented to breeding animals, especially gestating and lactating mares that foal during early spring after being wintered on stored roughages low in natural ß-carotene.

References

Ahlswede, L., and H. Konermann. 1980. Erfahrungen mit der Oralen und Parenteralen Applikation von Beta-Carotin beim Pferd. Prakt. Tierarzt 61:47.

Baker, H., S.M. Schor, B.D. Murphy, B. DeAngelis, S. Feingold, and D. Frank. 1986. Blood vitamin and choline concentrations in healthy domestic cats, dogs, and horses. Am. J. Vet. Res. 47:1468.

Barton, L. 1997. (Personal communication).

Bondi, A., and P. Sklan. 1984. Vitamin A and carotene in animal nutrition. Prog. Food Nutr. Sci. 8: 165.

Brief, S., and B.P. Chew. 1985. Effect of vitamin A and ß-carotene on reproductive performance in gilts. J. Anim. Sci. 60:998.

Chew, B.P., O. Szenci, T.S. Wong, V.L. Gilliam, P.P. Hoppe, and M.B. Coehlo. 1994. Uptake of ß-carotene by plasma, follicular fluid, granulose cells, luteal cells, and endometrium in pigs after administering injectable ß-carotene. J. Anim. Sci. 72 (Suppl 1):100.

Chew, B.P., J.S. Park, T.S. Wong, H.W. Kim, B. C. Weng, K.M. Byrne, M.G. Hayek, and G.A. Rinehart. 2000a. Dietary ß-carotene stimulates cell-mediated and humoral immune response in dogs. J. Nutr. 130:1910.

Chew, B.P., J.S. Park, B.C. Weng, T.S. Wong, M.G. Hayek, and G.A. Rinehart. 2000b. Dietary ß-carotene is taken up by blood plasma and leukocytes in dogs. J. Nutr. 130:1788.

Chew, B.P., J.S. Park, B.C. Weng, T.S. Wong, M.G. Hayek, and G.A. Rinehart. 2000c. Dietary ß-carotene absorption by blood plasma and leukocytes in domestic cats. J. Nutr. 130:2322.

Coffey, M.T., and J.M. Britt. 1993. Enhancement of sow reproductive performance by ß-carotene or vitamin A. J. Anim. Sci. 71:1198.

DRI. 2000. Dietary reference intakes for vitamin C, vitamin E, selenium and the carotenoids. National Academy Press. Washington, DC.

Eitzer, P., and H.J. Rapp. 1985. Zur Oralen Anwendung von Synthetischen ß-Carotin bei Zuchstuten. Prakt. Tierarzt 66:123.

Ferraro, J., and J.F. Cote. 1984. Broodmare management techniques improve conception rates. Standardbred 12:56.

Fonnesbeck, P.V., and L.D. Symons. 1967. Utilization of carotene of hay by horses. J. Anim. Sci. 26:1030.

Furr, H.C., and R.M. Clark. 1997. Intestinal absorption and tissue distribution of carotenoids. J. Nutr. Biochem. 8:364.

Garton, C.L., G.W. Van der Noot, and P.V. Fonnesbeck. 1964. Seasonal variation in carotene and vitamin A concentrations of the blood of broodmares in New Jersey. J. Anim. Sci. 23:1233 (Abstract).

Goodman D.S., R. Blomstrand, B. Werner, H.S. Huang, and T. Shiritori. 1966. The intestinal absorption and metabolism of vitamin A and beta-carotene in man. J. Clin. Invest 45:1615.

Greiwe-Crandell, K.M, D.S. Kronfeld, L.S. Gay, D. Sklan, W. Tiegs, and P.A. Harris. 1997. Vitamin A repletion in Thoroughbred mares with retinyl palmitate or ß-carotene. J. Anim. Sci. 75:2684.

Guilbert, H. R., C.E. Howell, and G.H. Hart. 1940. Minimum vitamin A and carotene requirements of mammalian species. J. Nutr. 19:91.

Hughes, D.A., A.J. Wright, P.M. Finglas, A.C. Peerless, A.L.Bailey, S.B. Astley, A.C. Pinder, and S. Southon. 1997. The effect of beta-carotene supplementation on the immune function of blood monocytes from healthy male non-smokers. J. Lab. Clin. Med. 129:309.

Iwanska S., and D. Strusinska. 1997. The effect of beta-carotene and vitamins A, D3 and E on some reproductive parameters in cows. Acta Vet Hung. 45:95.

Kienzle, E., C. Kaden, P. Hoppe, and B. Opitz. 2002. Serum response of ponies to ß-carotene fed by grass meal or a synthetic beadlet preparation with and without added dietary fat. J. Nutr. 132:1774S.

Kim, H.W., B.P. Chew, T.S. Wong, J.S. Park, B.C. Weng, K.M. Byrne, M.G. Hayek, and G.A. Reinhart. 2000a. Modulation of humoral and cell-mediated immune response by dietary lutein in cats. Vet. Immun. Immunopath. 73:331.

Kim, H.W., B.P. Chew, T.S. Wong, J.S. Park, B.C. Weng, K.M. Byrne, M.G. Hayek and G.A. Reinhart. 2000b. Dietary lutein stimulates immune response in the canine. Vet. Immun. Immunopath. 74:315.

Kramer, T.R., and B.J. Burri. 1997. Modulated mitogenic proliferative responsiveness of lymphocytes in whole blood cultures after a low-carotene diet and mixed carotenoid supplementation in women. Am. J. Clin. Nutr. 65:871.

Mäenpää, P.H., T. Koskinen, and E. Koskinen. 1988. Serum profiles of vitamins A, E and D in mares and foals during different seasons. J. Anim. Sci. 66:1418.

Michal, J.J., L.R. Heirman, T.W. Wong, B.P.Chew, M. Frigg and L. Volker. 1994. Modulatory effects of dietary beta-carotene on blood and mammary leukocyte function in periparturient dairy cows. J. Dairy Sci. 77:1408.

NRC. 1961. Nutrient Requirements of Horses. National Academy Press. Washington, DC.

NRC. 1989. Nutrient Requirements of Horses (5th Ed.). National Academy Press. Washington, DC.

O'Fallon, J.V., and B.P. Chew. 1984. The subcellular distribution of ß-carotene in the bovine corpus luteum. Proc. Soc. Exp. Biol. Med. 177:406.

Olson, J.A. 1999. Carotenoids. In: Shils, M.E., J.A. Olson, M. Shike, and A.C. Ross (Eds.) Modern Nutrition in Health and Disease (9th Ed.). p. 525. Williams & Wilkens. Baltimore.

Parrish, D.B., G.H. Wise, and J.S. Hughes. 1947. The state of vitamin A in colostrum and milk. J. Biol. Chem. 167:673.

Pres, J., B. Fuchs, and A. Schleicher. 1993. The effect of carotene and vitamins A and E supplementation on reproduction of sows. Arch. Vet. Pol. 33:55.

Ralston, S.L., S.A. Jackson, V.A. Rich, and E.L. Squires. 1985. Effect of vitamin A supplementation on the seminal characteristics and sexual behavior of stallions. In: Proc. 9th Equine Nutr. Physiol. Soc. Symp. p. 74. Michigan State University, East Lansing, Mich.

Santos, M.S., S.N. Meydani, L. Leka, D. Wu, N. Fotouhi, M. Meydani, C.H. Hennekens, and J.M. Gaziano. 1996. Natural killer cell activity in elderly men is enhanced by beta-carotene supplementation. Am. J. Clin. Nutr. 64:772.

Schweigert, F.J., and C. Gottwald. 1999. Effect of parturition on levels of vitamins A and E and of beta-carotene in plasma and milk of mares. Equine Vet. J. 31:319.

Simpson, K.L., and C.O. Chichester. 1981. Metabolism and nutritional significance of carotenoids. Ann. Rev. Nutr. 1:351.

Slifka, K.A., P.E. Bowen, M. Stacewicz-Sapuntsakis, and S.D. Crissey. 1999. A survey of serum and dietary carotenoids in captive wild animals. J. Nutr. 129:380.

Stowe, H.D. 1968. Experimental equine avitaminosis A and E. In: Proc. 1st Equine Nutr. Res. Soc. p. 27. University of Kentucky. Lexington.

Straub, O. 1987. Key to Carotenoids. Birkhauser Verlag, Basel, Boston.

Van der Noot, G.W., P.V. Fonnesbeck, and C.L. Garton. 1964. Seasonal variation in carotene and vitamin A concentration of the blood of brood mares in New Jersey. J. Anim. Sci. 23:12.

Van der Holst, M. 1984. Experiences with oral administration of beta-carotene to pony mares in early spring. p. 6 in Proc. 35th Annu. Meet. Eur. Assoc. Anim. Prod.

Waite, R., and K.N.S. Sastry. 1949. The carotene content of dried grass. J. Agr. Sci. 39:174.

Weng, B.C., B.P. Chew, T.S. Wong, J.S. Park, H.W. Kim, and A.J. Lepine. 2000. ß-carotene uptake and changes in ovarian steroids and uterine proteins during the estrous cycle in the canine. J. Anim. Sci. 78:1284.

VITAMIN E: AN ESSENTIAL NUTRIENT FOR HORSES?

ED KANE
Stuart Products, Bedford, Texas

Vitamin E is an essential nutrient for horses and is beneficial in combating the many effects of free radical production that can damage membranes and components of cells. As such, vitamin E appears to be most beneficial to young rapidly growing foals, pregnant mares, stallions, and especially equine athletes. Natural and synthetic sources of vitamin E, unlike other vitamins, have different structures and the natural form is transported quickly and retained in tissues approximately twice as long as that of synthetic vitamin E.

Introduction

Vitamin E (alpha-tocopherol) is a critically important nutrient for all horses, and supplementation is especially important for horses with limited or no access to lush pastures. This vitamin is not synthesized by the horse; therefore, it is an essential dietary nutrient. It is the primary lipid-soluble antioxidant that maintains cell membrane integrity and enhances humoral and cell-mediated immunity. Other metabolic roles of vitamin E have been reviewed by Brigelius-Flohe and Traber (1999).

Changes in husbandry practices and ingredients used to formulate equine diets have dramatically increased the need for supplementing diets with this critically important vitamin in all segments of the horse industry. The first NRC for horses was published in 1949 and the most recent revision was published in 1989. The second revision published in 1961 devoted only one paragraph to vitamin E and concluded that "dietary supplementation of vitamin E has not been shown unequivocally to be beneficial for either prevention of reproductive troubles or muscular dystrophy in the horse" (NRC, 1961). The 1989 revision reviewed studies in horses and published minimum requirements for horses ranging from 50 to 80 IU per kg dry matter (DM) (NRC, 1989). Gestating and lactating mares, young growing horses, and performance horses have the greatest need for vitamin E supplementation, especially those that do not have access to lush, green pasture.

Free Radicals May Harm Cells

Free radicals or reactive oxygen species are unstable atoms with unpaired numbers of electrons that are formed when oxygen interacts with other molecules in all cells. Once formed, these reactive radicals can initiate chain reactions resulting in a cascading negative effect on many other molecules within cells and cell walls resulting in oxidative stress within the animal. Free radicals are commonly produced as part of normal cell metabolism, but also can become excessive following injury or disease. Left uncontrolled, free radicals can cause considerable irreparable damage to cells and cell membranes. They can alter the structure of cell membranes, and create havoc to polyunsaturated fatty acids (PUFA), proteins, and DNA within cells. The more active the cell, the greater the potential risk of cellular damage. Excessive free radical production or oxidative stress results when the formation of free radicals overwhelms the body's ability to break the chain reactions that take place and an imbalance between production and removal of free radicals occurs. Uncontrolled oxidative stress can overpower the horse's ability to fight back and may result in tissue damage, thus possibly impairing life.

In several species, including humans, this damage has recently been linked to degenerative diseases such as rheumatoid arthritis, cancer, cardiovascular disease, inflammatory bowel disease, renal disease, Parkinson's disease, and cataracts. It may have a deleterious effect on the immune system (NRC Dietary Reference Intakes for Vitamin C, Vitamin E, Selenium and Carotenoids, 2000).

Antioxidants Help Prevent Cell Damage Caused by Oxidative Stress

Antioxidants are the horse's major defense system against the scourge of free radicals and oxidative stress. Enzymatic antioxidants are synthesized in the body to neutralize free radical production. Key enzymatic antioxidants include superoxide dismutase, glutathione peroxidase, and catalase (Table 1). Other major sources of antioxidants available to the horse are nonenzymatic or nutritional antioxidants. Nonenzymatic antioxidants, like vitamin E, carotenoids, vitamin C, and others, scavenge and convert free radicals to relatively stable compounds and stop the chain reaction of free radical damage (Table 1). Therefore, all antioxidants are critically important to protect horses from tissue damage and disease, and may enhance immunity during these processes. The critical phases of reproduction in mares and stallions, growth of foals, and exercise of equine athletes are all especially important. Thus, for the horse, vitamin E appears to be the most important dietary fat-soluble nonenzymatic antioxidant to assist in combating free radical production and propagation. Because horses synthesize vitamin C, vitamin E and possibly carotenoids appear to be the major antioxidant vitamins required from dietary sources.

Vitamin E is unique among vitamins in that it is not required for a specific metabolic function. As alpha-tocopherol (α-tocopherol), vitamin E's major function appears to

Table 1. Important enzymatic and nonenzymatic antioxidants.

Enzymatic antioxidants	Location	Properties
Superoxide dismutase (SOD)	Mitochondria and cytosol	Dismutase superoxide radicals, contains Cu and Zn
Glutathione peroxidase (GSH)	Mitochondria and cytosol	Removes hydrogen peroxide and organic hydroperoxide, contains Se
Catalase (CAT)	Mitochondria and cytosol	Removes hydrogen peroxide, contains Fe

Nonenzymatic antioxidants	Location	Properties
Vitamin E	Cell membrane	Major chain-breaking fat-soluble antioxidant in cell membrane
Vitamin C	Aqueous phase of cell	Acts as free radical scavenger and recycles vitamin E
Carotenoids	In membrane tissue	Scavengers of reactive oxygen species, singlet oxygen quencher
Uric acid	Product of purine metabolism	Scavenger of -OH radicals
Glutathione	Non-protein thiol in cell	Serves multiple roles in cellular antioxidant defense
Alpha-lipoic acid	Endogenous	Effective in recycling vitamin C, may also be an effective glutathione substitute
Bilirubin	Blood	Extracellular antioxidant
Ubiquinones	Mitochondria	Reduced forms are efficient antioxidants
Transferrin, ferritin, lactoferrin	Systemic	Chelating of metals ions, responsible for Fenton reactions

be the body's major fat-soluble antioxidant. Thus, vitamin E is notably essential for the proper function of the reproductive, muscular, nervous, circulatory, and immune systems. Figure 1 shows how vitamin E and vitamin C work in concert to protect cell membranes from being oxidized. Since selenium is in glutathione peroxidase, an enzymatic antioxidant, it is often difficult to distinguish between the signs of vitamin E and selenium deficiencies.

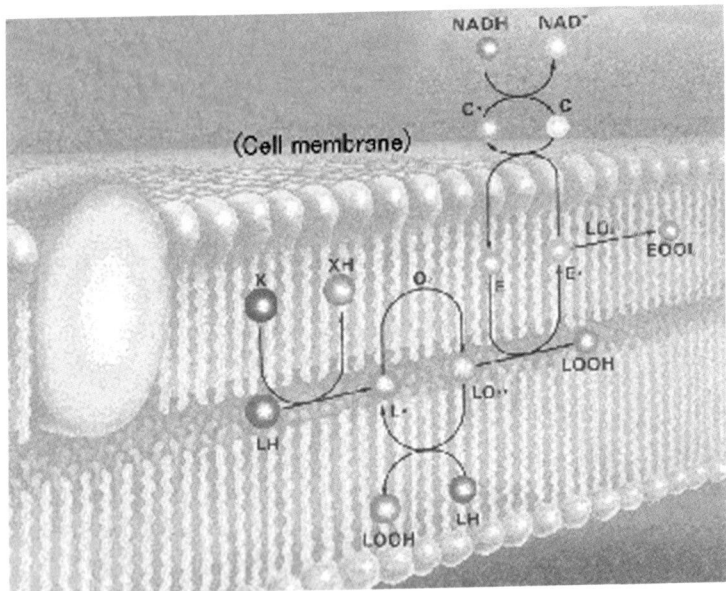

Figure 1. Mechanism of action of vitamin E and vitamin C (Eisai). The mechanism by which vitamin E (E) inhibits the chain reaction of lipid peroxidation in the membrane and the generated tocopheroxyl radical is recovered by vitamin C (C) on the membrane surface.

Vitamin E Deficiency Symptoms

Signs representing possible deficiencies of vitamin E have been extensively described in the foal and in adult horses (Schougaard et al., 1972; Wilson et al., 1976; NRC, 1989). Muscle degeneration was the most common symptom affecting both skeletal and cardiac muscle. Tongue muscles may also be affected. The latter defect may interfere with normal nursing. Steatitis has also been reported.

Vitamin E status is determined by measuring plasma or serum alpha-tocopherol levels. Low blood levels of alpha-tocopherol appear to be the first indication of vitamin E deficiencies in horses. Serum alpha-tocopherol levels above 4 µg/ml appear to be adequate for horses and levels below 2 µg/ml appear to be deficient (Schryver and Hintz, 1983). Prolonged low serum levels will lead to clinical deficiency symptoms. In order to assess vitamin E status in horses, serum or plasma alpha-tocopherol levels can be measured by HPLC.

Liu et al. (1983) reported degenerative myelopathy (spinal cord degeneration) in six Przewalski horses up to 14 years of age maintained in a zoo. They had been fed commercial horse pellets containing 22 IU vitamin E and 0.3 mg selenium/kg, timothy hay, and fresh grass in the summer. Plasma alpha-tocopherol concentrations were low and ranged from less than 0.3 to 0.8 µg/ml. Ataxia (incoordination) was evident in all, including abnormal movement of the hind limbs and abnormal wide-based gaits and stances.

Equine degenerative myeloencephalopathy (EDM) is a diffuse degenerative disease of the brain and spinal cord, a form of wobbler syndrome. Young horses affected by EDM first show signs of incoordination and clumsiness, which deteriorates over time to outright ataxia. These horses also showed low vitamin E levels in blood. Mayhew et al. (1987) found that supplementing mares with 1500 IU vitamin E per day decreased the incidence of EDM in foals born the following year from 40% to 10%. The researchers also found that horses from 3 to 30 months of age responded to vitamin E supplementation. The mean serum alpha-tocopherol concentration of 13 ataxic weanlings was 0.62 ± 0.13 µg/ml (range 0.47 to 0.84). A number of nonataxic weanlings had similar serum values, although vitamin E supplementation markedly reduced the incidence of the syndrome on affected farms. Based on these observations, horses prone to EDM due to genetics responded to vitamin E supplementation. Blythe and Craig (1993) found that young foals showing signs of incoordination and supplemented with 6000 IU vitamin E per day appeared normal by two years of age.

Clinical deficiency symptoms have been reported primarily in horses with limited vitamin E intake. However, subclinical vitamin E deficiencies most often go unrecognized in horses. Symptoms such as an impaired immune system or reproduction problems may often go undiagnosed and may be attributed to other causes besides inadequate vitamin E supplementation.

Determining Vitamin E Availability and Requirements

Vitamin E (alpha-tocopherol) is abundant in lush, green pastures (45 to 400 IU/kg DM), particularly in alfalfa (McDowell, 1989), and diminishes with maturation. Harvesting and length of storage diminish the quantity of vitamin E about tenfold below levels in fresh forages (Schingoethe et al., 1978). Vitamin E is abundant in the germ of grains and oils pressed from the germ (wheat germ oil, 1330 IU/kg). Vegetable oils, such as corn and soybean oil, are relatively high in vitamin E (50-300 IU/kg), but also contain higher levels of gamma- and delta-tocopherol, that have little or no vitamin E activity. Due to such variability in vitamin E content in processed feedstuffs, nutritionists typically do not rely on the diet to provide any vitamin E activity and depend totally upon supplementation to meet horse requirements. Though horses grazing lush pasture may obtain sufficient vitamin E, it is common practice to supplement horse feeds with vitamin E at the NRC recommended levels. This is especially important for mares and working horses maintained in confinement and consuming stored roughages.

In one of the first vitamin E studies in horses, Stowe (1968) found that foals deficient in vitamin E required 27 µg of parenteral (intramuscular) or 233 µg of oral alpha-tocopherol/kg of bodyweight/day to maintain erythrocyte stability. Prior to

Vitamin E

HPLC methodology, erythrocyte fragility was a means to measure cell wall integrity and indirectly vitamin E status since vitamin E helps maintain cell wall integrity.

Roneus et al. (1986) suggested that vitamin E supplements be provided daily and concluded that to ensure nutritional adequacy, adult Standardbred horses fed a diet low in vitamin E should receive a daily oral supplement of 600 to 1,800 IU synthetic vitamin E acetate, equivalent to 1.5 to 4.4 IU/kg bodyweight.

Mäenpää et al. (1988) observed seasonal differences in serum alpha-tocopherol concentrations in mares and foals kept on pasture from early June until early October, then fed timothy hay and oats through the winter. Serum alpha-tocopherol concentrations were highest in August and September (2.7 µg/ml for mares and 2.1 µg/ml for foals) and lowest in April or May (1.5 µg/ml for mares and 1.2 µg/ml for foals) after being fed hay during the winter months. When mares were given winter supplements of 100 to 400 IU of vitamin E/day, no significant increases in serum alpha-tocopherol concentrations occurred and seasonal differences persisted. However, when foals were supplemented with 400 IU vitamin E daily during winter months, serum alpha-tocopherol concentrations increased from 1.3 µg/ml to approximately 2 µg/ml in April and May. Blakley and Bell (1994) observed similar seasonal variation in plasma vitamin E (Figure 2).

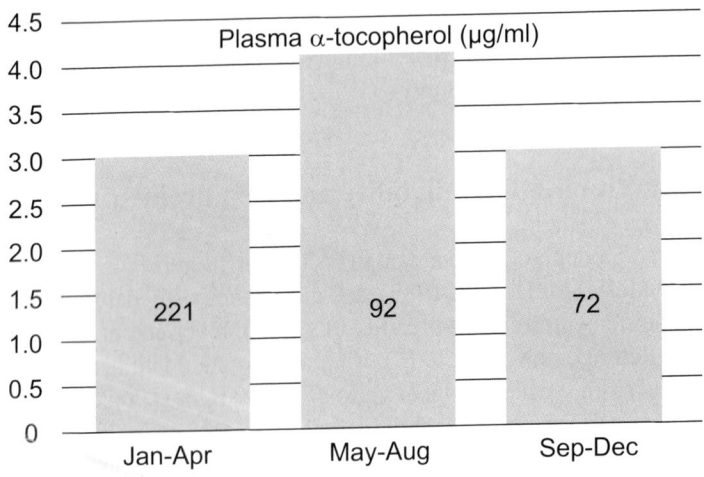

Numbers in columns represent number of observations

Figure 2. Seasonal variation in vitamin E status of horses in western Canada (Blakley and Bell, 1994).

Janssen and Ullrey (1986) observed that the capture and restraint of zebra and Przewalski horses for hoof trimming resulted in temporary to persistent muscle soreness and lameness. They found that plasma alpha-tocopherol concentrations were commonly below 1 µg/ml in animals consuming diets supplemented with 50

IU vitamin E/kg DM. When supplemental levels were increased to 100 IU/kg DM, no signs of muscle pathology were seen, and plasma alpha-tocopherol concentrations ranged from 1.5 to 3 µg/ml after increasing vitamin E supplemental levels.

Butler and Blackmore (1983) reported that the mean plasma alpha-tocopherol concentration for 140 samples from stabled Thoroughbreds in training was 3.3 ± 1.29 µg/ml. Barton (1997) measured alpha-tocopherol, beta-carotene, and selenium status in horses in confinement and pasture. Serum tocopherol values ranged from 0.9 to 7.0 µg/ml in horses on pasture (Figure 3), and the range was not as great in confined horses (3.1 to 5.1). Beta-carotene levels varied dramatically in horses on grass and the average beta-carotene was much lower in confined horses. These results obtained in pastured horses are similar to results obtained by Maylin et al. (1980), who reported a range of 1.7 to 9.5 µg/ml in pastured horses.

	Alpha-tocopherol (µg/ml)	Beta-carotene (µg/dl)	Selenium (ppm)
Pastured (n=8)	3.1 (0.9-7.0)	54.7 (3.3-293.1)	0.173 (0.05-0.24)
Stabled (n=3)	3.9 (3.1-5.1)	8.4 (1.8-16.0)	0.187 (0.9-0.24)
All horses (n=21)	3.2	48.1	0.174

Survey conducted by Barton and Blakeslee (1997).
Seven farms were pastured and one farm stabled.
Values in parentheses are ranges.

Figure 3. Alpha-tocopherol, beta-carotene, and selenium status in pastured and confined horses.

The NRC maintenance requirement for vitamin E is 50 IU per kg DM or 0.75-1.0 IU per kilogram body weight (1989). For growing horses, pregnant and lactating mares, and performance horses, the requirement is raised to 80 IU per kilogram DM. A dietary concentration of 100 IU of vitamin E per kg DM provides the equivalent of about 1.5 to 2 IU vitamin E per kg of body weight daily. Based on daily intake of 3% body weight, the NRC daily recommendations range from 375 IU for maintaining a 500-kg horse to 1200 IU per day for a 500-kg lactating mare and 500-kg working horse.

Research in other species indicates that vitamin E requirements to prevent frank deficiency symptoms are considerably lower than those levels needed to improve immune status and prevent free radical damage. The amount of vitamin E required for optimum immune function has not been thoroughly studied in horses, but has been shown to be much higher than normally fed in other species (Nockels, 1979; Tengerdy, 1981). Baalsrud and Overnes (1986) supplemented a basal diet daily with 600 IU vitamin E, 5 mg selenium, or both. They observed an improved humoral immune response to tetanus toxoid or equine influenza virus in adult horses supplemented with selenium alone or selenium plus vitamin E. No improvement was seen with vitamin E alone, possibly due to an inadequate level being fed.

Vitamin E Benefits Horses During All Life Stages and Performance Levels

MARES AND FOALS

It is beneficial to provide supplemental vitamin E to breeding horses. Green pasture, generally high in vitamin E, is not always available to gestating and lactating mares that often foal during winter months. It is advantageous to feed mares in late pregnancy and early lactation higher levels of vitamin E in order to assure that vitamin E levels will be adequate in colostrum and milk. It has been suggested (Harper, 2002) that mares known to have poor-quality colostrum, or that had foals with failure of passive immunity transfer in previous years, should be supplemented with twice the vitamin E normally fed for at least a month before and after foaling. It was also recommended that pregnant mares fed lower quality hay should be given vitamin E supplementation a month before and after foaling. In a Swedish demonstration, Gard (2003) showed that gestating mares supplemented with 1500 IU vitamin E per day as water-soluble natural vitamin E for 21 days before foaling had higher plasma alpha-tocopherol at foaling, and their foals also had higher vitamin E status at 12-36 hours after birth (Figure 4). The higher plasma tocopherol levels in foals nursing supplemented mares was attributed to higher colostrum transfer of vitamin E. Mares supplemented with vitamin E have shown increased passive transfer of antibodies to foals, which greatly enhances the immune system (Hoffman et al., 1999). This study showed an advantage of feeding vitamin E during late gestation and early lactation. Serum and colostrum IgG levels were greater in mares supplemented with 160 IU of vitamin E per kg feed (along with a mixed grass hay and grain ration), than those receiving 80 IU vitamin E per kg feed. The foals from all mares had similar levels of IgG, IgA, and IgM at birth prior to nursing. After nursing, foals from mares fed the high level of vitamin E were found to have higher serum levels of IgG and IgA, which were reflected in the dam's colostrum.

EXERCISING HORSES

Decreased vitamin E status is implicated in the etiology of exercise-induced muscle damage in horses (i.e., "tying up") (Snow & Valberg, 1994). Siciliano et al. (1997) showed that supplemental synthetic vitamin E levels of 80 IU and 300 IU per kg dry matter were necessary to maintain blood and skeletal muscle concentrations in horses

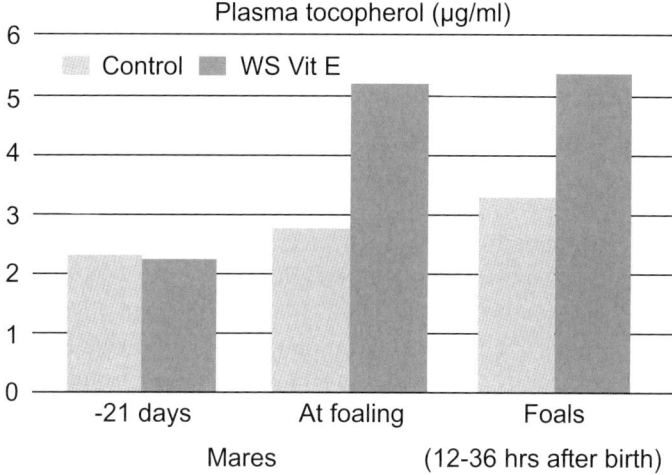

Each value represents the mean of 14 breeding mares and foals at three different locations in Sweden. Mares were supplemented with 1,500 IU vitamin E as d-alpha-tocopherol (water-soluble tocopherol).

Figure 4. Vitamin E supplementation improves status in late gestating mares and foals (Ekeby Gard, Bälinge, Sweden, 2003).

undergoing exercise conditioning. Serum tocopherol levels did not affect the integrity of skeletal muscle following repeated submaximal exercise, as measured by changes in creatine kinase (CK) and aspartate amino transferase (AST) activities, nor did vitamin E level of supplementation affect thiobarbituric acid reactive substances (TBARS). In a study performed at KER, exercising horses supplemented with 2000 IU daily for six weeks with natural vitamin E acetate (d-alpha-tocopheryl acetate) had higher plasma alpha-tocopherol levels pre- and post-exercise compared to horses receiving an equal amount of synthetic vitamin E acetate (dl-alpha-tocopheryl acetate) (Pagan, 2004).

Natural Vitamin E Differs from Synthetic Vitamin E

While grazing pasture, the only source of vitamin E consumed by the horse is natural vitamin E. In nature, most plants and oils contain a mixture of tocopherols (alpha-, beta-, gamma- and delta-). Of the four tocopherols, alpha-tocopherol is the only isomer recognized to have vitamin E activity (Traber, 1999; Dietary Reference Intakes, 2000).

The two commercial sources of vitamin E are natural-source tocopherol and synthetic-source tocopherol and their corresponding acetate-esters. Synthetic vitamin sources are for the most part identical in efficacy and structure to the natural source of that vitamin. Not so for vitamin E. The source of vitamin E with the highest biological activity is natural vitamin E, which is officially recognized to have 36% greater biological activity than synthetic source. The two sources have different structures and the natural isomer has been shown to be transported to and retained in tissues at levels approximately twice that of synthetic vitamin E (Traber et al., 1992). Natural vitamin E is one isomer (RRR-alpha-tocopherol or d-alpha-tocopherol). Synthetic vitamin E (all-rac(emic)-alpha-tocopherol or dl-alpha-tocopherol) is a racemic mixture of eight isomers, of which one or 12.5% is identical to the natural isomer and the other seven isomers are different than the natural RRR-isomer. Studies have clearly shown preferential uptake, transport, and tissue retention of the natural isomer in humans compared to synthetic sources (Ingold et al., 1987; NRC Dietary Reference Intakes for Vitamin C, Vitamin E, Selenium and Carotenoids, 2000). In addition, research in humans and swine has shown that milk transfer of the natural isomer is greater than for the synthetic source (Stone et al., 2003; Mahan et al., 2000).

In a study by KER, horses fed natural vitamin E had higher plasma vitamin E levels than horses supplemented with equal IU of synthetic vitamin E (Pagan, 2004). Horses were initially bled, then fed graded levels of either synthetic or natural-source vitamin E for two weeks. The initial daily supplements provided 500 IU and were doubled every two weeks until the maximum levels of 8000 IU were fed. After two weeks at 8000 IU, supplementation ended and the last two weeks was a depletion phase in the study. Figure 5 shows the responses obtained in the study. There was no difference in serum alpha-tocopherol when 500 IU of either natural or synthetic vitamin E was fed. As levels of supplementation increased, horses fed the natural vitamin E had progressively higher serum tocopherol levels that continued during the withdrawal period. Figure 6 shows that natural vitamin E, when fed at less than one-half the IU level of synthetic, had similar plasma tocopherol levels (Gansen et al., 2001). These studies in horses show that the present IU values for natural and synthetic vitamin E underestimate the value of natural vitamin E. Had the published IU values been correct then there should have been no difference in blood tocopherol levels when equal amounts were fed. In human studies, natural vitamin E is recognized to have 100% the activity of an equal amount of synthetic, not 36% that was determined utilizing the rat fetal resorption assay (NRC Dietary Reference Intakes, 2000).

Importance of Form of Vitamin E-Tocopherol Utilized Better Than Tocopheryl-Ester

Horses must be able to efficiently absorb fat-soluble nutrients. Because natural and synthetic vitamins E are antioxidants, in order for them to be included into rations, and not lose their potency, esters are added to provide stability. In order for supplemental vitamin E-ester to be utilized, two steps are necessary. The ester has to be removed and the alpha-tocopherol has to be made water-soluble by the action of bile salts (Gallo-Torres, 1980) (Figure 7).

Ralston, S.L., and S. McKenzie. 1992. Effect of carbohydrate intake on behavioral reactivity and activity levels in horses. J. Anim. Sci. 70(Suppl. 1):159. (Abstr.).

Sandstead, H.H. 2000. Causes of iron and zinc deficiencies and their effects on the brain. J. Nutr. 130:347S-349S.

Smith, K.A., C.G. Fairburn, and P.J. Cowen. 1997. Relapse of depression after rapid depletion of tryptophan. The Lancet 349:915-919.

Smyth, G.B., D.W. Young, and L.S. Hammond. 1988. Effects of diet and feeding on post-prandial serum gastrin and insulin concentrations in adult horses. Equine Vet. J. Suppl. 7:56-59.

Sweeting, M.P., C.E. Houpt, and K.A. Houpt. 1985. Social facilitation of feeding and time budgets in stabled ponies. J. Anim. Sci. 60:369-374.

Werbach, M.R. 1992. Nutritional influences on aggressive behavior. J. Orthomolecular Med. 7:45-51

Willard, J.G., J.C. Willard, S.A. Wolfram, and J.P. Baker. 1977. Effect of diet on cecal pH and feeding behavior of horses. J. Anim. Sci. 45:87-93.

Winskill, L.C., N.K. Waran, and R.J. Young. 1996. The effect of a foraging device (a modified "Edinburgh Foodball") on the behaviour of the stabled horse. Appl. Anim. Behav. Sci. 48:25-35.

NUTRITION AND MANAGEMENT OF THE PERFORMANCE HORSE

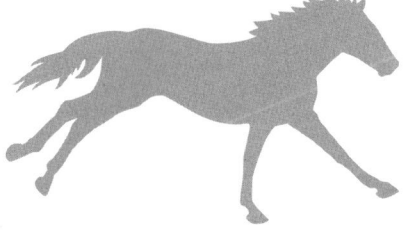

THE EFFICIENCY OF UTILIZATION OF DIGESTIBLE ENERGY DURING SUBMAXIMAL EXERCISE

JOE D. PAGAN, GEMMA COWLEY, DELIA NASH, AMY FITZGERALD, LINDSEY WHITE, AND MELISSA MOHR
Kentucky Equine Research, Versailles, Kentucky

Introduction

Two methods can be employed to calculate energy requirements for work: the factorial (analytical method) and the global method (feeding experiments) (Martin-Rosset and Vermorel, 2004). The factorial method estimates the energy cost of a specific bout of exercise based on its intensity and duration. This energy cost is then converted into a feeding recommendation based on an estimation of the efficiency of utilization of feed energy for exercise. The global method measures the amount of feed energy required by horses to maintain constant body weight while performing a specific amount of daily exercise.

The 1989 NRC uses both methods to describe the energy requirements for exercise. The global method of calculation was used by Anderson et al. (1983), where Quarter Horses were fed to maintain constant body weight while exercising at different intensities on a treadmill. These data were incorporated into an equation that estimates digestible energy requirements based on body weight and distance traveled. The NRC also cited a factorial equation from Pagan and Hintz (1986) that estimated digestible energy (DE) requirements based on measurements of energy costs at different speeds that were calculated from calorimetry measures made on horses walking, trotting, and cantering on a track. In this equation, DE requirements above maintenance were estimated assuming that the efficiency of utilization of DE for work was 57%. This value was based on the assumption that, since body fat is the primary substrate for energy generation in horses during low-intensity exercise, the DE efficiency value for fattening was also appropriate for exercise.

Both methods of calculating energy requirements have weaknesses. The exercise performed in the Anderson et al. (1983) study took place on an inclined treadmill, so translating it to other forms of work is questionable. The Pagan and Hintz (1986) study used oxygen consumption in horses exercised with and without riders, so its exercise intensity can be more easily applied to other types of exercise where VO2 has been measured or to horses ridden on flat ground. However, its predication of DE requirements was based on an assumption of efficiency of utilization of DE for work that was not validated with body weight measurements. Therefore, we designed a study to utilize both factorial and global methods to 1) determine the DE requirements for a measured amount of exercise; 2) determine the efficiency with which DE was utilized for work; and 3) develop a new equation to predict digestible energy requirements for exercise.

Materials and Methods

Three Thoroughbred geldings (520 kg ± 3.6 kg) were used in a 3x3 Latin square design. Each 35-day period was divided into a rest phase (14 days) and an exercise phase (21 days). During the rest phase of each period the horses were housed in box stalls with a minimum of 5 hours of turnout per day in a small paddock. Horses were muzzled while turned out to prevent grazing. During the exercise phase of each period, the horses performed a standardized regime of exercise on a high-speed treadmill and a mechanical horse walker. During this exercise phase, the horses continued to receive the same amount of turnout as during the rest phase.

EXERCISE SCHEDULE

During the exercise phase of each period, the horses performed an identical schedule of exercise on a high-speed treadmill and mechanical walker. The weekly exercise schedule consisted of 6 days of exercise on either the treadmill or the walker followed by a day with no forced exercise. The horses exercised every other day on the high-speed treadmill. This exercise bout consisted of a 5-min walk, 20-min trot (4 m/s), 6-min canter (7 m/s), 20-min trot (4 m/s), 6-min canter (7 m/s), and 5-min walk followed by a 15-min warmdown period on the walker. The trot and canter work was done at a 3-degree incline. On the alternate three days the horses exercised at 1.5 m/s for 1 hour on the mechanical walker.

NET ENERGY EXPENDITURE

During the third week of each exercise period, oxygen consumption was measured using indirect calorimetry during the last day of treadmill exercise. The amount of oxygen consumed above maintenance was estimated by subtracting 3 ml/kg BW/min from each oxygen consumption measurement. This is the amount of oxygen that horses would normally consume at rest. Oxygen consumption on the walker was assumed to be the same as when the horses walked at the same speed on the flat treadmill. Net energy expended during exercise was calculated by multiplying total oxygen consumption above maintenance by 4.863. This is the known energy equivalent per liter of O2 consumed at a respiratory quotient of 0.85 (Maynard and Loosli, 1969).

DIETS AND DE INTAKES

The horses were fed a diet of unfortified sweet feed (45% cracked corn, 45% whole oats, and 10% molasses) and grass hay at a forage-to-grain ratio of 65:35. The horses also received 120 g of a vitamin-mineral supplement (Micro-Phase, KPP), 50 g loose salt, and 60 g electrolytes (Summer Games, KPP) daily. The digestible energy content of the diets was determined in each horse in a 5-day complete collection digestibility trial prior to the beginning of the first experimental period. The DE content of the diets equaled 2.26 ± .01 Mcal/kg on an as-fed basis.

During each period the horses were fed one of three feed intakes that supplied digestible energy intakes that ranged from near maintenance (16-17 Mcal DE/d) to 200% maintenance (Table 1). The sweet feed and supplements were fed in two meals at 6:30 AM and at 4 PM. Nosebags were used to prevent feed wastage. The grass hay was offered in three portions, two fed with the sweet feed and the third portion fed at 10 PM. All hay fed throughout the trial was taken from the same batch.

Table 1. Feed and DE intakes during each period.

	Period	Sweet feed intake (kg)	Hay intake (kg)	Caloric intake (Mcal DE/day)
Horse 1	1 Rest	4.0	8.0	27.2
	1 Exercise	4.0	8.0	27.2
	2 Rest	3.0	6.0	20.4
	2 Exercise	3.0	6.0	20.4
	3 Rest	2.5	5.0	17.0
	3 Exercise	3.5	7.0	23.0
Horse 2	1 Rest	5.0	10.0	33.6
	1 Exercise	5.0	10.0	33.6
	2 Rest	3.8	7.5	25.3
	2 Exercise	3.8	7.5	25.3
	3 Rest	2.5	5.0	16.8
	3 Exercise	4.0	8.0	26.9
Horse 3	1 Rest	4.0	8.0	27.4
	1 Exercise	4.0	8.0	27.4
	2 Rest	3.0	6.0	20.5
	2 Exercise	3.0	6.0	20.5
	3 Rest	2.5	5.0	17.1
	3 Exercise	3.5	7.0	23.9

BODY WEIGHT MEASUREMENTS

Horses were weighed daily before their 6:30 AM feeding. Average daily body weight changes during each phase of each period were estimated by regression analysis of body weight vs. days on trial. Weights from the first three days of each phase were not included in the analysis because weights may have fluctuated during this time due to changes in feed intake from the previous period.

Results

Body weight changes vs. caloric intake are listed in Table 2 and depicted graphically in Figure 1. When the horses were unexercised, they gained weight at every level of energy intake. During exercise the horses lost weight at all but the highest DE intake. Regression analysis of these data suggests that these horses would require 30.57 kcal DE/kg BW/d to maintain body weight at rest and 61.46 kcal DE/kg BW/d to maintain body weight during exercise. For a 500-kg horse this translates to 15.3 Mcal DE/d for maintenance and 30.7 Mcal DE/d for exercise.

Table 2. Body weight changes and DE intake.

	Period	Avg BW (kg)	Avg BW change (kg/d)	Caloric intake (Mcal DE /day)	Avg BW change (g/kg BW/d)	Caloric intake (kcal DE/kg BW/d)
Horse 1	1 Rest	522	1.112	27.24	2.130	52.2
	1 Exercise	525	-0.200	27.24	-0.381	51.9
	2 Rest	531	0.264	20.43	0.497	38.5
	2 Exercise	532	-0.475	20.43	-0.893	38.4
	3 Rest	522	0.097	17.025	0.186	32.6
	3 Exercise	516	-0.415	23.835	-0.804	46.2
Horse 2	1 Rest	522	1.288	33.6	2.468	64.4
	1 Exercise	525	0.037	33.6	0.070	64.0
	2 Rest	533	0.479	25.312	0.899	47.5
	2 Exercise	531	-0.346	25.312	-0.652	47.7
	3 Rest	523	0.325	16.8	0.621	32.1
	3 Exercise	517	-0.194	26.88	-0.375	52.0
Horse 3	1 Rest	508	1.147	27.36	2.258	53.9
	1 Exercise	510	-0.037	27.36	-0.073	53.6
	2 Rest	510	0.054	20.52	0.105	40.2
	2 Exercise	510	-0.353	20.52	-0.692	40.2
	3 Rest	503	0.114	17.1	0.227	34.0
	3 Exercise	501	-0.279	23.94	-0.557	47.8

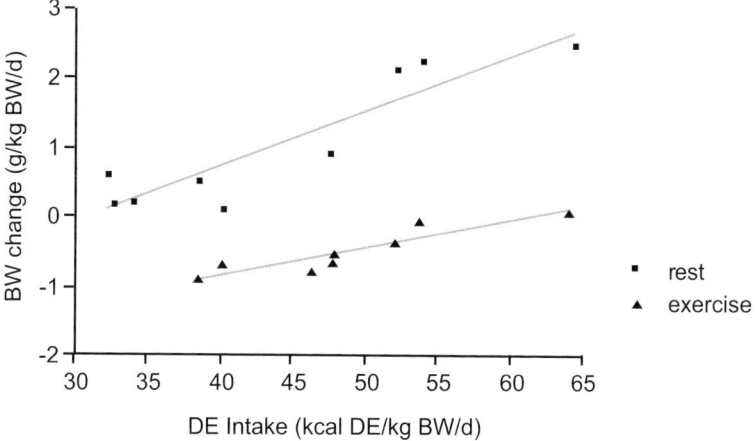

Figure 1. Body weight changes and DE intake.

Table 3 illustrates the quantity of oxygen consumed and NE expended by a horse during one day of treadmill exercise and one day of exercise on the walker. Average daily NE expenditure was calculated by multiplying these values by 3 (the number of days of each type of exercise) and dividing by 7 (number of days in a week). Table 4 contains the average daily NE expended by each horse during each exercise period. The horses expended an average of 7.87 ± .26 kcal NE/kg BW/d above maintenance during exercise. This equals 3.94 Mcal NE/d for a 500-kg horse.

Table 3. Oxygen consumed and NE expended by one horse during one day of treadmill exercise and one day of exercise on the walker.

	Type of exercise	Speed (m/s)	VO_2 ml/kg/ min	Extra O_2 consumed ml/kg/min	BW	Extra O_2 consumed l/min	NE Kcals/ min	Exercise duration (min)	NE expended per exercise period (Kcals)
Treadmill day	walk (flat)	1.5	16.25	13.25	510	6.76	32.87	5	164.33
	trot (3°)	4.0	45.87	42.87	510	21.86	106.32	5	531.58
	trot (3°)	4.0	40.16	37.16	510	8.95	92.15	5	460.75
	trot (3°)	4.0	44.41	41.41	510	21.12	102.70	5	513.48
	trot (3°)	4.0	46.65	43.65	510	22.26	108.27	5	541.34
	canter (3°)	7.0	71.41	68.41	510	34.89	169.67	6	1018.02
	trot (3°)	4.0	44.39	41.39	510	21.11	102.65	5	513.27
	trot (3°)	4.0	43.62	40.62	510	20.71	100.73	5	503.67
	trot (3°)	4.0	40.16	37.16	510	18.95	92.15	5	460.75
	trot (3°)	4.0	43.73	40.73	510	20.77	101.02	5	505.08
	canter (3°)	7.0	72.79	69.79	510	35.59	173.09	6	1038.57
	walk (flat)	1.5	17.06	14.06	510	7.17	34.87	5	174.34
	walk (walker)	1.5	16.66	13.66	510	6.96	33.87	15	508.00
Walker day	walk	1.5	16.66	13.66	510	6.96	33.87	60	2032.01

Table 4. Daily NE expenditure above maintenance during exercise.

Horse	Period	NE (kcal/d)	BW (kg)	NE (kcal/kg BW/d)
Horse 1	1	4473	525	8.52
	2	4433	532	8.33
	3	4795 5	516	9.29
Horse 2	1	4298	525	8.19
	2	3954	531	7.45
	3	3501	517	6.77
Horse 3	1	3824	510	7.50
	2	3842	510	7.53
	3	3635	501	7.26

One way to calculate the efficiency of utilization of DE for work is to divide the extra amount of DE required for work ($DE_{work} - DE_{maintenance}$) by the NE expended for that work. Using this method, the DE from this study would have been used with an efficiency of just 25.5% (Table 5). This is a much lower efficiency than the value of 57% used in the equation of Pagan and Hintz (1986). Martin-Rosset and Vermorel (2004) suggested that exercise increased the maintenance energy requirement by 10-20%. Increasing the maintenance DE requirement by 10% results in an efficiency of DE for work of around 28% (Table 5).

Table 5. Efficiency of utilization of DE for work.

	Maintenance DE (kcal/kg BW/d)	Exercise DE (kcal/kg BW/d)	DE (work) (kcal/kg BW/d)	NE (kcal/kg BW/d)	DE efficiency
Maintenance	30.57	61.46	30.89	7.87	25.5%
110% Maintenance	33.63	61.46	27.83	7.87	28.0%

The amount of DE required per kg of body weight gain was very different at rest vs. during exercise. Horses required 25.6 Mcal DE per kg of gain during exercise, but only 12.8 Mcal DE/kg of gain at rest. If the efficiency of utilization of DE for gain during rest equaled 57%, then each kg of gain would equal 7.3 Mcal/kg. If the same energy content of gain was used for exercise, then the efficiency of DE for gain would equal 28.5%. This study suggests that the efficiency of utilization of DE by horses for work is significantly lower than during rest. This is contrary to the assumptions currently used to calculate energy requirements for work factorially. More research is needed to determine the various factors that affect this efficiency. Particularly, the effects of breed, diet composition, and exercise duration and intensity warrant further investigation. Until these factors can be quantified, the global method of calculating energy requirements is preferable in developing practical feeding standards for performance horses participating in different disciplines.

References

Anderson, C.E., G.D. Potter, J.L. Kreider, and C.C. Courtney. 1983. Digestible energy requirements for exercising horses. J. Anim. Sci. 56:91.

Martin-Rosset, W., and M. Vermorel. 2004. Evaluation and expression of energy allowances and energy value of feeds in the UFC system for the performance horse. In: EAAP publication No. 111. Julliand, V., and W. Martin-Rosset (Eds.).

Maynard, L.A., and J.K. Loosli. 1969. Animal Nutrition (6th Ed.). McGraw-Hill Book Company.

NRC. 1989. Nutrient Requirements of Horses. (5th Ed.). National Academy Press. Washington, DC.

Pagan, J.D., and H.F. Hintz. 1986. Equine energetics. II. Energy expenditure in horses during submaximal exercise. J. Anim. Sci. 63:822.

EFFICACY OF AN HERBAL FEED SUPPLEMENT IN REDUCING EXERCISE-RELATED STRESS IN HORSES

VANESSA E. WILKINS, HOLLY M. GREENE, AND STEVEN J. WICKLER
California State Polytechnic University, Pomona, California

Introduction

Ergogenic aids are often used in horses to enhance performance without adequate scientific validation. These supplements, which might contain herbal components, are not required by law in the United States to provide evidence supporting manufacturers' claims. The present study investigated an herbal supplement containing *Withania somnifera* (ashwaghanda), *Ocimum sanctum* (holy basil), *Phyllanthus emblica* (Indian gooseberry), *Asparagus racemosus* (asparagus), *Glycyrrhiza glabra* (licorice), *Mangifera indica* (mango), *Tribulus terrestris* (puncture vine), and shilajit (mineral pitch).

Literature suggests that various herbs in the supplement have anti-stressor (Archana and Namasivayam, 1999) and "adaptogenic" properties (Bhattacharya et al., 2002), as well as the ability to affect the hypothalamic-pituitary-adrenal axis (Al-Qarawi et al., 2002). More specifically, the supplement investigated in the study contains herbs which have been found to decrease stress-induced plasma cortisol concentrations (Archana and Namasivayam, 1999), heart rate (Dhulcy, 2000), and lactate concentrations (Dadkar et al., 1987).

Methods and Materials

Six horses (three Thoroughbreds, three Arabians) were used in a crossover design with animals serving as their own controls. Animals were fed the supplement or placebo for 15 days and a standardized exercise test (SET) was conducted followed by a 15-day clearance period. Feeds were then switched and protocols repeated. Samples were taken at rest, at speeds of 3.5, 4.0, 4.5, 5.0, and 5.5 m/s on a 10% incline, and 15, 30, 45, and 60 minutes and 24 hours post SET. Samples were analyzed for plasma cortisol, blood lactate, neutrophil:lymphocyte ratio, white blood cell count, packed cell volume (PCV), and hemoglobin. Heart rates (HR) were measured continuously during the SET.

Results

ANOVA indicated there was an interaction (p=0.026) of treatment and recovery time on cortisol concentrations during the recovery period. The cortisol concentrations were decreased in the supplement group an average of 11% in the 15, 30, and 45 minutes post-SET samples (p=0.001, p=0.010, and p=0.045, respectively).

There was an effect of supplement on PCV during the SET (p=0.007) and during the recovery period (p=0.009). PCV was decreased in supplemented horses at rest and 3.5 m/s samples (p=0.009 and p=0.001, respectively) during the SET and during the recovery period at 15, 30, and 45 minutes post-SET samples (p=0.009, p<0.001, and p<0.001, respectively).

ANOVA indicated there was an interaction of treatment and recovery time (p=0.038) on hemoglobin concentrations. Hemoglobin concentrations were decreased during the recovery period at 15 and 30 minutes post-SET samples (p=0.048 and p=0.018, respectively).

The supplement did not have an effect on blood lactate concentrations during the SET. Although the supplement did not decrease blood lactate concentrations during the recovery period, the data support that there was an interaction (p=0.063) between supplement and recovery time. Blood lactate concentrations were lowered during the recovery period at 30 minutes post-SET samples (p=0.011).

There was no effect of the supplement on white blood cell counts and neutrophil:lymphocyte ratio at rest, during exercise, or during the recovery period, or on average HR during exercise and HR recovery time.

Discussion

Cortisol is often used as an indicator of stress due to stimulation of the hypothalamic-pituitary-adrenal axis, which is a common physiological response to various stressors. The attenuation of cortisol during the recovery period in the supplemented animals is interpreted as a reduction of stress (Stull and Rodiek, 2002).

During exercise, the sympathetic nervous system stimulates splenic contractions, which increase circulating red blood cell (RBC) numbers, assessed here as either PCV or hemoglobin concentrations. The decreased RBC at rest, when running at lower speeds during the SET, and during the recovery period suggests that the supplement is affecting sympathetic tone. A decreased sympathetic tone could account for the decreased release of red cells at rest and increased sequestering of RBC during the recovery period, supporting the claims of reduced stress, at least at lower concentrations of sympathetic activity (Rose and Allen, 1985).

Although the lowered lactate concentrations produced by the supplement during the recovery period in the present study do not support the claims of increased metabolic performance, they are perhaps indicative of increased speed of recovery, which may increase performance potential for a subsequent exercise bout (Wickler and Anderson, 2000).

Take-Home Message

Although the mechanism is unknown, the data from the present study support the hypothesis that the supplement reduced exercise-related stress (as assessed by plasma cortisol) in horses. Although the supplement had no effect on cardiovascular or metabolic performance during an exercise bout (as assessed by heart and blood lactate), it appeared to increase the speed of recovery following a moderate intensity exercise bout.

References

Al-Qarawi, A.A., H.A. Abdel-Rahman, B.H. Ali, and S.A. El Mougy. 2002. Liquorice (*Glycyrrhiza glabra*) and the adrenal-kidney-pituitary axis in rats. Food Chem. Toxicol. 40(10):1525-7.

Archana, R., and A. Namasivayam. 1999. Antistressor effect of *Withania somnifera*. J Ethnopharmacol 64(1):91-3.

Bhattacharya, A., A.V. Muruganandam, V. Kumar, and S.K. Bhattacharya. 2002. Effect of polyherbal formulation, EuMil, on neurochemical perturbations induced by chronic stress. Indian J. Exp. Biol. 40(10): 1161-3.

Dadkar, V.N., N.U. Ranadive, and H.L. Dhar. 1987. Evaluation of antistress (adaptogen) activity of *Withania somnifera* (ashwagandha). Indian J. Clin. Biochem. 2:101-108.

Dhuley, J.N. 2000. Adaptogenic and cardioprotective action of ashwagandha in rats and frogs. J. Ethnopharmacol. 70(1):57-63.

Rose, R.J., and J.R. Allen. 1985. Hematologic response to exercise and training. Vet. Clin. of North Am.: Equine Prac. 1(3):461-475.

Stull, C.L., and A.V. Rodiek. 2002. Effects of cross-tying horses during 24 h of road transport. Equine Vet. J. 34(6):550-5.

Wickler, S.J., and T.P. Anderson. 2000. Hematological changes and athletic performance in horses in response to high altitude (3,800 m). Am. J. Physiol. Regul. Integr. Comp. Physiol. 279(4):R1176-81.

UPDATE ON BONE DISEASE: THE IMPACT OF SKELETAL DISEASE ON ATHLETIC PERFORMANCE

C. WAYNE MCILWRAITH

Colorado State University, Fort Collins, Colorado

Introduction

Bone is a critical component of the equine musculoskeletal system. It not only provides strength to the legs, but also acts as the foundation for cartilage in the moveable joints. Much of the clinical disease in the horse associated with bone involves the subchondral bone immediately under the articular cartilage leading to problems in the joint. These conditions can be divided into developmental problems of bone and traumatic problems of bone. They will be considered separately.

Developmental Problems of Bone

The term developmental orthopedic disease (DOD) was coined in 1986 to encompass all orthopedic problems seen in the growing foal and is a term that encompasses all general growth disturbances of horses and is therefore nonspecific (McIlwraith, 1986). The term should not be used synonymously with osteochondrosis, and it is inappropriate for subchondral cystic lesions, physitis, angular limb deformities, and cervical vertebral malformations, all to be presumed as manifestations of osteochondrosis. When the term developmental orthopedic disease was first coined, it was categorized to include the following:

1. Osteochondrosis. Osteochondrosis is a defect in endochondral ossification that can result in a number of different manifestations depending on the site of the endochondral ossification defect. These manifestations include osteochondritis dissecans (OCD) and some subchondral cystic lesions. Not all subchondral cystic lesions or osseous cyst-like lesions are necessarily manifestations of osteochondrosis. Another manifestation is some physitis (but we now recognize that most clinical swelling associated with the physis has no pathologic change involving the physis itself).
2. Acquired angular limb deformities.
3. Physitis.

4. Subchondral cystic lesions.
5. Flexural deformities.
6. Cuboidal bone malformation.

Osteochondrosis

Osteochondrosis (dyschondroplasia) was initially defined as a disturbance of cellular differentiation in the growing cartilage (Olsson, 1978). Osteochondrosis is considered to be the result of a failure of endochondral ossification and therefore may affect either the articular epiphyseal cartilage complex or the metaphyseal growth cartilage. It is usually in the articular epiphyseal cartilage. It can have three consequences: (1)These areas of retained cartilage, due to a lack of endochondral ossification, can heal; (2) They can break out and form flaps of cartilage and bone or fragments of cartilage and bone (called osteochondritis dissecans or OCD); or (3) The retained cartilage can undergo necrosis and form a subchondral cystic lesion (subchondral bone cyst).

The majority of cases of OCD and subchondral bone cysts are considered to be the result of necrosis occurring in the basal layers of the thickened retained cartilage with subsequent pressure and strain within the joint giving rise to fissures in the damaged cartilage.

OSTEOCHONDRITIS DISSECANS

There is a general agreement that this condition involves a dissecting lesion with the formation of a chondral or osteochondral flap. Flaps may become detached and form joint mice. In some instances, lesions have been found at arthroscopy that consist of cartilage separated from bone, and the cartilage does not appear to be thickened (McIlwraith, 1993). Based on these observations, the author questions whether persistence of hypertrophied cartilage is a necessary event prior to the development of an OCD lesion. This question is based on instances seen at arthroscopic examination or in follow-up histologic examination where dissection or separation occurs close to the cartilage-bone interface, rather than in the underlying cancellous bone between normal cartilage and a normal bone-cartilage junction, as it commonly does in humans. The clinical manifestations and treatment of the common entities of OCD are discussed in a separate lecture.

SUBCHONDRAL CYSTIC LESIONS

Subchondral bone cysts were first reported as a clinical entity in 1968 (Pettersson, 1968). Subchondral cystic lesions have also been proposed as manifestations of osteochondrosis by a number of authors (Rooney, 1975; Stromberg, 1979), and there is some pathologic support for this (Rejno and Stromberg, 1978). However, more recent work has demonstrated that subchondral cystic lesions can be produced from a small defect in the bone, and other work has shown that the lining of clinical subchondral cystic lesions contained increased quantities of neutral metalloproteinases, PGE-2, and interleukin-1, and also are capable of osteoclastic resorption of bone.

The Cause of OCD

Despite the instances where there is no evidence of thickened cartilage, it is generally accepted that most OCD lesions are manifestations of osteochondrosis. In the one- to two-year-old horse, most cases of subchondral cystic lesions are also related to osteochondrosis. For that reason, the following discussion is on various etiologic factors associated with osteochondrosis.

GENETIC PREDISPOSITION

There have been a number of genetic studies on the heredity of OCD in the hock in Standardbreds and Scandinavian cold-blooded horses. A radiographic survey by Hoppe and Phillipson in Standardbred trotters and Swedish Warmbloods showed that one stallion of each breed had a significantly higher frequency of OCD among its progeny, compared with the progeny groups of the other stallions ($p < 0.001$) (1985). In another study, Schougaard et al. (1990) showed radiographic evidence of a significantly higher proportion of OCD in the progeny of one of eight stallions, even though the stallion itself did not show radiographic signs of OCD. Since that time, there have been two additional studies on the heritability of osteochondrosis in the tibiotarsal joint (Grondahl and Dolvik, 1993; Phillipsson et al., 1993). Both of these studies were in Standardbred trotters but did show significant heritability with OCD. Studies in other breeds are markedly lacking. In the Dutch Warmblood, there has been a protocol preventing breeding of stallions with any OCD for ten years, but whether this has lowered the incidence of the disease is questionable.

GROWTH AND BODY SIZE

An association has been made between body weight and OCD by Pagan and Jackson (1996). Foals in Kentucky that had to have arthroscopic surgery for OCD were significantly heavier than foals that did not have OCD.

MECHANICAL STRESS AND TRAUMA

It has long been recognized clinically that mechanical stresses precipitate the onset of clinical signs, presumably by avulsing an OCD flap or fragment (Pagan and Jackson,

1996). The role of trauma as a primary initiator of a lesion is more controversial. Pool pointed out that there are no unique histologic features that will consistently distinguish the lesion of osteochondrosis from that of trauma at a developing osteochondral junction, and that the radial vessels supplying the chondrocytes in the epiphyseal physis may be sheared and cause a primary osteochondrosis lesion (1986). He felt that biomechanical forces are an important factor and are superimposed upon an idiopathic lesion to produce defective cartilage. Reflection back to the classic paper by Konig in 1887 is appropriate in considering the potential role of trauma in the pathogenesis. He claimed that loose bodies in the knee joints of young people had three causes: (1) very severe trauma, (2) lesser trauma causing contusion and necrosis, and (3) minimal trauma acting on an underlying lesion, for which he suggested the name "osteochondritis dissecans" (and for which he is considered the originator) (Barrie, 1987). I feel that these three different syndromes can be seen in the horse.

DEFECTS IN VASCULARIZATION

OCD was initially described as being caused by a vascular or ischemic necrosis of the subchondral bone (Adams, 1974). Although recent work in the pig suggested that the viability of epiphyseal cartilage in the articular-epiphyseal cartilage complex is highly dependent on an adequate blood supply from cartilage canal vessels, and strongly implicates a defect in blood supply in the pathogenesis of osteochondrosis, there is no evidence yet documented in the horse (Carlson et al., 1991).

NUTRITION

Osteochondrosis-like lesions have been induced in horses by feeding 130% of National Research Council (NRC) carbohydrate and protein (Glade and Belling, 1986). More recently, further work has defined that 130% of NRC digestible energy will certainly significantly increase the incidence of osteochondrosis lesions, but increasing the protein content does not (Savage et al., 1993).

MINERAL IMBALANCES

Various mineral imbalances have been implicated in the pathogenesis, including high calcium, high phosphorus, low copper, and high zinc. There is no good equine-specific support for high calcium causing problems, but three times the NRC levels of phosphorus significantly increased the number of OCD lesions (Savage et al., 1993).

Low copper has been implicated as a cause. In experimental studies, it has been reported that a marked copper deficiency (1.7 ppm) produced both flexural deformities and osteochondrosis-like lesions (Bridges and Harris, 1988). Bridges and Harris also noticed a softening of articular cartilage and suggested that the low copper status may lead to reduced cross-linking of collagen by lysyl oxidase, predisposing to physeal and articular fractures. Hurtig et al. conducted a controlled experiment with high (30 ppm) and low (7 ppm) copper diets (1990). A much higher incidence of lesions of osteochondrosis was seen in the foals fed the low copper diet. Many of the changes were present in the cervical spine. Hurtig and coworkers considered the cause as one of reduced structural strength rather than arrested or abnormal endochondral ossification (1990). Further work has been done in copper by Pearce and coworkers in New Zealand (Pearce et al., 1998a; Pearce et al., 1998b; Pearce et al., 1998c). The absolute levels of copper at which OCD can be produced have been questioned, or at least it appears clear that there are differences between different countries. Pearce and coworkers (1998a) failed to produce significant clinical OCD with low copper diets. They also showed that, while oral supplementation of mares could enhance the foals' copper status, parental administration could not.

Excessive zinc intake has been related to equine osteochondrosis (Messer, 1981). The effects of environmental exposure to zinc and cadmium were studied in pregnant pony mares following observations of lameness, swollen joints, and unthriftiness, particularly in foals (Gunson et al., 1982).

ENDOCRINE FACTORS

It has been postulated by Glade (1986) that the production of osteochondrosis lesions in association with overfeeding is mediated by the endocrine system. Glade has proposed that feeding initiates increased concentrations of insulin and T4 and high concentrations of insulin could inhibit growth hormone, although the exact mechanism is not known (Glade et al., 1983). A long-term administration of dexamethasone has been associated with the production of osteochondrosis-like lesions (Glade et al., 1983). More recent work showing an association between high-glycemic feed, insulin secretion, and osteochondrosis has been made by Ralston and Pagan.

SITE VULNERABILITY

Because the lesions of equine osteochondrosis occur at specific anatomic sites, this does suggest vulnerability that could be related back to trauma or excessive stress and interference with blood supply as originally suggested by Pool (1986). Lesions are frequently bilateral in the femoropatellar and tarsocrural joints and quadrilateral in the fetlock joint, although they infrequently involve different joints in the same animal. This observation could perhaps suggest a "window of vulnerability" in the endochondral ossification of that specific joint at that specific location.

Natural History of Osteochondrosis Lesions

Recent work done by the workers at Utrecht has shown that many lesions in the stifle and the hock will heal. In this study, foals were radiographed every month, and lesions developed (defects developed, signifying a lack of endochondral ossification) and then the lesions healed (Dik et al., 1999). Relatively few of them became clinical, but the times at which they were going to persist were established. This study emphasized that we need to be careful of radiographic surveys in deciding that we have a problem with OCD. This author feels that only when we have clinical signs associated with it should we be intervening. This study also clarified the age at which surgical treatment was appropriate. If surgical intervention is carried out at a very young age, it is likely that it is unnecessary in many instances.

Further work by McIntosh and McIlwraith (1993) showed that it was certainly possible to have lesions heal beyond this time if foals were confined. Definition of what lesions can heal with conservative management has greatly progressed treatment, and this is discussed elsewhere.

Management of OCD Lesions and Subchondral Bone Cysts that Do Not Respond to Conservative Management

OSTEOCHONDRITIS DISSECANS OF THE (STIFLE) JOINT

The stifle joint is one of the principal joints affected with OCD. Although stifle OCD can be diagnosed in almost any breed, it seems to be more common in Thoroughbreds than in other breeds. Approximately 60% of affected horses will be one year of age or less at the time the condition becomes symptomatic, and younger animals that develop clinical signs often have more severe damage within the joint. However, incidental lesions are sometimes identified in older horses where no clinical signs have ever been observed.

Clinical and radiographic signs

Animals usually present with a sudden onset of joint swelling and lameness. A recent increase in the level of exercise is sometimes part of the history. Lameness sometimes may be very mild, with a stiff action and shortened stride being observed, rather than the horse having a prominent lameness. Some more severely affected horses will have a "bunny hop" action behind that can initially be confused with a neurologic problem.

Joint distention, however, is the most consistent sign seen with OCD of the stifle. Careful palpation of the joint may identify free bodies, or the surface irregularity associated with the damage within the joint. Bilateral involvement is common in the stifle, so careful examination of both stifles should be completed. In one study, 57% of affected animals had bilateral involvement.

Breed Distribution of 161 Horses Presented for Femoropatellar OCD

Breed	Number	Percentage
Thoroughbred	82	50.9
Quarter Horse	39	24.2
Arabian	16	9.9
Warmblood	9	5.6
Crossbred	5	3.1
Paint Horse	3	1.9
Appaloosa	3	1.9
Other	4	2.5

Age Distribution of 161 Horses Presented for Femoropatellar OCD

Age (yr)	Number	Percentage
<1	22	13.7
1	68	42.2
2	36	22.4
3	21	13
>4	14	8.7

Flexion of the limb will usually exacerbate the lameness, and anesthetic placed into the joint will improve or eliminate the lameness. However, intra-articular anesthesia is usually not necessary to confirm a diagnosis.

Lateral to medial radiographs provide the most useful information regarding specific lesion location and size. The most common defect identified is a variably sized irregularity or flattening of the lateral trochlear ridge of the femur. The area of the ridge that comes in contact with the bottom portion of the patella is most commonly involved. Partial calcification of the tissue within the defect is sometimes seen, and free bodies are also occasionally identified. It is rare to see OCD primarily affecting the patella, but secondary radiographic change in the patella resulting from the trochlear ridge damage can be seen. The medial ridge of the femur is much less commonly involved.

Generally, the extent of damage to the joint identified at surgery is more extensive than would be predicted from radiographs. Although other joints can be involved concurrently, this is uncommon. In one study of 161 horses with stifle OCD, five horses also had OCD affecting the rear fetlocks, four had hock OCD, and one had OCD of a shoulder joint.

Treatment

It is generally accepted that surgical debridement of the lesions using arthroscopic technique is the treatment of choice. However, smaller lesions identified in younger horses may respond to rest and resolve radiographically. These are generally lesions that are not causing severe clinical signs. If lameness and swelling are prominent, arthroscopic surgery is indicated.

As for all joint surgery, the joint is thoroughly explored, and suspicious lesions are probed. Loose or detached tissue is elevated and removed. Loose bodies are also removed. The defect site is then debrided down to healthy tissue. Care must be taken to not be overly aggressive with bone debridement in young animals having soft subchondral bone.

Animals are usually stall-rested for 2 weeks after surgery, at which time hand-walking is started. Restricted exercise is usually continued for 2-3 months after surgery, at which time training is started or the horse is turned out.

Prognosis

In one study of 252 stifle joints in 161 horses, follow-up information was available for 134 horses (McIlwraith et al., 1991). Of these 134 horses, 64% returned to their previous use, 7% were in training, 16% were unsuccessful, and 13% were unsuccessful due to reasons unrelated to the stifle. The success rate was higher in horses having smaller lesions, and it was also higher for older horses. However, this age factor was considered to be due to the fact that the most severe lesions were generally identified in the younger horses.

OSTEOCHONDRITIS DISSECANS OF THE TARSOCRURAL (HOCK) JOINT

Hock OCD usually affects the intermediate ridge of the tibia in the proximal and cranial portion of the joint. However, lesions can also develop along the trochlear ridges (lateral ridge much more common than medial ridge) and the medial malleolus of the tibia. Hock OCD is very common in Standardbreds but can be diagnosed in most breeds.

Clinical and radiographic signs

The most common clinical sign of hock OCD is effusion of the tarsocrural joint. This is manifested clinically as a "bog" spavin, which simply refers to the prominent in the degree of lameness. However, for more localized lesions, the prognosis is favorable for a successful outcome.

The shoulder is probably the most difficult joint on which to perform arthroscopic surgery, due to the depth of the joint below the muscles in the area. Surgery is easier on younger animals due to their relative muscle mass. Problems encountered in the shoulder are inaccessibility of lesions due to their location within the joint, and extravasation or leakage of fluid outside the joint, which impairs visibility within the joint.

Prognosis

A large series of cases having surgery has not yet been reported although preliminary results from such a series being compiled at CSU suggest that the overall prognosis is approximately 50%. The prognosis seems to be less favorable if lesions are present on both the humeral head and the glenoid cavity. In unsuccessful cases, further deterioration of the joint surfaces on radiographs is common.

Traumatic Lesions of the Subchondral Bone

In recent years, good evidence has been provided that intra-articular fractures are preceded by subchondral bone disease. This subchondral bone disease consists of a spectrum of microcracks, diffuse microdamage, cell loss (apoptosis or necrosis), and accompanying subchondral bone sclerosis.

CAUSE OF SUBCHONDRAL BONE DISEASE

The development of microdamage is presumed to be associated as a consequence of cyclic trauma. The repeated wear and tear has been noted with radiographic study and, more recently, CT to contribute to subchondral bone sclerosis. However, the direct association between sclerosis leading to the necrosis of bone has not been totally demonstrated. The development of lytic lesions in the subchondral bone, however, is presumed to be associated with microdamage. Factors involved in the predisposition of horses to damage based on the cyclic trauma of an athletic career include racetrack or arena surface, conformation, genetic predisposition, and a destabilizing traumatic injury.

CONSEQUENCES OF TRAUMATIC SUBCHONDRAL BONE DISEASE

Subchondral bone disease creates an environment for pathologic fractures. The most common manifestations are osteochondral chip fractures, which can be career-ending if not treated successfully. However, the overall success with arthroscopic surgery is high. Slab fractures represent a more severe injury requiring internal fixation. Some of these cases can return to athletic activities. However, in other instances such as collapsing slab fractures in the carpus, the failure to treat adequately can lead to loss of life. The third level of fracture injury in terms of severity is made up of catastrophic injuries that can be life-threatening. Surgical treatments of such conditions are salvage procedures.

Diagnosis

Early diagnosis is critical. The recognition that early disease in the subchondral bone can lead to fractures has resulted in research efforts to diagnose bone disease early.

Treatment

By 1975 the arthroscope began to achieve real clinical use in human orthopedics, and diagnostic arthroscopy of equine carpal joints in three horses was reported in 1975 (Hall and Keeran, 1975). Experience with the limitations of what could be achieved with arthroscopy surgery has fed back into attempts to develop novel treatment techniques, as well as recognizing the need for early diagnosis and prevention of injury (McIlwraith, 1990a; McIlwraith and Bramlage, 1996).

The application of arthroscopic techniques to the horse has revolutionized the treatment of traumatic joint injuries. The first detailed paper on diagnostic arthroscopy in the horse was published in 1978 (McIlwraith and Fessler, 1978), and it is important to recognize that arthroscopic surgery is the diagnostic method of choice to evaluate articular cartilage and remains the gold standard for assessing pathologic joints. As in human orthopedics, use of the arthroscope in horses extended into surgical practice as technology and techniques of triangulation developed. These techniques were first detailed in textbook form in 1984 (McIlwraith, 1984). Diagnostic arthroscopy is especially valuable when response to medical treatment of a joint is suboptimal. In many instances, articular cartilage lesions are more extensive than what is insinuated on radiographs, but these lesions can sometimes be better related to physical examination and the extent of clinical signs.

By 1990, arthroscopy in the horse had gone from being a diagnostic technique used by a few veterinarians to the accepted way of performing joint surgery (McIlwraith, 1990a). Prospective and retrospective data substantiated the value of the technique in the treatment of carpal chip fractures (McIlwraith et al., 1987), fragmentation of the dorsal margin of the proximal phalanx (Yovich and McIlwraith, 1986), carpal slab fractures (Richardson, 1986), osteochondritis dissecans (OCD) of the femoropatellar joint (Martin and McIlwraith, 1985; McIlwraith and Martin, 1985), OCD of the shoulder (Bertone et al., 1987), and subchondral cystic lesions of the femur (Lewis, 1987). The results with tarsocrural OCD were published in 1991 (McIlwraith et al.,

1991). During this period, the use of diagnostic arthroscopy led to the recognition of previously undescribed articular lesions, many of which are treated using arthroscopic techniques.

Since 1990 there has been further sophistication of techniques. New ones have been developed and treatment principles have been changed based on new pathobiologic knowledge and further prospective and retrospective studies defining the success of various procedures. Many of these advances have been recorded in a recent publication (McIlwraith, 2002). For example, there has been further documentation of success rates following arthroscopic removal of fragments from the dorsoproximal margin of the proximal phalanx (Kawcak and McIlwraith, 1994; Colon et al., 2000). Advances and understanding of the pathogenesis of osteochondral disease and fragmentation in the carpus and fetlock have been reported (Norrdin et al., 1998; Kawcak et al., 2001), which naturally led to progression and diagnosis and treatment. Parameters for the surgical treatment of joint injury have been carefully defined (McIlwraith and Bramlage, 1996). Arthroscopic treatment of fractures in the previously considered inaccessible palmar aspect of the carpus have been described (Wilke et al., 2001), together with arthroscopy of the palmar aspect of the distal interphalangeal joint (Brommer et al., 2001; Vacek et al., 1992). Arthroscopy has also led to understanding of the contribution of soft tissue lesions to joint disease. In the carpus, tearing of the medial palmar intercarpal ligament (MPICL) was first reported in 1992 (McIlwraith, 1992) and its implications discussed by Phillips and Wright (1994) and others (Whitton and Rose, 1997; Whitton et al., 1997a,b).

In the fetlock joints, success rates following arthroscopic removal of osteochondral fragments of the palmar/plantar aspect of the proximal phalanx have now been documented (Foerner et al., 1987; Fortier et al., 1995). Results for arthroscopic treatment of osteochondritis dissecans for the distal/dorsal aspect of the third metacarpal/metatarsal bones (McIlwraith et al., 1990) and results of arthroscopic surgery to treat apical, abaxial, and basilar fragments of the sesamoid bones have also been reported (Southwood et al., 1998; Southwood and McIlwraith, 2000).

The results of arthroscopic surgery for the treatment of OCD in the tarsocrural joint have been documented (McIlwraith et al., 1991), and the arthroscopic approach and intra-articular anatomy of the plantar pouch of this joint have also been described (Zamos et al., 1994).

Considerable advances have been made in arthroscopic surgery of the stifle joint. Results of arthroscopic surgery for the treatment of OCD of the femoropatellar joint were reported in 1992 (Foland et al., 1992), and the syndrome of fragmentation of the distal apex of the patellar was recognized and its treatment reported in the same year (McIlwraith, 1990b). The use of arthroscopic surgery for treating certain patellar fractures was discussed in 1990 and reported in the refereed literature in 2000 (Marble and Sullins, 2000).

In the femorotibial joints, the use of arthroscopic surgery to treat subchondral cystic lesions of the medial condyle of the femur and proximal tibia has been reported

(Howard et al., 1995; Textor et al., 2001). Research has led to alternative methods of treating subchondral cystic lesions. After an initial demonstration that subchondral cystic lesions could develop on the medial condyle after 3 mm deep, 5 mm wide penetration of the subchondral bone plate (Ray et al., 1996), examination of the fibrous tissue of subchondral cystic lesions in horses demonstrated that it produced local mediators and neutral metalloproteinases and caused bone resorption in vitro (von Rechenberg et al., 2000a). Production of nitric oxide (NO), PGE2, and MMPs in media of explant cultures of equine synovial membrane and articular cartilage has also been demonstrated in normal and osteoarthritic joints (von Rechenberg et al., 2000b). Injection of corticosteroids into the lining membrane of subchondral cysts has therefore been carried into the clinical arena.

Cartilage lesions of the medial femoral condyle have been described (Schneider et al., 1997). Arthroscopy has allowed great advances in the recognition and treatment of meniscal tears and cruciate injuries (Walmsley, 1995; Walmsley, 2002; Walmsley et al., 2003). Successful treatment of grade I and grade II meniscal tears has been achieved and documented as well as lack of success recognized with lesions that are not completely accessible. Arthroscopy has also been used to remove fragments from the intercondylar eminence of the tibia (Mueller et al., 1994), and internal fixation of one case has been reported (Walmsley, 1997). Techniques have also been developed for diagnostic and surgical arthroscopy of the caudal pouches of the femorotibial joints (Stick et al., 1992; Hance et al., 1993; Trumble et al., 1994; Walmsley, 2002).

Diagnostic and surgical arthroscopy of the coxofemoral joint has been described, lesions identified, and some surgical treatments performed (Honnas et al., 1993; Nixon, 1994). The use of the arthroscope is no longer confined to the limbs and the arthroscopic anatomy of the temporomandibular joint has been described recently (Weller et al., 2002).

References

Adams, O.R. 1974. Lameness in Horses (3rd Ed.) Lea and Febiger, Philadelphia.

Barrie, H.J. 1987. Osteochondritis dissecans: 1887-1987-A Centennial look at Konig's memorable phrase. J. Bone Joint Surg. Br. 69B:693-695.

Bertone, A.L., C.W. McIlwraith, B.E. Powers, G.W. Trotter, and T.S. Stashak. 1987. Arthroscopic surgery for the treatment of osteochondrosis in the equine shoulder joint. Vet. Surg. 16:303-311.

Bridges, C.H., and E.D. Harris. 1988. Experimentally induced cartilaginous fractures (osteochondritis dissecans) in foals fed low-copper diets. J. Amer. Vet. Med. Assoc. 193:215-221.

Brommer, H., A.M. Rijkenhuizen, H.A.M. van den Belt, et al. 2001. Arthroscopic removal of an osteochondral fragment at the palmaroproximal aspect of the distal interphalangeal joint. Equine Vet. Educ. 13:294-297.

Carlson, C.S., D.J. Meuten, and D.C. Richardson. 1991. Ischemic necrosis of cartilage in spontaneous and experimental lesions of osteochondrosis. J. Orthop. Res. 9:317-329.

Colon, J.L., L.R. Bramlage, S.R. Hance, and R.M. Embertson. 2000. Qualitative and quantitative documentation of the racing performance of Thoroughbred racehorses after arthroscopic removal of dorsoproximal first phalanx osteochondral fractures (1986-1995). Equine Vet. J. 32:475-481.

Dik, K.J., E. Enzerink, and R. van Weeran. 1999. Radiologic development of osteochondral abnormalities in the hock and stifle of Dutch Warmblood foals from age 1 to 11 months. Equine Vet. J. Suppl. 31:9-15.

Foerner, J.J., W.P. Barclay, T.N. Phillips, et al. 1987. Osteochondral fragments of the palmar/plantar aspect of the fetlock joint. In: Proc. Amer. Assoc. Equine Practnr. 33:739-744.

Foland, J.W., C.W. McIlwraith, and G.W. Trotter. 1992. Arthroscopic surgery for osteochondritis dissecans of the femoropatellar joint. Equine Vet. J. 24:419-423.

Fortier, L.A., J.J. Foerner, and A.J. Nixon. 1995. Arthroscopic removal of axial osteochondral fragments of the plantar/palmar proximal aspect of the proximal phalanx in horses: 119 cases (1988-1992). J. Amer. Vet. Med. Assoc. 206:71-74.

Glade, M.J. 1986. Control of cartilage growth in osteochondrosis: A review. J. Equine Vet. Sci. 6:175-187.

Glade, M.J., and T.H. Belling. 1986. A dietary etiology for osteochondrotic cartilage. J. Equine Vet. Sci. 6:151-155.

Glade, M.J., L. Krook, H.F. Schryver, et al. 1983. Morphologic and biochemical changes in cartilage of foals treated with dexamethasone. Cornell Vet. 73:170-192.

Grondahl, A.M., and N.I. Dolvik. 1993. Hereditability estimations of osteochondrosis in the tibiotarsal joint and of bony fragments in the palmar/plantar portion of the metacarpophalangeal and metatarsophalangeal joints of horses. J. Amer. Vet. Med. Assoc. 203:101-104.

Gunson, D.E., D.F. Kowalczyk, C.R. Shoop, et al. 1982. Environmental zinc and cadmium pollution associated with generalized osteochondrosis, osteoporosis and nephrocalcinosis in horses. J. Amer. Vet. Med. Assoc. 180:295-299.

Hall, M.E., and R.J. Keeran. 1975. Use of the arthroscope in the horse. Vet. Med. Small Animal Clin. 70:705-706.

Hance, R., R.K. Schneider, R.M. Embertson, et al. 1993. Lesions of the caudal aspect of the femoral condyles in foals: 20 cases (1980-1990). J. Amer. Vet. Med. Assoc. 202:637-646.

Honnas, C.M., D.T. Zamos, and T.S. Ford. 1993. Arthroscopy of the coxofemoral joint of foals. Vet. Surg. 22;115-121.

Hoppe, F., and J. Phillipsson. 1985. A genetic study of osteochondrosis in Swedish horses. Equine Pract. 7:7-15.

Howard, R.D., C.W. McIlwraith, and G.W. Trotter. 1995. Arthroscopic surgery for subchondral cystic lesions of the medial femoral condyle in horses: 41 cases (1988-1991). J. Amer. Vet. Med. Assoc. 206:846-850.

Hurtig, M.B., S.L. Green, H. Dobson, et al. 1990. Defective bone and cartilage in foals fed a low copper diet. In: Proc. Amer. Assoc. Equine Practnr. 35:637-643.

Kawcak C.E., and C.W. McIlwraith. 1994. Proximodorsal first phalanx osteochondral chip fragments in 320 horses. Equine Vet. J. 26:392-396.

Kawcak, C.E., C.W. McIlwraith, R.W. Norrdin, R.D. Park, and S.D. James. 2001. The role of subchondral bone in joint disease: A review. Equine Vet. J. 33:120-126.

Lewis, R.B. 1987. Treatment of subchondral bone cysts of the medial condyle of the femur using arthroscopic surgery. In: Proc. Amer. Assoc. Equine Pract. 33:887-893.

Marble, G.P., and K.E. Sullins. 2000. Arthroscopic removal of patellar fracture fragments in horses: 5 cases (1989-1998). J. Amer. Vet. Med. Assoc. 216:1799-1801.

Martin, G.S., and C.W. McIlwraith. 1985. Arthroscopic anatomy of the equine femoropatellar joint and approaches for treatment of osteochondritis dissecans. Vet. Surg. 14:99-104.

McIlwraith, C.W. 1984. Diagnostic and surgical arthroscopy in the horse. Veterinary Medicine Publishing Co.

McIlwraith, C.W. 1986. AQHA Developmental Orthopedic Disease Symposium. American Quarter Horse Association. Amarillo, TX. 1-77.

McIlwraith, C.W. 1990a. Diagnostic and Surgical Arthroscopy in the Horse (2nd Ed.) Lea and Febiger, Philadelphia.

McIlwraith CW. 1990b. Osteochondral fragmentation or the distal aspect of the patella in horses. Equine Vet. J. 22:157-163.

McIlwraith, C.W. 1992. Tearing of the medial palmar intercarpal ligament in the equine mid-carpal joint. Equine Vet. J. 24:367-371.

McIlwraith, C.W. 1993. What is developmental orthopedic disease, osteochondrosis, osteochondritis, metabolic bone disease? In: Proc. Amer. Assoc. Equine Practnr. 39:35-44.

McIlwraith, C.W. 2002. Arthroscopy: An Update. In: Clinical Techniques in Equine Practice. p. 199-281. WB Saunders, Philadelphia.

McIlwraith, C.W., and L.R. Bramlage. 1996. Surgical treatment of joint injuries. In: C.W. McIlwraith and G.W. Trotter (Eds.) Joint Disease in the Horse. WB Saunders, Philadelphia.

McIlwraith, C.W., and J.F. Fessler. 1978. Arthroscopy in the diagnosis of equine joint disease. J. Amer. Vet. Med. Assoc. 172:263-268.

McIlwraith, C.W., and G.S. Martin. 1985. Arthroscopic surgery for the treatment of osteochondritis dissecans in the equine femoropatellar joint. Vet. Surg. 14:105-116.

McIlwraith, C.W., and M. Vorhees. 1990. Management of osteochondritis dissecans of the dorsal aspect of the distal metacarpus and metatarsus. In: Proc. Amer. Assoc. Equine Practnr. 35:547-550.

McIlwraith, C.W., J.J. Foerner, and D.M. Davis. 1991. Osteochondritis dissecans of the tarsocrural joint: Results of treatment with arthroscopic surgery. Equine Vet. J. 23:155-162.

McIlwraith, C.W., J.V. Yovich, and G.S. Martin. 1987. Arthroscopic surgery for the treatment of osteochondral chip fractures in the equine carpus. J. Amer. Vet. Med. Assoc. 191:531-540.

McIntosh, S.C., and C.W. McIlwraith. 1993. Natural history of femoropatellar osteochondrosis in three crops of Thoroughbreds. Equine Vet. J. 16:54-61.

Messer, N.T. 1981. Tibiotarsal effusion associated with chronic zinc intoxication in three horses. J. Amer. Vet. Med. Assoc. 178:294.

Mueller, P.O.E., D. Allen, E. Watson, et al. 1994. Arthroscopic removal of a fragment from an intercondylar eminence fracture of the tibia in 2-year-old horse. J. Amer. Vet. Med. Assoc. 204:1793-1795.

Nixon, A.J. 1994. Diagnostic and operative arthroscopy of the coxofemoral joint in horses. Vet. Surg. 23:377-385.

Norrdin, R.W., C.E. Kawcak, B.A. Capwell, and C.W. McIlwraith. 1998. Subchondral bone failure in an equine model of overload arthrosis. Bone 22:133-139.

Olsson, S.E. 1978. Introduction. Acta. Radiol. Supp. 358:9-14.

Pagan, J.D., and S.G. Jackson. 1996. The incidence of developmental orthopedic disease on a Kentucky Thoroughbred farm. World Equine Vet. Rev. 20-26.

Pearce, SG., E.C. Firth, N.D. Grace, and P.F. Fennessy. 1998a. Effect of copper supplementation on the evidence of developmental orthopaedic disease in pasture-fed New Zealand Thoroughbreds. Equine Vet. J. 30:211-218.

Pearce, S.G., N.D. Grace, E.C. Firth EC, et al. 1998b. Effect of copper supplementation on the copper status of pasture-fed young Thoroughbreds. Equine Vet. J. 30:204-210.

Pearce, S.G., N.D. Grace, J.I. Wichtel, et al. 1998c. Effect of copper supplementation on copper status of pregnant mares and foals. Equine Vet. J. 30:200-203.

Pettersson, H., and F. Sevelius. 1968. Subchondral bone cysts in the horse: A clinical study. Equine Vet. J. 1:75.

Phillips, T.J., and I.M. Wright. 1994. Observations on the anatomy and pathology of the palmar intercarpal ligaments in the middle carpal joints of Thoroughbred racehorses. Equine Vet. J. 26:486-491.

Phillipsson, J., E. Andreasson, B. Sandgren, et al. 1993. Osteochondrosis in the tarsocrural joint and osteochondral fragments in the fetlock joints in Standardbred trotters. II Hereditability. Equine Vet. J 16:38-41.

Pool, R.R. 1986. Pathologic manifestations of osteochondrosis. In: C.W. McIlwraith (Ed.) p. 3-7. AQHA Developmental Orthopedic Disease Symposium. American Quarter Horse Association. Amarillo, TX.

Ray, C.S., G.M. Baxter, C.W. McIlwraith, et al. 1996. Development of subchondral cystic lesions after articular cartilage and subchondral bone damage in young horses. Equine Vet. J. 28:225-232.

Rejno, S., and B. Stromberg. 1978. Osteochondrosis in the horse. II. Pathology. Acta Radiol. Suppl. 358:153-178.

Richardson, D.W. 1986. Technique for arthroscopic repair of third carpal bone slab fractures in horses. J. Amer. Vet. Med. Assoc. 188:288-291.

Rooney, J.R. 1975. Osteochondrosis in the horse. Mod. Vet. Pract. 56:41-43, 113-116.

Savage, C.J., R.N. McCarthy, and L.B. Jeffcott. 1993. Effects of dietary phosphorus and calcium on induction of dyschondroplasia in foals. Equine Vet. J. 516:80-83.

Schneider, R.K., P. Jenson, and R.M. Moore. 1997. Evaluation of cartilage lesions on the medial femoral condyle as a cause of lameness in horses: 11 cases (1988-1994). J. Amer.Vet. Med. Assoc. 210:1649-1652.

Schougaard, H., J. Falk-Ronne, and J. Phillipsson. 1990. A radiographic survey of tibiotarsal osteochondrosis in a selected population of trotting horses in Denmark and its possible genetic significance. Equine Vet. J. 22:288-289.

Southwood, L.L., and C.W. McIlwraith. 2000. Arthroscopic removal of fracture fragments involving a portion of the base of the sesamoid bone in horses. J. Amer. Vet. Med. Assoc. 217:236-240.

Southwood, L..L., G.W. Trotter, and C.W. McIlwraith. 1998. Arthroscopic removal of abaxial fracture fragments of the proximal sesamoid bone in horses: 47 cases (1989-1997). J. Amer. Vet. Med. Assoc. 213:1016-1021.

Stick, J.A., L.A. Borg, F.A. Nickels, et al. 1992. Arthroscopic removal of osteochondral fragment from the caudal pouch of the lateral femorotibial joint in a colt. J. Amer. Vet. Assoc. 200:1695-1697.

Stromberg, J. 1979. A review of the salient features of osteochondrosis in the horse. Equine Vet. J. 11:211-214.

Textor, J.A., A.J. Nixon, J. Lumsden, et al. 2001. Subchondral cystic lesions of the proximal extremity or the tibia in horses: 12 cases (1983-2000). J. Amer. Vet. Med. Assoc. 218:408-413.

Trumble, T.N., A.J. Stick, S.P. Arnoczky, et al. 1994. Consideration of anatomic and radiographic features of the caudal pouches of the femorotibial joints of horses for the purpose of arthroscopy. Amer. J. Vet. Res. 55:1682-1689.

Vacek, J.R., R.D. Welch, and C.M. Honnas. 1992. Arthroscopic approach and intra-articular anatomy of the palmaroproximal and plantaroproximal aspect of distal interphalangeal joints. Vet. Surg. 4:257-260.

von Rechenberg, B., H. Guenther, C.W. McIlwraith, et al. 2000a. Fibrous tissue of subchondral cystic lesions in horses produce local mediators in neutral metalloproteinases and cause bone resorption in vitro. Vet. Surg. 29:420.429.

von Rechenberg, B., C.W. McIlwraith, and M. Akens. 2000b. Spontaneous production of nitric oxide (NO) prostaglandins (PGE2) in neutral metalloproteinases based on what the intended use is for the horse. If vigorous athletic activity is planned, prophylactic surgery is justified. If less rigorous pursuits are planned, most horses will not require surgery and the fragment will not lead to further arthritic changes within the joint.

Surgery is rarely indicated for Type II fragments, and most of these fragments will unite with the parent bone over a period of many months. However, Type I and II fragments can occasionally occur together in the same joint, and the Type I fragment may require surgery. The prognosis for Type I fragments with surgery is favorable. Most Type II fragments are self-limiting.

OSTEOCHONDRITIS DISSECANS OF THE SHOULDER JOINT

OCD involving the shoulder joint is probably the most debilitating type of OCD affecting horses. Generally, large areas of the joint surfaces are involved, and secondary joint disease is common. However, it is unusual to have free or loose bodies develop. OCD of the shoulder is less common than for the other joints described, and seems to affect Quarter Horses and Thoroughbreds with a similar incidence.

Clinical and radiographic signs

Most horses with shoulder OCD present at one year of age or younger with a history of forelimb lameness of variable severity. Many of these horses will have prominent lameness. If lameness has been present for many weeks, muscle atrophy will also be seen. Because of the altered gait and use of the limb, many cases develop an upright or club-footed appearance to the foot, and the foot may appear smaller on the affected limb. Deep pressure over the shoulder joint will often cause discomfort, and forced flexion/extension of the limb will sometimes accentuate the lameness that is seen. Intra-articular anesthesia will improve or eliminate the lameness.

On radiographs, the most common sign is flattening or indentation of the humeral head. Often, cystic type lesions are also identified in the glenoid cavity of the scapula. Productive remodeling changes are also commonly identified along the caudal border of the glenoid cavity.

Treatment

Conservative treatment is rarely associated with a successful outcome, and sufficient numbers having surgery have not yet been accumulated to accurately identify the prognosis with surgery. However, there is little doubt that surgery dramatically improves the clinical signs in most cases. If extensive degenerative arthritic change is present on radiographs at the time of initial examination, the prognosis for an athletic career is unfavorable, and surgery should only be considered for relative improvement or without a fragment in place but also have free or loose bodies within the joint (Type III OCD).

Treatment

A conservative approach is initially recommended where only flattening without fragmentation is identified. Many of these cases will have resolution of clinical signs, as well as improvement or disappearance of radiographic signs; however, surgery will eventually be necessary in some of these cases. Surgical debridement is recommended for lesions where fragmentation or loose bodies are present. The prognosis is quite favorable for Type I lesions using conservative treatment but more guarded for Type II and Type III lesions (McIlwraith and Vorhees, 1990). Horses having other signs of articular cartilage erosion or wear lines within the joint had a less favorable prognosis. If the lesion extended out onto the condyle of the metacarpus/metatarsus from the sagittal ridge, the prognosis was also less favorable. It was determined that clinical signs would persist in approximately 25% of cases.

PROXIMAL PALMAR/PLANTAR FRAGMENTS OF THE FIRST PHALANX

Two types of fragments have been identified in this location. Type I fragments usually involve the hind fetlock joints and are located between the midline of the bone and its caudomedial (most common) or caudolateral (less common) borders. Type II fragments are also called ununited proximoplantar tuberosities of the proximal phalanx, as these lesions occur almost exclusively in the hind limb. These fragments are located at the most lateral (most common) or medial (much less common) borders of the bone.

Both of these entities have been identified frequently in radiographic surveys completed on yearling Standardbreds, supporting a developmental concept.

Clinical and radiographic signs

With Type I fragments, effusion is uncommon, and typically lameness is identified only as a somewhat vague problem at racing speeds or at the upper levels of performance. Flexion tests are often positive and anesthetic placed within the joint will usually eliminate any clinical signs that may be present. Regular oblique radiographs will usually demonstrate the lesions, although a special view is often used to highlight their location. Most fragments are present medially. Lameness and effusion are rare with Type II fragments.

Treatment

Arthroscopic surgery is recommended for Type I fragments where clinical signs are present. If these lesions are identified incidentally on fetlock radiographs, treatment is may be decreased. Maintenance of good bandages is more difficult for the hocks and must be taken in the early postoperative period to avoid subsequent infection in the joint through the small surgical incisions.

Prognosis

In a study involving 183 horses, 76% raced successfully and performed at their intended use after surgery (McIlwraith et al., 1991). If degenerative changes were identified at surgery in the cartilage surrounding the OCD lesion, the prognosis was less favorable. Resolution of effusion was inferior for lesions involving the lateral trochlear ridge compared to the intermediate ridge of the tibia; however, this seemed to have no effect on subsequent performance.

OSTEOCHONDRITIS DISSECANS OF THE FETLOCK JOINT

The most common manifestation of OCD in the fetlock joint is fragmentation and irregularity that occurs on the dorsal aspect of the sagittal ridge and the condyles of the metacarpus or metatarsus (cannon bone). A second condition involving the fetlock that may be OCD is fragmentation of the proximal palmar-plantar aspect of the first phalanx or long pastern bones. Debate continues as to whether these fragments are truly OCD-related or whether they represent small avulsion fractures. A final entity is OCD of the palmar aspect of the metacarpal condyles, which does seem to be a trauma-related condition of racehorses. Although this condition has been referred to as OCD, it does not fit with the developmental etiology. The remainder of this discussion will include the first two entities.

OSTEOCHONDRITIS DISSECANS OF THE DORSAL ASPECT OF THE DISTAL METACARPUS/METATARSUS (FETLOCK JOINT)

Clinical and radiographic signs

Joint swelling (effusion) is the most common clinical sign, with lameness being variable in both appearance and severity. Fetlock flexion tests are usually positive. It is not unusual for all four fetlocks to be involved, and bilateral forelimb or hind limb involvement is quite common.

The diagnosis is confirmed on radiographs, and clinically silent lesions (no effusion or baseline lameness) are often identified along with the lesions causing clinical signs. Lameness can sometimes be induced by flexion in these clinically silent joints. A variety of radiographic presentations are seen with fetlock OCD. Some joints will show only flattening of the sagittal ridge (Type I OCD), others will have a fragment in place within the area of flattening (Type II OCD), and others have flattening with swelling seen most readily along the medial or inside aspect of the joint. Lameness can also be seen but it is not common and is rarely prominent. Racehorses usually present as two-year-olds, but non-racehorses usually present as yearlings prior to going into training.

On radiographs, most attention is paid to the intermediate ridge of the tibia, followed by the lateral trochlear ridge, and then the medial malleolus of the tibia. Lesions are identified as fragments still in place (intermediate ridge) or surface irregularities of the trochlear ridge(s) or malleolus. The radiographic appearance often underestimates the extent of damage identified at surgery, particularly for lateral trochlear ridge lesions. The hock is also a joint where radiographically silent lesions (lesions identified at surgery where no abnormality was seen on radiographs) occur more commonly than in other joints.

Location of OCD Lesions in 318 Tarsocrural Joints

Number of Joints	Location
244	Intermediate ridge (dorsal aspect) of distal tibia
37	Lateral trochlear ridge of talus
12	Medial malleolus (dorsal aspect) of tibia
11	Intermediate ridge of tibia plus lateral trochlear ridge of talus
4	Intermediate ridge plus medial malleolus of tibia
3	Intermediate ridge plus medial trochlear ridge of talus
3	Medial trochlear ridge of talus
3	Lateral trochlear ridge of talus plus medial malleolus of tibia
1	Lateral and medial trochlear ridge of talus
318	**Total**

Treatment

Although lameness is usually minimal with hock OCD, surgery is the recommended treatment. Lameness may only be a problem at racing speeds or at upper levels of performance that cannot be observed during a clinical examination. As well, resolution of the effusion cannot be expected without removal of the abnormal tissue. That is not to say, however, that all horses having hock OCD need to have surgery. Horses with small lesions, minimal effusion, no lameness, and a potential career as a pleasure horse or light-use horse may not require surgery. Surgery should be considered early enough in the course of the disease so that the joint capsule is not unduly stretched, making resolution of the joint effusion less likely.

Arthroscopic identification and removal of fragments is recommended, although an arthrotomy (surgical incision into the joint) can be used successfully and is preferred by some for certain OCD lesions in this joint. Postoperative management is similar to that for OCD of the stifle, and for small lesions the time period for restricted exercise

(MMPs) in media of explant cultures of equine synovial membrane and articular cartilage from normal and osteoarthritic joints. Equine Vet. J. 32:140-150.

Walmsley, J.P. 1995. Vertical tears in the cranial horn of the meniscus and its cranial ligament in the equine femorotibial joint: 7 cases and their treatment by arthroscopic surgery. Equine Vet. J. 27:20-25.

Walmsley, J.P. 1997. Fracture of the intercondylar eminence of the tibia treated by arthroscopic internal fixation. Equine Vet. J. 29:148-150.

Walmsley, J.P. 2002. Arthroscopic surgery of the femorotibial joint. Clin. Tech. Equine Pract. 1:226-233.

Walmsley, J.P., T.J. Phillips, and H.G. Townsend. 2003. Meniscal tears in horses: An evaluation of clinical signs and arthroscopic treatment of 80 cases. Equine Vet. J. 35:402-406.

Weller, R.R., L.J. Maieler, I.M. Bowen, S.A. May, and H.G. Liebich. 2002. The arthroscopic approach and intra-articular anatomy of the equine temporomandibular joint. Equine Vet. J. 34:421-424.

Whitton, R.C., and R.J. Rose. 1997. The intercarpal ligaments of the equine mid-carpal joint. Part II: the role of the palmar intercarpal ligaments in the restraint of dorsal displacement of the proximal row of carpal bones. Vet. Surg. 26:367-373.

Whitton, R.C., N.J. Kannegieter, and R.J. Rose. 1997a. The intercarpal ligaments of the equine mid-carpal joint. Part III: clinical observations in 32 racing horses with mid-carpal joint disease. Vet. Surg. 26:374-381.

Whitton, R.C., P.H. McCarthy, and R.J. Rose. 1997b. The intercarpal ligaments of equine mid-carpal joint. Part I: the anatomy of the palmar and dorsomedial intercarpal ligaments of the mid-carpal joint. Vet. Surg. 26:359-366.

Wilke, M., A.J. Nixon, and J. Malark. 2001. Fractures of the palmar aspect of carpal 7 bones in horses: 10 cases (1984-2000). J. Amer. Vet. Med. Assoc. 219:801-804.

Yovich, J.V., and C.W. McIlwraith. 1986. Arthroscopic surgery for osteochondral fractures of the proximal phalanx of the metacarpophalangeal and metatarsophalangeal (fetlock) joints in horses. J. Amer. Vet. Med. Assoc. 188:243-279.

Zamos, D.T., C.M. Honnas, and A.G. Hoffman. 1994. Arthroscopic approach and intra-articular anatomy of the plantar pouch of the equine tarsocrural joint. Vet. Surg. 23:161-166.

NUTRITION AND MANAGEMENT OF THE BROODMARE

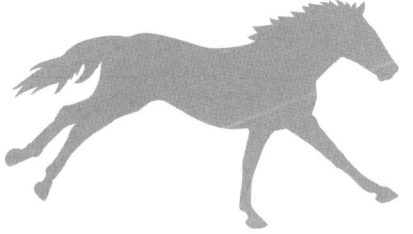

THE NEW NRC: UPDATED REQUIREMENTS FOR PREGNANCY AND GROWTH

LAURIE LAWRENCE

University of Kentucky, Lexington, Kentucky

Introduction and Brief History of *Nutrient Requirements of Horses*

The National Research Council (NRC) appointed a committee to revise the publication *Nutrient Requirements of Horses* in March of 2004. The committee consisted of 11 members from diverse geographical and educational backgrounds. When the publication is printed, it will represent the sixth revision under the current title. Prior to the first edition of *Nutrient Requirements of Horses*, the NRC produced a publication titled *Recommended Nutrient Allowances for Horses*. This book was published in 1949 and could be purchased for fifty cents. Many of the concepts used to predict nutrient requirements in past versions of *Nutrient Requirements of Horses* are also used in the sixth revised edition. However, the sixth revised edition of *Nutrient Requirements of Horses* will include some new approaches to estimating requirements and new combinations of methods used in previous publications. A variety of approaches have been used to estimate requirements in the sixth revised edition of *Nutrient Requirements of Horses*. Although it would have been preferable to use one system for estimating requirements for all nutrients, this was not possible due to a lack of information in some areas. Therefore, some requirements have been estimated using data derived solely in horses, whereas other estimates have incorporated information derived for other species.

The sixth revised edition of *Nutrient Requirements of Horses* will include nutrient requirements for maintenance, pregnancy, lactation, growth, and work (regular, imposed exercise). A Web-based computer program will be available to calculate requirements and compare dietary supply to the requirements for a number of nutrients. Nutrient requirements are expressed in amounts per day rather than nutrient concentrations/densities. The Web-based program will calculate nutrient densities if the user specifies a level of intake. In addition to the written explanation of the derivation of the requirements, there will be chapters on feeds and feed processing, feed additives, feeding management, feed analysis, unique aspects of equine nutrition (including discussion of the nutritional management of horses with special needs), and nutrition of donkeys and other equids.

This paper reviews the methods used to develop the protein and energy requirements for pregnant mares and growing horses. As in past versions of *Nutrient Requirements of Horses*, protein requirements are expressed as crude protein. However, crude protein requirements are generally derived from estimates of digestible protein requirements and dietary protein digestibility. Energy requirements are expressed in units of digestible energy. Some requirements have been derived from studies that reported digestible energy intakes, whereas other requirements have been derived from estimates of recovered energy (tissue or milk) and/or measures of heat production.

The Pregnant Mare

The nutritional requirements of pregnant animals are difficult to study, and thus the nutritional requirements of pregnant mares have received little attention from researchers. There are several reasons the nutrient requirements of pregnant mares have not been extensively studied. Mares have a relatively long gestation period, so the appropriate experimental period is long. Conducting even short-term nutritional balance studies with mares can be challenging. Mares can use body tissue to meet the demands of fetal development, making it hard to observe the effects of marginal nutrient intakes. It is often difficult to ascertain whether foals are born with "normal" or "optimal" nutritional and health status. Furthermore, it may take several months or years to realize any impacts of maternal nutrition on the offspring, so data must be collected on foals for several years after birth. Given these challenges, it is not surprising that there are fewer studies dealing with nutrition of the pregnant mare compared to other classes of horses.

The nutrients needed by pregnant animals can be partitioned into the following categories: (1) nutrients needed by the dam to maintain her body; (2) nutrients needed by the dam to synthesize fetal tissue; (3) nutrients needed by the dam to synthesize the accessory tissues of conception (the placenta, enlargement of the uterus, enlargement of the mammary gland); (4) nutrients needed to maintain the newly synthesized tissues of the fetus, placenta, uterus, and mammary gland.

To accurately calculate the nutrient needs of pregnant mares, it would be necessary to know the rate of accumulation of fetal and accessory tissues, the efficiency of nutrient use for the synthesis of this tissue, and the maintenance costs of these tissues. Very little of this information was available for use in the sixth revised edition of *Nutrient Requirements of Horses*. As a result, the requirements suggested in the sixth revised edition are based on limited data from horses, assumptions from previous editions of *Nutrient Requirements of Horses*, and some data from other species.

Slaughter of pregnant females at various stages of gestation has produced estimates of the rates of fetal and placental tissue accretion in other species. Bell et al. (1995) reported on the accretion of energy and protein in the gravid uterus of dairy cows slaughtered between 190 and 270 d of gestation. Ji and coworkers (2005) measured the weight and composition of the fetus, uterus, and mammary gland of gilts slaughtered at 0, 45, 60, 75, 90, 102 and 112 d of gestation. Similar studies have not been conducted in horses. Information from papers published by Meyer and Ahlswede (1976; 1978) was used as a basis for several of the recommended intakes for pregnant mares that were reported in the 1989 edition of *Nutrient Requirements of Horses*. Meyer and Ahlswede (1976; 1978) determined the composition of aborted fetuses or foals that died at birth. Gestational age of the fetuses ranged from 161 to 354 days. Most of the fetuses were produced by Thoroughbred or Warmblood-type mares. Platt (1978) also reported fetal weights of aborted Thoroughbred foals. More recently, in an experiment designed to investigate equine fetal cardiovascular function, Giussani and coworkers (2005) reported the weights of several aborted fetuses and prematurely delivered foals from Welsh pony mares that had been instrumented between 143 and 328 days of gestation. Ideally, data from normal fetuses should be used to develop curves for fetal tissue accretion. However, in the absence of data from normal horses, data from the studies of Meyer and Ahlswede (1978), Platt (1978), and Giussani et al. (2005) were used to develop an equation to predict fetal weight during gestation. Meyer and Ahlswede (1978) had previously suggested that weight of Thoroughbred fetuses during late gestation could be calculated using the equation:

Fetal wt (kg) = $0.00067(X^2) - 20.7$; where X = days of gestation.

Although this equation may be useful for Thoroughbreds, it cannot be applied to horses with larger or smaller body sizes. To produce an estimate that would apply to more types/breeds of horses, fetal weights reported by each of the studies cited above were converted to a percentage of expected birth weight. These fetal weights as a percentage of mature weight were then used to develop an equation that could be used to estimate fetal tissue accretion across all mature body weights. In the study by Meyer and Ahlswede (1978), the protein and lipid contents of fetal tissue were relatively constant during the last 5 months of gestation at 60% protein and 10% lipid on a dry matter basis. Mineral content of the fetal tissue was more variable. Meyer and Ahlswede (1978) reported that calcium content of the fetal tissue in the seventh month of gestation was 59.5 +/- 14.8 g/kg DM. In the tenth month of gestation the value was 75.6 +/- 11.9 g Ca/kg DM.

An estimate of the nutrient accretion in the fetus is the first step in calculating a daily requirement. The next step is to estimate the efficiency of incorporating absorbed nutrients into fetal tissue. The efficiency of incorporation varies by nutrient. For example, the efficiency of digestible energy use for fetal tissue has been suggested to be 60% (NRC, 1966), whereas the efficiency of digestible protein use for fetal tissue deposition has been estimated at 45% (NRC, 1973). The efficiency of use of absorbed minerals is usually considered to be 100%. Finally, for nutrients such as protein and minerals, dietary availability must be considered.

In addition to the nutrients needed to deposit new tissue associated with conception, nutrients must also be used to maintain the newly deposited tissue. For example, during the tenth month of gestation, the fetus requires nutrients for growth plus nutrients to meet the metabolic demands of the existing tissues. Researchers at the University of Cambridge have developed sophisticated instrumentation techniques to study fetal metabolism in utero. These techniques have produced estimates of oxygen utilization by the fetus and associated tissues (Fowden et al., 2000). Their data suggest that rate of oxygen utilization by the tissues of conception is approximately double the average rate of oxygen utilized by the horse at maintenance. Very few data are available to assess the maintenance requirements of fetal tissue for other nutrients.

Although the fetus comprises the largest portion of the tissue accumulated during gestation, the other tissues of conception must also be considered. Placental weight at foaling is correlated with foal birth weight (Oulton et al., 2004; Whitehead et al., 2004). In a study of Standardbreds, average birth weight was 53 kg and placental weight was 4.4 kg. No data could be found on the increase in tissue weight sustained by the uterus during pregnancy in mares, so studies with other species were reviewed. It was estimated that uterine tissue accretion was equal to, and paralleled, placental tissue accretion. Data reported in a textbook (Ginther, 1992) suggest that accumulation of uterine and placental tissues begins in mid-gestation. In swine, combined fetal and placental tissues reach more than 50% of final weight by mid-gestation (Ji et al., 2005). At 190 days of gestation in cows, the non-fetal tissues and fluids of conception have attained more than 40% of final weight, whereas the fetus has attained less than 25% of birth weight at the same time (Bell et al., 1995). Studies in cattle and swine also suggest that the accretion of placental and uterine tissues follows linear functions. Therefore, it was concluded that placental and uterine development begins prior to the last trimester in horses and that it follows a linear function. In the fourth edition of *Nutrient Requirements of Horses* (1978), requirement estimates were given for mares in early gestation and during the last 90 days of gestation. In the subsequent edition (1989) of the publication, estimates were given for early gestation and the ninth, tenth, and eleventh months of gestation. In the sixth edition, requirements will be estimated for pregnant mares at less than 5 months of gestation and then at 5, 6, 7, 8, 9, 10, and 11 months of gestation. The crude protein and digestible energy requirements for mares in late gestation in the sixth revised edition of *Nutrient Requirements of Horses* are similar to, or slightly higher than, previous estimates (NRC, 1989). Another addition to this version of *Nutrient Requirements of Horses* will be estimates of the expected body weight of pregnant mares during the fifth through eleventh months of gestation.

Growing Horses

The nutrient requirements of growing horses have been estimated from a variety of methods. In the 1966 version of *Nutrient Requirements of Horses*, the protein requirement for gain was derived from studies with cattle. However, in the third and fourth editions (1973; 1978), protein requirements for gain were derived from estimates of the amount of protein deposited in each kilogram of gain using body composition data from horses. In 1989 the protein requirements of growing horses were calculated from feeding studies with growing horses. In addition, the recommended crude protein and lysine intakes were linked to the daily digestible energy intake of the horses (NRC, 1989). The crude protein and lysine requirements for weanlings were 50 and 2.1 g/Mcal DE/day, respectively (NRC, 1989). The requirements for yearlings were 45 g CP/Mcal DE/d and 1.9 g lysine/Mcal DE/day (NRC, 1989). Possibly as a result of the different methods used to calculate the crude protein requirement, some of the estimates in 1989 and 1978 were quite different. For example, the recommended crude protein intake for a 12-month-old yearling with an expected mature body weight of 500 kg was 760 g/d in 1978 compared to 851-956 g/d in 1989 (depending on rate of growth). In the sixth edition of *Nutrient Requirements of Horses*, the committee chose to calculate crude protein and lysine requirements in a manner similar to that used in 1978, and protein requirements were no longer calculated from energy intakes. The text of the sixth edition provides information on the digestible protein needs of growing horses as well as the crude protein requirements. The recommended daily amounts of crude protein and lysine in the sixth edition are somewhat lower than in the 1989 edition, partly because protein digestibility in common feeds used for growing horses was estimated to be higher than in previous editions.

In the third and fourth revised editions (1973; 1978) of *Nutrient Requirements of Horses*, the digestible energy required for a kilogram of gain was estimated using the following equation:

$$\text{Kcal DE/kg gain} = 3.8 + 12.3X - 6.6X^2;$$
$$\text{where } X = \text{fraction of mature weight (NRC, 1978)}$$

The source of the equation to derive the amount of energy needed for a kilogram of gain was not given, but it may have been extrapolated from a previous equation developed from data for beef cattle described in the second edition of the publication (NRC, 1966). In 1989, estimates of the digestible energy needed per kilogram of gain were derived from the summarization of feeding studies with horses (NRC, 1989). The amount of digestible energy required per kilogram of gain was estimated by the following equation:

$$\text{Mcal DE/kg gain} = 4.81 + 1.17X - 0.023X^2;$$
$$\text{where } X = \text{age in months (1989)}$$

In the previous editions of *Nutrient Requirements of Horses*, the daily digestible energy intake of growing horses was calculated by adding the requirement for gain to the requirement for maintenance. In 1978, the digestible energy required for maintenance was calculated using the following equation:

Kcal DE/day = 155 $W^{0.75}$; where W = body weight in kilograms (NRC, 1978)

In 1989, the NRC committee abandoned the concept of expressing energy requirements on a metabolic body size and used an equation developed by Pagan and Hintz (1986) to estimate the digestible energy requirement for maintenance. The equation used in the 1989 NRC to estimate the digestible energy requirement for maintenance was:

Mcal DE/d = 1.4 + 0.03W; where W = weight in kilograms

When the equations for estimating the digestible energy needed for maintenance and gain were combined, the daily digestible energy intakes of horses were calculated in the 1989 NRC using the following equation:

Mcal DE/d = (1.4 + 0.03W) + (4.81 + 1.17X - 0.023X^2)(ADG);
where W = weight in kg; X = months of age; and ADG = daily gain in kg

A comparison of predicted and actual weight gains of growing horses fed at or near NRC (1989) recommended digestible energy levels suggests that the equation developed in 1989 may have slightly overestimated the amount of digestible energy needed for the specified rates of gain (Lawrence, 2000). In the sixth revised edition of *Nutrient Requirements of Horses*, the committee considered whether the equation developed in 1989 to estimate energy requirements of growing horses should be modified. An important consideration was the method of determining the maintenance requirements of growing horses.

In 1978 and 1989, the NRC committee concluded that the equations for calculating maintenance requirements should apply to both adult animals and growing animals. Therefore, the amount of energy needed to maintain the body weight (no growth) of a 200-kg weanling Thoroughbred would be the same as the amount of energy needed to maintain the weight (no gain) of a 200-kg 10-year-old pony. Given the probable differences in body composition and potential differences in voluntary activity between an adult pony and a Thoroughbred weanling, it seems likely that maintenance requirements would also be different. In addition, when the 1989 NRC equation and assumptions about the composition of gain (NRC, 1978) are used to calculate the partial efficiency of digestible energy use for gain, the resulting value is relatively low, especially for horses 12 months of age and older. These considerations caused the committee to consider whether the equations developed in 1978 and 1989 correctly partitioned the energy for maintenance and the energy for gain in growing horses.

Limited data are available on the maintenance requirements of growing horses. Cymbaluk et al. (1989) determined mean maintenance values for growing horses (6 to 24 months of age) of 37.8 and 35.6 kcal/kg BW depending on the amount of diet that was fed. The horses in that experiment were turned out for 6 hours per day during the study. These data would suggest that the maintenance requirements of 15-month-old horses (average age during the study) would be approximately 36.5 kcal/kg BW. The

1989 NRC maintenance equation predicts a slightly lower digestible energy intake of 34 kcal/kg BW for a 350-kg yearling. Therefore, the maintenance equation suggested by Pagan and Hintz (1986) and later adopted by the NRC (1989) appears to slightly underestimate the maintenance needs of yearling horses. The discrepancy between actual and predicted maintenance requirements might be greater for younger horses. In one study of neonatal foals, the digestible energy for maintenance was close to 70 kcal/kg BW (Ousey et al., 1997). Coenen (2000) suggested that the maintenance requirement for 3- to 6-month-old horses was 210 kcal/W0.75, which would be approximately 55 kcal/kg BW. For the sixth revised edition of *Nutrient Requirements of Horses*, the available data on maintenance requirements of growing horses were summarized and an equation was derived to predict maintenance energy as a function of body weight and age. Several studies reporting age, body weight, digestible energy intake, and weight gain of growing horses were then used to calculate the digestible energy needed above maintenance for gain as a function of age. A new equation that combines the maintenance component and the gain component of the digestible energy intake was developed. This equation is similar in concept to the equation developed in 1989, but differs in that it tends to partition more energy towards maintenance and less energy towards gain.

The final step in calculating the energy needs of growing horses is to estimate average daily gain. The total amount of digestible energy required each day will vary with rate of gain. The committee appointed to revise *Nutrient Requirements of Horses* in March of 2004 received several requests to include growth curves for a variety of horse breeds in the publication. In previous editions of the publication, nutrient requirements and growth data were categorized by expected mature weight, not breed. Growth curves were shown in a figure in the 1978 edition of *Nutrient Requirements of Horses*, but no source for the information was cited and specific breeds were not identified. The sixth revised edition of *Nutrient Requirements of Horses* will not include breed-specific growth curves. The absence of breed-specific growth curves is partly due to an absence of data for many breeds. In addition, within some breeds there is a great deal of variation among horses. For example, a growth curve derived using halter-type Quarter Horses might not apply very well to cutting-bred Quarter Horses, even though they are members of the same breed.

The 1989 *Nutrient Requirements of Horses* provided estimates of body weights and average daily gains for horses at 4, 6, 12, 18, and 24 months of age. The source of the data used to develop these estimates was not given, and there were some inconsistencies between the body weight estimates and the average daily gain estimates. The body weight of a weanling expected to mature at 500 kg was predicted to be 175 kg at 4 months and 215 kg at 6 months (NRC, 1989). Based on these two weights, the expected average daily gain would have been 0.66 kg/d (40 kg in 60 days). However, the suggested rates of daily gain were 0.85 kg/d for the 4-month-old, and 0.65 to 0.85 kg/d for the 6-month-old horses. A goal of the committee appointed to revise *Nutrient Requirements of Horses* was to develop a method to predict the growth rate of all types of horses. The method that was developed can be applied across breeds to calculate weight at a specific age. Once body weight is estimated, average daily gain can be calculated.

A number of researchers have studied growth characteristics of Thoroughbred horses including Green (1969), Hintz et al. (1979), Jelan et al. (1996), Pagan et al. (1996), and Kavazis and Ott (2003). Fewer or less comprehensive studies are available for other breeds. Therefore, to obtain a continuous growth curve that would apply to all horses, the committee to revise *Nutrient Requirements of Horses* took an approach of expressing growth as a function of mature weight. This is not a new concept and has been described by others including Austbo (2004) and Coenen (2000). To obtain an equation to predict body weight at any age from mature weight, growth data from the following breeds or types of horses were summarized: Thoroughbred, Morgan, Quarter Horse, pony, Arabian, Belgian, Hanoverian, and Swedish Standardbred. Once data for each breed were summarized by age, body weights were expressed as a percentage of mature body weight. Mature body weights were obtained from values given in the reviewed papers or from a search of the literature. The data from all breeds/types were combined, and a single growth curve was developed. The resulting growth curve can be applied to any breed or type of horse, if an estimate of expected mature weight is available. There were insufficient data to generate separate curves for colts, fillies, and geldings. However, different estimates of body weight at any age will be obtained if users estimate different mature weights for stallions, geldings, and mares. There were also insufficient data to generate separate curves for ponies, light horses, and draft horses. Although representatives of each type of horse were included in the data used to generate the final equation, the data set for Belgian horses included only foals/weanlings.

The committee recognizes that there are some limitations to the method developed to predict equine growth in the sixth revised edition of *Nutrient Requirements of Horses*. First, the method that was developed was based on body weight data and did not incorporate any factor for optimal skeletal growth. The committee did not find sufficient data to quantify an optimal growth rate. Therefore, the method that was developed provides information only about the average rate of gain and does not account for growth rates that might be preferred in order to meet specific production goals of an individual horse owner. Second, the equation developed to predict body weight suggests that rate of gain continuously decreases with age, a situation which may not occur in practice. Real-world data sets suggest that average daily gain varies with environment and that the rate of gain of yearlings on high-quality pasture in the spring may exceed the rate of gain of weanlings/yearlings during the prior winter (Pagan et al., 1996; Asai, 2000; Staniar et al., 2004). Therefore the method suggested in the sixth revised edition of *Nutrient Requirements of Horses* probably overestimates average daily gain of weanlings/yearlings in the winter and underestimates their growth rate the following spring. Finally, the method to estimate growth rate in the sixth revised edition of *Nutrient Requirements of Horses* was developed primarily with data from horses with mature body weights of 400 to 600 kg. Therefore it is not known how well this method will apply to miniature horses, small ponies, or draft and provide a confidence interval for the mean response at a specified foal age within each foal-age category. When gender was being considered, it was included as an explanatory variable. When a significant (p<0.05) main effect or interaction was found, multiple comparisons were made (P<0.05) using the Tukey-Kramer test (NCSS software package, NCSS, Kaysville, Utah).

Results are expressed as mean and 95% confidence interval and significance is reported at the 5% level.

Results and Discussion

FOALS

Colts were between 1.7 and 3.0 kg heavier and 0.6 and 1.3 cm taller than fillies (p < 0.05) throughout the study. Fillies and colts exhibited similar BCS from birth to 7 days of age (p > 0.05); however, at 1 month of age fillies were fatter than colts (p < 0.05) and remained so until the end of the study (Table 1 and Figure 1).

Table 1. Body weight, height, and BCS ± 95% confidence intervals of Kentucky fillies and colts.

Days	Body weight (kg)			Height (cm)			BCS		
	Colts	Fillies	p	Colts	Fillies	p	Colts	Fillies	p
1	57.24 ± 1.04	55.12 ± 1.02	<0.05	103.20 ± 0.44	102.19 ± 0.43	<0.05	5.21 ± 0.03	5.20 ± 0.0	3n/s
7	67.28 ± 0.71	65.16 ± 0.69	<0.01	105.60 ± 0.30	104.59 ± 0.29	<0.01	5.39 ± 0.02	5.38 ± 0.02	n/s
30	100.46 ± 0.61	98.75 ± 0.60	<0.01	112.98 ± 0.19	112.42 ± 0.18	<0.01	5.65 ± 0.02	5.68 ± 0.02	<0.05
60	137.81 ± 0.75	135.16 ± 0.74	<0.01	120.38 ± 0.19	119.65 ± 0.19	<0.01	5.66 ± 0.02	5.73 ± 0.02	<0.01
90	171.83 ± 0.88	168.94 ± 0.88	<0.01	126.02 ± 0.20	125.04 ± 0.20	<0.01	5.62 ± 0.02	5.71 ± 0.02	<0.01
120	202.21 ± 1.06	199.38 ± 1.04	<0.01	130.25 ± 0.21	129.54 ± 0.21	<0.01	5.56 ± 0.02	5.65 ± 0.02	<0.01
150	230.56 ± 1.61	227.59 ± 1.59	<0.01	133.90 ± 0.29	133.09 ± 0.29	<0.01	5.55 ± 0.02	5.63 ± 0.02	<0.01

January, February, and March foals had lower body weights than April or May foals during the first month of age. January and February foals remained lighter than foals born in March, April, and May until 3 months of age, and January foals remained lighter than all other foals until 4 months of age (Table 2). By 150 days of age, there was no difference in body weight between birth months.

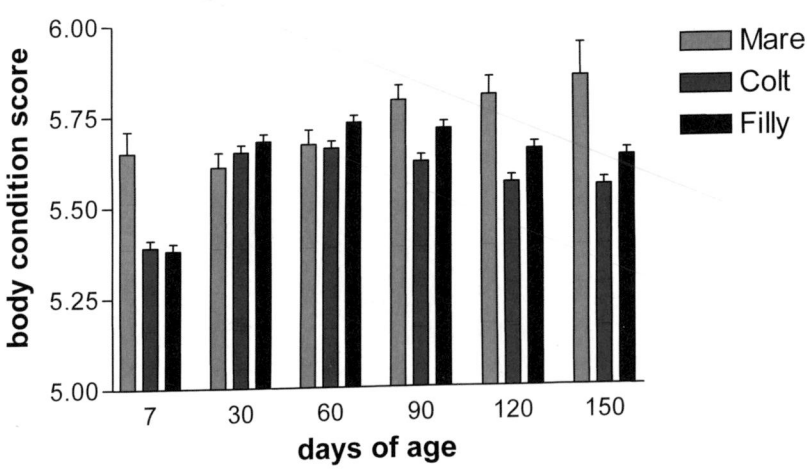

Figure 1. Body condition score ± 95% confidence intervals of Kentucky mares, fillies and colts.

Table 2. Foal body weight (kg) ± 95% confidence interval. Differing superscripts within rows indicate significant differences (p < 0.05).

Days	January	February	March	April	May
1	53.69 ± 3.67[a]	54.86 ± 1.57[a]	55.21 ± 1.91[a]	57.76 ± 2.11[ab]	60.17 ± 2.60[b]
7	62.86 ± 1.99[a]	64.36 ± 0.88[a]	65.71 ± 0.84[a]	68.18 ± 1.16[b]	69.96 ± 1.43[b]
30	93.50 ± 1.37[a]	96.27 ± 0.80[b]	100.80 ± 0.78[c]	102.74 ± 0.84[d]	102.11 ± 1.18[d]
60	128.48 ± 1.75[a]	133.72 ± 1.05[b]	138.90 ± 0.96[c]	138.82 ± 0.99[c]	137.31 ± 1.62[c]
90	163.85 ± 2.24[a]	169.03 ± 1.18[b]	172.61 ± 1.12[c]	171.26 ± 1.28[bc]	170.92 ± 1.70[bc]
120	195.66 ± 2.53[a]	199.46 ± 1.31[ab]	201.98 ± 1.47[b]	202.24 ± 1.50[b]	202.55 ± 2.32[b]
150	226.00 ± 3.07[a]	228.74 ± 1.83[a]	230.63 ± 2.24[a]	230.92 ± 3.31[a]	227.11 ± 4.18[a]

January and February foals had lower ADG than March, April, and May foals at 7 days and 1 month of age. January foals had greater ADG than all foals at 3 months of age coinciding with rapid spring pasture growth beginning in April. May foals had the lowest ADG of all foals at 2, 3, and 4 months, which coincides with July, August, and September when late summer pasture is losing its quality, suggesting a seasonal effect on foal ADG (Figure 2).

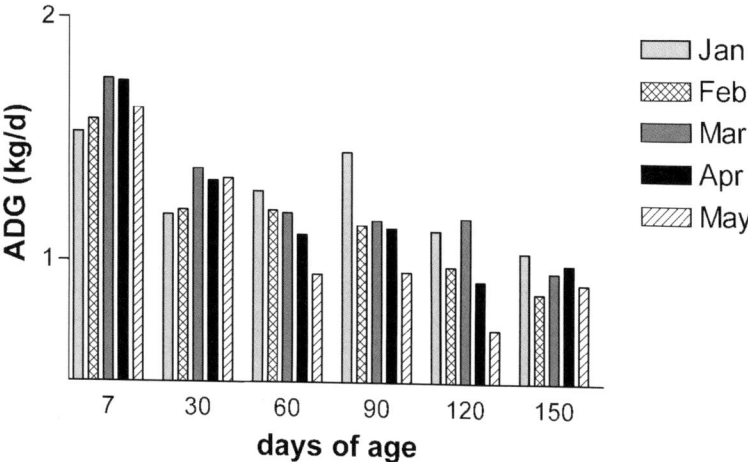

Figure 2. ADG (kg/d) of Kentucky foals separated by month of birth.

Month of birth had no effect on foal BCS at 7 days as well as 4 and 5 months of age. In all foals BCS was lowest at 7 days and increased between 7 and 30 days. May foals had lower BCS than all other foals at 1 and 2 months of age. January and February foals had significantly greater BCS than March, April, and May foals at 3 months (Table 3 and Figure 3).

Table 3. BCS (scale 1-9) ± 95% confidence interval of Kentucky foals born in January, February, March, April, and May. Differing superscripts within a row indicate significant differences ($p < 0.05$).

Days	January	February	March	April	May
7	5.39 ± 0.06[a]	5.36 ± 0.03[a]	5.39 ± 0.03[a]	5.41 ± 0.03[a]	5.37 ± 0.04[a]
30	5.68 ± 0.04[a]	5.65 ± 0.02[ab]	5.67 ± 0.02[a]	5.69 ± 0.02[a]	5.61 ± 0.03[b]
60	5.74 ± 0.04[a]	5.71 ± 0.03[a]	5.73 ± 0.02[a]	5.68 ± 0.02[b]	5.63 ± 0.03[c]
90	5.72 ± 0.05[a]	5.73 ± 0.03[a]	5.66 ± 0.02[b]	5.62 ± 0.02[b]	5.60 ± 0.04[b]
120	5.64 ± 0.04[a]	5.61 ± 0.03[a]	5.59 ± 0.02[a]	5.59 ± 0.03[a]	5.60 ± 0.05[a]
150	5.61 ± 0.04[a]	5.59 ± 0.03[a]	5.57 ± 0.03[a]	5.58 ± 0.05[a]	5.66 ± 0.07[a]

MARES

Winter foaling mares (January and February) had lower body weights in the first 2 months postpartum than mares which foaled in March, April, or May. By months 4 and 5 of lactation, there was no difference in mare body weight between any of the groups (Figure 4).

142 *Body Weight and Condition*

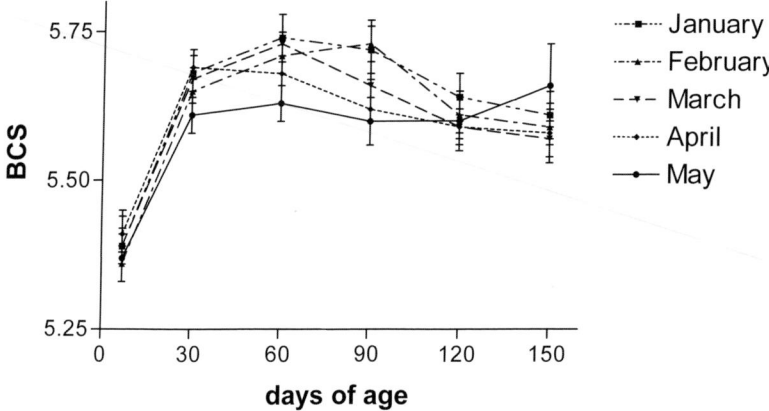

Figure 3. BCS (scale 1-9) ± 95% confidence interval of Kentucky foals separated by month of birth.

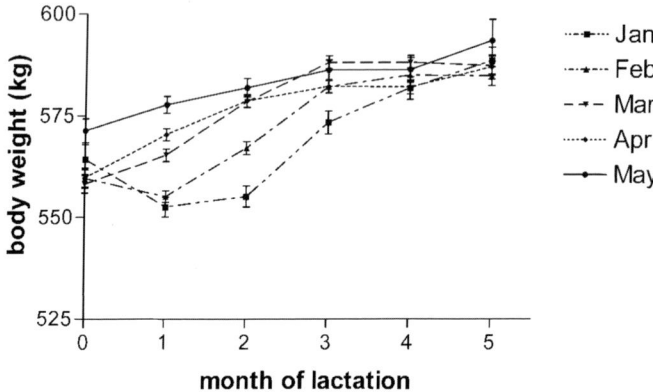

Figure 4. Mare body weight (kg) ± 95% confidence interval in relation to month of lactation.

Winter-foaling mares showed negative daily weight change in the first month postpartum compared with mares which foaled in spring (March, April, and May). January-foaling mares had the lowest daily weight change during month 2 and the highest daily weight change during months 4 and 5 compared to all other mares, and during month 3 of lactation, January- and February-foaling mares exhibited greater daily weight change than all other mares (Figure 5).

Mare body weight, daily weight change, and BCS increased in the spring (March through June) in all mares regardless of stage of lactation (Figures 6, 7, and 8). Mares that foaled in the winter months showed a negative daily weight change during January and February, which then increased to approximately 0.5 kg/d in March, where it remained positive until the completion of the study (Figure 7). Changes in mare body weight and BCS appeared to be related to seasonal and management factors. Winter-

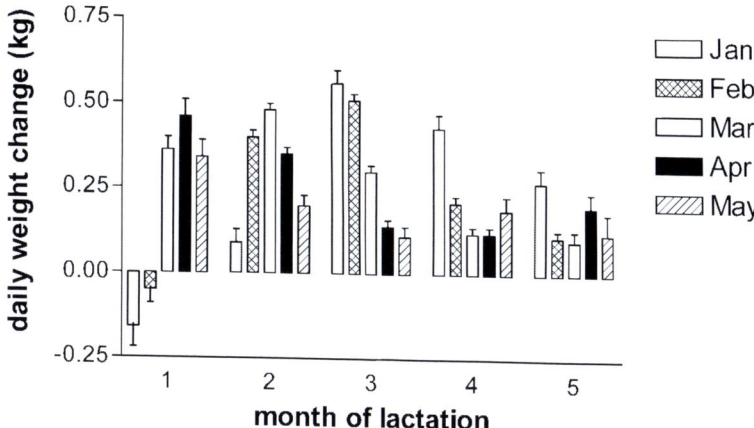

Figure 5. Daily weight change (kg/d) ± 95% confidence interval of Kentucky mares in relation to month of lactation.

foaling mares that showed decreased body weight, negative daily weight gain, and lower BCS after foaling are likely to spend more time indoors with restricted access to pasture until the spring.

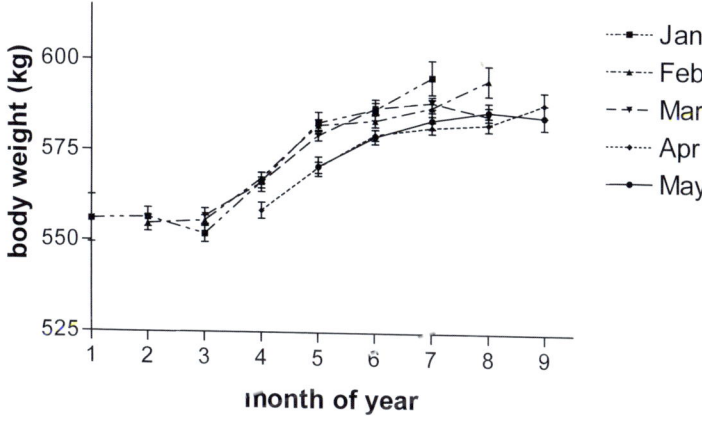

Figure 6. Body weight (kg) ± 95% confidence intervals of Kentucky mares in relation to month of the year (1 represents January, 2 represents February, etc.).

RELATIONSHIPS BETWEEN MARE AND FOAL DATA

Foal body weight was positively correlated to mare body weight ($p < 0.05$), foal ADG was positively associated with mare ADG ($p < 0.05$), and foal BCS was positively related to mare BCS during months 1-5. These relationships indicate that heavier mares

144 Body Weight and Condition

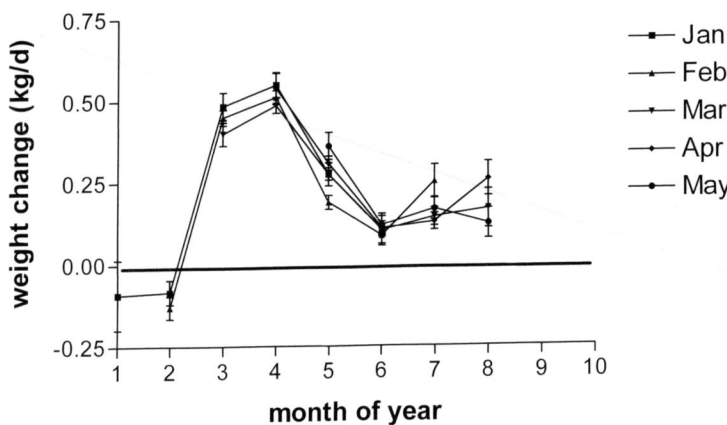

Figure 7. Daily weight change (kg/d) ± 95% confidence intervals of Kentucky mares in relation to month of the year (1 represents January, 2 represents February, etc.).

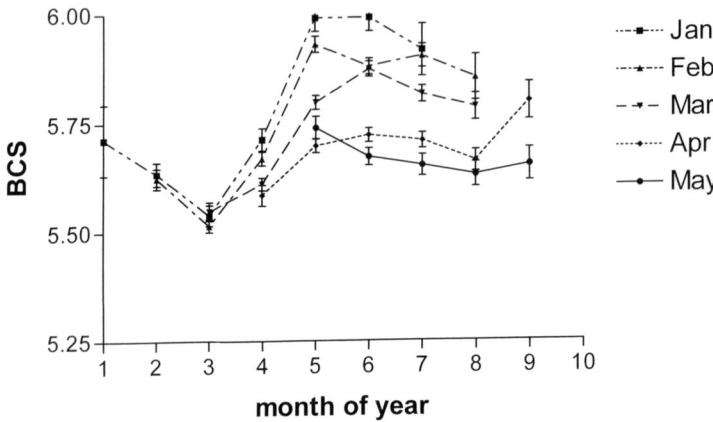

Figure 8. Body condition score (scale 1-9) ± 95% confidence intervals of Kentucky mares in relation to month of the year (1 represents January, 2 represents February, etc.).

produce heavier foals, faster-growing foals are from mares that are gaining weight, and fatter foals are produced from fatter mares. There was a positive relationship between foal BCS and mare daily weight change at 2 and 3 months (peak lactation), indicating that mares that are gaining weight during the first 3 months of lactation have fatter foals.

Regardless of month of birth, mares that exhibited a negative energy balance postpartum (losing weight or negative daily weight change) had foals that did not gain as much weight as mares that were in a positive energy balance at any age ($p < 0.05$).

These data clearly demonstrate that season of the year affects growth in suckling foals. Foals born in January and February were smaller at birth and grew slower during the first two months than foals born later in the year. January- and February-foaling mares tended to lose weight in early lactation, suggesting that their caloric intakes were insufficient to meet their energy requirement for early lactation. Later in lactation when there was access to adequate pasture, these early-foaling mares gained more weight and supported faster growth rates in their foals than later-foaling mares. It is unclear whether the faster growth rates in these 3- to 4-month-old foals was due to greater milk production, greater pasture consumption by the foals, or a combination of both factors.

In Kentucky, growth rate of suckling foals was affected by birth month and season of year. Foals born in the winter grew slower during the first two months, but compensated by growing faster later in lactation so that the net result was that by 5 months of age there was no difference between body weights in any of the groups. This is different than in Canada (Hintz et al., 1979), where foals born early in the year remained smaller throughout their yearling year, or in the UK (Jones and Hollands, 2005), where growth rate was not different between birth months for the first 200 days of age. In Canada, pasture availability in the spring may not have been enough to allow for compensatory weight gain in early-born foals. In the UK, perhaps winter pasture availability was sufficient to meet mare energy requirements and support foal growth.

References

Henneke, D.R., G.D. Potter, and J.L. Kreider. 1981. A condition score relationship to body fat content of mares during gestation and lactation. In: Proc. Equine Nutr. Physiol. Soc. 7:105-110.

Hintz, H.F., R.L. Hintz, and L.D. van Vleck. 1979. Growth rate of Thoroughbreds: Effect of age of dam, year and month of birth and sex of foal. J. Anim. Sci. 48:480-487.

Jones, L., and T. Hollands. 2005. Estimation of growth rates in UK Thoroughbreds. Pferdeheilkunde 21;121-123.

Pagan, J.D., S.G. Jackson, and S. Caddel. 1996. A summary of growth rates of Thoroughbred horses in Kentucky. Pferdeheilkunde 123:285-289.

THE EFFECT OF DIETARY CALCIUM ON INDICATORS OF BONE TURNOVER IN BROODMARES

BRYAN CASSILL, SUSAN HAYES, JENNIFER RINGLER, KRISTEN JANICKI, AND LAURIE LAWRENCE

University of Kentucky, Lexington, Kentucky

Introduction

Preliminary studies in our laboratory have found that serum ICTP, an indicator of bone turnover, is increased shortly after foaling. This increase may indicate that mares mobilize bone mineral during lactation. In addition, Glade (1993) reported that estimated metacarpal bone breaking strength decreased in lactating mares fed a diet containing the recommended NRC (1989) levels of calcium and phosphorus. In that study, bone breaking strength rebounded after weaning. This study was conducted to determine whether dietary calcium and phosphorus concentration would affect indicators of bone turnover in mares during late lactation and after weaning.

Materials and Methods

The study used 12 mares (average age 10 ± 4.8 y) split into two groups (control and high-calcium). Groups were balanced for age and parity. The study was initiated at 2.5 mo of lactation and lasted for 16 wk. Foals were weaned at 4.5 mo of lactation. Mares were kept on cool-season grass pastures and were fed a concentrate containing 0.6% Ca and 0.5% P (DM basis). When pasture availability declined, mares were offered timothy hay (0.5% Ca, 0.4% P, DM basis). The high-calcium group was fed the same as the control except dicalcium phosphate was added to the concentrate to increase total estimated calcium intake to 150% of the control group while maintaining a balanced calcium to phosphorus ratio. All mares were fed the concentrate at 1% of body weight until the sixth week of the study. At that time concentrate intake was reduced to 0.8% of body weight. During the seventh week, concentrate intake was reduced to 0.7% of body weight, and in the final week before weaning, the concentrate intake was reduced to 0.6% of body weight. At weaning, concentrate intake was dropped to 0.3% of body weight.

Collection of Data

Body weights were obtained every 14 d and blood samples were collected every 28 d for the duration of the study. Milk samples were collected every 28 d for the first 56 d. Calcium concentrations of milk and serum were determined using atomic absorption spectrophotometry. The serum was analyzed for osteocalcin, a protein that is a marker for bone formation, and ICTP, a type I carboxy-terminal pyridinoline crosslink telopeptide that is a marker for bone resorption. Serum ICTP was measured using a radioimmunoassay (DiaSorin, Stillwater, MN). Serum osteocalcin was determined using an enzyme-linked immunosorbent assay (ELISA) (Quidel, San Diego, CA). All samples were assayed in duplicate using the supplied set of standards along with a high and low control that had been previously analyzed in our laboratory.

Results

Calcium concentration in milk decreased over time ($P < 0.005$) with an average concentration of 593.0 ± 77.6 µg/g at 2.5 mo and 476.2 ± 113.6 µg/g at 4.5 mo. Milk calcium concentration was not affected by diet. Total daily milk production was not measured, but average daily gain of foals from mares fed the high-calcium diet ± 1.01 (0.2 kg) was not different from average daily gain of foals from mares in the control group ± 0.97 (0.08 kg). Calcium concentration in serum averaged 105.6 ± 11.2 mg/L at the beginning of the study (2.5 mo of lactation) and 109.6 ± 10.4 mg/L at the end of the study (2.0 mo after weaning). There was no effect of diet or time on serum calcium concentration. Serum ICTP concentration decreased over time ($P < 0.05$) from an average concentration of 3.82 ± 0.84 µg/L at the beginning of the study (2.5 mo of lactation) to 3.17 ± 0.60 µg/L at the end of the study (2.0 mo after weaning). Osteocalcin concentration in serum was 17.23 ± 3.88 ng/L at the beginning of the study (2.5 mo of lactation) and 16.16 ± 3.33 ng/L at the end of the study (2.0 mo after weaning) and was not affected by time ($P > 0.10$). There was no effect of diet on serum osteocalcin or serum ICTP concentration.

Discussion

Estimated calcium intakes for 500-kg mares through the first 5 wk of the study were 58 g of Ca and 46 g of P for the control diet, and 86 g of Ca and 71 g of P for the high-calcium diet. The NRC (1989) recommends 56 g of Ca and 36 g of P for 500-kg mares in early lactation. There was no effect of diet on milk calcium, serum ICTP, or serum osteocalcin, suggesting that these variables are not responsive to dietary calcium or phosphorus at levels above the NRC (1989) recommendations. Average milk calcium concentration in this study was 548.1 (104.2 µg/g, which is lower than the value of 800 (µ/g used in the NRC (1989) to calculate calcium requirements of mares in late lactation. If the NRC (1989) overestimates the calcium concentration in milk during late lactation, it is possible that the calcium requirement in late lactation is also overestimated. Serum ICTP concentrations decreased with time suggesting that mares mobilized less bone mineral in later lactation and after weaning. However, serum osteocalcin concentrations did not change over time suggesting that the rate at which bone mineral is deposited remained constant. Further research is needed to define changes in bone turnover in pregnant and lactating mares.

References

Glade, M.J. 1993. Effects of gestation, lactation, and maternal calcium intake on mechanical strength of equine bone. J. Amer. Coll. Nutr. 12(4):372-377.
NRC. 1989. Nutrient requirements of horses (5th Ed.). National Academy of Press, Washington, DC.

NUTRITION OF THE DAM INFLUENCES GROWTH AND DEVELOPMENT OF THE FOAL

LARRY A. LAWRENCE
Kentucky Equine Research, Versailles, Kentucky

Introduction

A 1996 Kentucky Equine Research (KER) study monitored the incidence of developmental orthopedic disease (Pagan and Jackson, 1996). The results of this study provided early evidence of the importance of nutrition of the mare to the proper growth and development of the foal. The farm in this study produced 271 foals. Ten percent of the foals showed signs of developmental orthopedic disease by radiography. The foals were weighed monthly from birth, and those weights were compared to a large data set of weights from other central Kentucky farms.

Foals with fetlock lesions tended to be small at 15 days, 3.2 kg below the average. Lesions were most often seen in foals born in January, February and March and were more prevalent in fillies than colts. Approximately 2% of the foals were affected and the average age of diagnosis was 102 days. Foals that developed lesions at a later age (379 days) tended to be normal-sized up to 120 days but grew faster than average and were heavier after weaning. Foals that developed hock osteochondritis dissecans (OCD) averaged 7 kg heavier than the Kentucky body weight (BW) average at 15 days. By 240 days of age these foals were 14 kg heavier than the population average. Average daily gains were significantly higher in the OCD group. Foals that developed stifle or shoulder lesions averaged 5.5 kg heavier than the Kentucky average at 25 days and 17 kg heavier at 120 days of age. Stifle and shoulder OCD lesions were diagnosed in approximately 2% of the foals at an average age of 336 days.

The mare has a tremendous effect on development of the foal through weaning. The size of the foal at birth is determined by genetics, nutrition, and uterine environment. Growth after birth is mostly a result of the mare's milk production. In utero growth of the foal is governed by actual placental size and competency and available area of healthy endometrium.

Fetal Nutrition

The placenta of the mare consists of fetal and maternal tissues in diffuse villous attachments. The villi are organized at around day 100-150 of gestation into complex tufts which cover the entire surface of the fetal membrane and fit into complex crypts of the endometrium. Health of the endometrium is important for the exocrine secretory glands that produce histotrophs that sustain the unimplanted embryo during the first 40 days of pregnancy. Inadequate "uterine milk" in early pregnancy or the development of an inadequate total area of functional microcotyledons on the surface of the allantochorion in later gestation will have deleterious effects on embryonic and/or fetal growth.

Allen (2006) listed three examples of nutritional restrictions and their effects on the equine fetus: (1) spontaneous embryonic death or resorption when twin conceptuses result in a reduction of fetal membrane absorption of "uterine milk;" (2) abortion of twin conceptuses around 7 to 9 months of gestation due to competition between fetal membranes and limited endometrial surfaces; and (3) age-related degenerative changes in the mare's endometrium, which result in the formation of fibrous tissue around groups of endometrial glands – called "gland nests" – that do not function, causing failure of lymph drainage and leading to development of lymph-filled endometrial cysts. The degeneration of the endometrium results in patchy areas where fewer and less well-developed microcotyledons results in a serious reduction in the level of nutrition available to the fetus.

Wilsher and Allen (2003) demonstrated that age and parity of Thoroughbred mares have a significant effect on the development of the microcotyledons on the placental surface. They reported a reduction in surface area of microcotyledons not only in older mares with age-related degenerative changes but also in young primigravid mares. The reduction in fetomaternal contact in the maiden mares resulted in lower birth weights compared to younger multiparous mares.

There appears to be a priming effect on the microcotyledon surface density after the first pregnancy. Placental weight was correlated with foal birth weight in a study of the effects of placental and fetal development in maiden Thoroughbred mares (Wilsher and Allen, 2003).

During the third trimester, mares become insulin resistant. This appears to be a mechanism designed to increase glucose uptake by the placenta. Williams et al. (2001) reported that during the third trimester approximately 40% of the insulin-stimulated glucose uptake was reduced. The crown-rump length of the equine fetus reaches its maximum length in mid-gestation. The growth in the last trimester is in body weight through development of muscle and increases in body fat.

Fetal development is dependent on maternal glucose supply. The increased transfer of oxygen and nutrients to support this high rate of metabolism is achieved by increased uterine blood flow, increases in weight and surface areas of the uteroplacental tissues, and a decrease in glucose consumption of uteroplacental tissue on a weight-specific basis.

Fetal energy metabolism is glucose-dependant and the maternal to fetal blood glucose concentration gradient is the most important factor for supplying energy. There is a direct relationship between glucose concentration and size and weight of the placenta, which correlates directly with foal weight (Allen et al., 2002).

Barron (1995) surveyed racetrack performance of Thoroughbred racehorses in the United Kingdom. Offspring from mares aged 7 to 11 years produced more successful offspring in terms of time-form-rating (an expression of racing merit) when compared to maiden mares or mares greater than 11 years of age. Finocchio (1986) reported that the third foal from a Thoroughbred mare was the most likely to be a stakes winner, followed closely by the fifth, second and fourth foals, respectively.

Cymbaluk and Laarveld weighed foals born to 13 primiparous and 19 multiparous draft-cross mares (1996). The mares were weighed and blood samples were drawn near delivery. Foals from primiparous mares were lighter with colts weighing an average of 169.2 kg and fillies an average of 145.2 kg while fillies and colts from multiparous mares were 177.8 and 173.3 kg, respectively.

Cymbaluk and Laarveld (1996) reported serum values of insulin-like growth factor (IGF-I) for foals born to primiparous and multiparous draft-cross mares. Foals born to multiparous mares had an average serum IGF-I of 386 ng/ml while foals born to primiparous mares averaged 237.5 ng/ml ($p < 0.065$). Colts (378 ng/ml) averaged higher ($p < 0.05$) serum IGF-I concentrations than fillies (254.5 ng/ml) regardless of dam parity. Colts also tended ($p < 0.12$) to be heavier than fillies (173.5 vs. 159.2 kg, respectively). Foals were weaned at 13 or 16 weeks of age, and in both cases growth rates and serum IGF-I concentrations were reduced. One to three weeks after weaning, growth rates returned to normal and IGF-I concentrations returned to preweaning values when weights rebounded.

Nutritional Status of Mares

When placental supply of nutrients is altered experimentally or by malnourishment, fetal growth and postnatal adaptive responses may be affected. Thoroughbred fetuses carried by pony mares after embryo transfer had low birth weight, took longer to stand and nurse, and had hypercortisolemia for 48 hours after foaling, indicating in utero stress. They also had precocious stimulation of the fetal hypothalamic-pituitary-adrenal axis (Ousey et al., 2004). In this study, pony foal embryos were transferred into Thoroughbred mares. These foals showed exaggerated pancreatic ß-cell responses possibly as a consequence of enhanced delivery of nutrients in utero (Forhead et al., 2004). These overgrown pony foals had higher basal insulin levels without insulin resistance, and glucose was removed from the blood at a faster rate than in the Thoroughbred-in-pony group.

Hay (1995) reported that acute maternal hyperglycemia produces an increase in uteroplacental glucose uptake with saturation kinetics that parallel those of the fetus. At mid-gestation there are developmental changes in placental glucose transport, and by the third trimester fetal growth demands more glucose.

Glucose diffuses down a concentration gradient from mare plasma to fetus. When the mare's diet is restricted for long periods and hypoglycemia becomes chronic, the fetus begins producing its own glucose. That in turn elevates the fetal glucose concentration relative to that of the mare and shifts the balance of glucose uptake by the uterus to placental metabolism and less to the fetus (Hay, 1995). The second adaptation to chronic hypoglycemia in late gestation is a reduction in placental weight.

154 *Nutrition of the Dam*

The reduction in placental weight does not appear to include a reduction in surface area or glucose transporter numbers or affinity (Aldoretta et al., 1994). The changes associated with reduced glucose supply result in reduced fetal and placental growth; however, rates of metabolism are maintained to insure normal fetal and placental tissue while reducing drain on maternal metabolism (Hay, 1995).

Milk Production

The nutrition of the mare affects growth and development of the foal both in utero and via milk production. These effects carry over through 12 months or more. In a study reported by Cymbaluk and Laarveld (1996), 15 one-day-old foals fed milk replacer for 7 weeks were compared with 5 foals that nursed their dams. During the first 2 weeks, replacer-fed foals did not gain (0.46 kg/d) as rapidly ($p < 0.03$) as mare-nursed foals (1.73 kg/d). The resulting IGF-I values for replacer-fed foals (139 ng/ml) were lower ($p < 0.0001$) than values for mare-nursed foals (317.4 ng/ml). After the first 2 weeks, gains were similar between the two groups; however, serum IGF-I concentrations of replacer-fed foals were only 36% and 60% of values obtained for mare-nursed foals at 8 and 18 weeks of age, respectively. The differences between mare-nursed and replacer-fed foals in serum IGF-I concentrations persisted to 1 year of age, when the serum IGF-I concentration of mare-nursed foals (1,203 ng/ml) was 48% higher than that of replacer-fed foals (815 ng/ml).

In 2001, Williams and coworkers fed lactating mares a sugar and starch diet (59.4% NSC, 18.5% NDF, 3.2% fat) or a fat and fiber diet (34.1% NSC, 36% NDF, 16.6% fat). The researchers reported higher glucose and insulin area under the curves for the sugar and starch diets after a meal. Mares use glucose for milk production (Williams et al., 2001). Energy demands for lactation are among the highest for horses.

Mares can produce 11.8 kg of milk per day or 2.3% of their body weight during the first 30 days of lactation (Gibbs et al., 1982). Pool-Anderson and coworkers (1994) determined milk yield in Quarter Horse mares for early lactation (2-29 days) and late lactation (60-120 days). Daily milk production was greater ($p < 0.05$) during early lactation compared to mid-lactation (12.1 vs 10.8 kg, respectively) and tended to be greater ($p = 0.08$) during mid-lactation (11.7 vs 10.4 kg, respectively) in multiparous mares compared to primiparous mares but was similar between groups in late lactation.

The extreme demands for glucose during early lactation may represent a time when feeds with higher glycemic responses would benefit the mare and foal. Foals can begin digesting grain within 10 days to 2 weeks of birth. It will be 6 to 8 weeks before a functional hindgut will be able to contribute to the overall nutrition of the foal with forage. Declines in milk production and nutrient concentrations after 2 months may represent a time when foals should be given supplemental feed (Gibbs, 1982).

Hoffman et al. (1998) reported on the effects of dietary carbohydrates and fat influence on milk composition and fatty acid profile of mare's milk. The sugar and starch diet (SS) was high in corn and molasses (62.4% NSC) while the fat and fiber diet

(FF) was high in corn oil, beet pulp, soy hulls, and oat straw (26.5% NSC). The findings revealed a 4.2-fold increase (p = 0.028) in IgG concentration from the colostrum of mares fed the FF diet versus the mares fed the SS diet 6 to 12 hours post foaling (3140 mg/dl vs 755 mg/dl IgG, respectively). The fatty acid profile was higher in linoleic omega-6 and trans-vaccenic fatty acids in the milk of mares fed the FF diet.

In 1999, Hoffman et al. supplemented a grain mix containing 80 IU/kg daily intake vitamin E with an additional 160 IU/kg of vitamin E (1999b). Mares were supplemented for 4 weeks. Within 2 weeks of foaling, serum IgG concentrations were greater (p = 0.064) and serum IgA tended to be greater (p = 0.13) in vitamin E supplemented mares. Presuckled colostrum of vitamin E supplemented mares was higher in IgG (p = 0.005) and tended to be in IgM and IgA (p = 0.12 and 0.12, respectively). Serum concentrations of IgG, IgM, and IgA of the foals reflected those of their dams' colostrum post-suckling.

The researchers suggested that the 4.2-fold increase in IgG in the colostrum collected 6 to 12 hours post foaling in the previous study was due to the vitamin E content of the corn oil (327 IU/kg). Corn oil is high in omega-6 fatty acids (linoleic acid). Hoffman et al. (1998) suggested that higher linoleic acid content of the milk would protect against gastric ulcers.

Kruglik et al. (2005) studied the effects of supplementation of 454 g of a marine-derived, protected omega-3 fatty acid source (PFA). The PFA supplement provided approximately 10.4 g of docosahexaenoic acid (DHA) and 8.6 g eicosapentaenoic acid (EPA) per mare daily. The control diet was top-dressed with corn oil. They reported mares fed PFA had elevated DHA (p < 0.05) for the first 3 weeks of supplementation, during foaling and 24 hours, 7 days, 14 days, and 21 days postpartum. EPA was greater for the PFA-supplemented mares at weeks 1 and 2 (p < 0.05) and at all times postpartum (p < 0.001). In milk, both DHA and EPA were higher (p < 0.001) in PFA-supplemented mares at all times. EPA and DHA were higher (p < 0.001) in PFA foals at all times.

Growth Regulators

Growth responds to energy availability. Energy for growth must be supplied in excess of maintenance requirements. Blood levels of glucose and insulin are key signals to the somatotropic axis. The most important hormones in the somatotropic axis are growth hormone (GH) and insulin-like growth factor 1 (IGF-I).

Growth hormone is necessary for normal postnatal bone growth and stimulates longitudinal bone growth in a dose-dependent manner (Cheek and Hill, 1974). The metabolic effects of GH include protein anabolism and enhanced utilization of fat by stimulating adipocytes to break down triglycerides and by suppressing their abilities to take up circulating fats. GH controls blood glucose by an anti-insulin effect suppressing the ability of insulin to stimulate the uptake of glucose into tissues and it enhances glucose synthesis in the liver. A major role of GH is to stimulate the liver and other tissues to secrete IGF-I.

156 Nutrition of the Dam

IGF-I stimulates whole body protein synthesis rates. GH and IGF-I increase lean body mass and decrease adipocytes. IGF-I has insulin-lowering effects that improve insulin sensitivity. IGF-I stimulates the proliferation of chondrocytes. GH stimulates the differentiation of chondrocytes while IGF-I also stimulates differentiation and proliferation of myoblasts. Somatostatin is another hormone in the somatotropic axis that inhibits GH in response to low blood glucose. GH secretion is also controlled by a negative feedback loop with IGF-I (Figure 1). High blood levels of IGF-I lead to decreased secretion of GH not only by directly suppressing the somatotroph but by stimulating release of somatostatin from the hypothalamus. Integration of all factors leads to a pulsatile secretion of GH (Martin et al., 1989).

Feeding a highly hydrolyzable carbohydrate meal to growing horses may create exaggerated glucose and insulin responses. As glucose increases in the blood, insulin increases and lowers blood glucose. Low blood glucose stimulates GH, which in turn stimulates IGF-I. If IGF-I is too high then GH is suppressed. If GH and IGF-I reach abnormal levels, overproliferation of cartilage may contribute to OCD (Staniar et al., 2002). Glade and Luba (1987) found changes in T3 and T4 were affected in horses fed high-carbohydrate meals by gastric infusion and suggested these active growth regulators may be involved with the development of DOD.

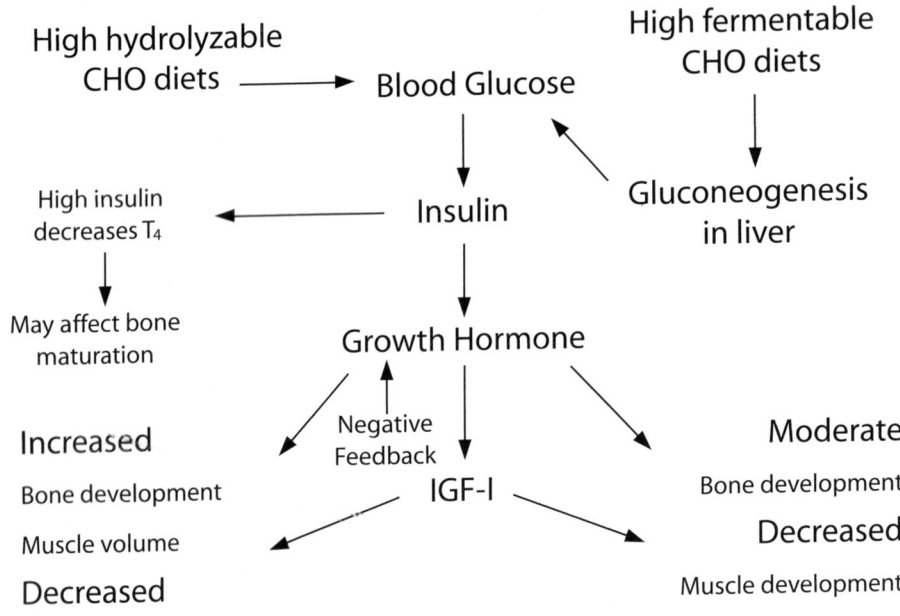

Figure 1. Growing horses fed highly soluble carbohydrate diets versus highly fermentable carbohydrate diets that provide the same DE may experience different growth patterns.

Ropp et al. (2003) fed a diet with 2.21% fat and 33.9% starch (CARB) and a diet with 10.3% fat and 24% starch (FAT) to weanlings for 60 days. On days 0, 30 and 60, blood samples were taken and analyzed for glucose, insulin, GH, IGF-I, and nonesterified fatty acids (NEFA). Over the 60-day period, the average daily gain (kg/d) was 0.85 for the CARB diet and 0.84 for the FAT diet.

On day 30 weanlings on the CARB diet had higher blood glucose concentrations and shorter duration in elevation postprandially. This was attributed to dietary fat sparing glucose and slowing down of gastric emptying. On day 60 there were no differences in blood glucose between treatments. There were no differences in serum insulin at 30 days, but at 60 days serum insulin was higher in the CARB group. Fat may have slowed gastric emptying and with adaptation the CARB group controlled blood glucose via higher insulin secretion. There was no consistent change in GH between diets. There was also no treatment effect on IGF-I. The authors concluded that neither the CARB diet nor the FAT diet had an effect on GH or IGF-I.

Savage et al. (1993) reported a higher incidence of dyschondroplasia in weanling foals fed 129% of NRC energy requirements to weanling foals for 16-18 weeks. The control feed was a rice-based pellet while the high-energy feed was the rice-based diet with 5% added corn oil. Hoffman et al. (1999a) developed a sugar and starch (SS) diet and a fat and fiber (FF) diet and fed them to mares and foals. The weanlings and yearlings were continued on the supplements for 16 months. The SS diet was partially composed of 61% corn and 10% molasses, a NSC content of 62.4%, a fat content of 2.4% and a DE of 3.00 Mcal/kg. The FF diet was oat-straw and beet-pulp based with 10.4% fat and 26.5% NSC and a DE of 2.98 Mcal/kg. All other nutrients met or exceeded NRC requirements.

Standardized subjective scores for evidence of developmental orthopedic disease (DOD), season and associated pasture growth, and hard ground during drought and freezing temperatures were more highly correlated with DOD than diet. In weanlings and yearlings fed the FF diet the bone mineral content (BMC) was lower from September to May between 140±5 days to 376±5 days of age.

Treiber et al. (2004, 2005) fed SS diets to Thoroughbreds raised on pasture that contained 49% NSC, 21% NDF, and 3% fat or FF diets with 12% NSC, 44% NDF, and 10% fat. As weanlings, the foals were tested by modified frequency intravenous glucose tolerance test. All samples were also analyzed for IGF-I. Insulin sensitivity was also estimated. Insulin sensitivity was 37% less in weanlings fed SS than those fed FF. The authors also tested acute response to glucose and developed a disposition index. They reported that decreased insulin sensitivity was compensated for by acute insulin response to glucose; therefore, there were greater insulin concentrations in the SS group. IGF-I was greater ($p = 0.001$) in SS weanlings.

Based on these studies, when fed at NRC nutrient requirements or above, there appears to be a range of interactive NSC, NDF, and fat that may alter glucose/insulin dynamics and affect GH and IGF-I in growing horses (Table 1). These ranges of NSC, NDF, and fat cannot be separated from energy balance. Staniar (2002) reported the greatest difference between IGF-I in diets similar to Treiber's SS or FF were greater during periods of rapid growth. He further reported that high correlations existed between ADG and temperature, suggesting pasture availability had a significant impact on ADG. ADG was also positively correlated with IGF-I.

Table 1. Lower glycemic diets for growing horses.

NSC, %	NDF, %	Fat, %
26-35	28-44	5-10

Further evidence of environmental effects was reported by Cymbaluk and Christison (1989) in which weanlings gaining 0.83 to 0.89 kg/d had maintenance DE requirements that were 27% and 57% higher than those reported for growing horses (Cymbaluk et al., 1989) and mature horses (Pagan and Hintz, 1986), respectively. While evidence exists that diets with high glycemic indices may be associated with DOD (Ralston, 1996; Pagan et al., 2001), there is no real evidence to support the claim that a low-glycemic diet will prevent this disease (Kronfeld et al., 2005).

Managers making decisions about feeding practices for growing horses must carefully consider pasture and forage quality, feeding frequency, environmental factors, genetic predisposition, and exercise before a complex decision is made concerning the glycemic properties of a supplemental grain source.

References

Aldoretta, P.W., T.D. Carver, and W.W. Hay, Jr. 1994. Ovine uteroplacental glucose and oxygen metabolism in relation to chronic changes in maternal and fetal glucose concentration. Placenta. 15:753-764.

Allen, W. R. 2006. Total feeding failures in the equine fetus. In: Proc. Workshop on Embryonic and Fetal Nutrition. Havenmeyer Foundation Monograph Series, No. 10. May 15-18. Ravello, Italy. 67-69. R&W Publications, Newmarket Limited, Suffolk, UK.

Allen, W.R., S. Wilsher, C. Turnbill, F. Stewart, J. Ousey, P.D. Rossdale, and A.L. Fowden. 2002. Influence of maternal size on placental, fetal and postnatal growth in the horse. Develop. in utero Repro. 123:445-453.

Barron, J.K. 1995. The effect of maternal age and parity on the racing performance of Thoroughbred horses. Equine Vet. J. 27,1:73.

Cheek, D., and D.E. Hill. 1974. Effect of growth hormone on cell and somatic growth. In: Handbook of Physiology (Fourth Volume). E. Knobil and W. Sawyer (Eds.). American Physiological Society. Washington, DC. 159-185.

Cymbaluk, N. F., and G. I. Christison.1989. Effects of diet and climate on growing horses. J. Anim. Sci. 67:48-59.

Cymbaluk, N.F., G.I. Christison, and D.A. Leach. 1989. Energy intake and utilization by limit- and ad libitum-fed growing horses. J. Anim. Sci. 67:403-413.

Cymbaluk, N.F., and B. Laarveld. 1996. The ontogeny of serum insulin-like growth factor-I concentration in foals: Effects of dam parity, diet, and age at weaning. Domes. Anim. Endocrinol. 3:197-209.

Finocchio, E.J. 1986. Race performance and its relationship to birth rank and maternal age. In: Proc. Amer. Assoc. Equine Pract. 31:571-578.

Forhead, A.J., J.C. Ousey, W.R. Allen, and A.L. Fowden. 2004. Postnatal insulin secretion and sensitivity after manipulation of fetal carbohydrate metabolism. Equine Vet. J. Suppl. 19-25.

Glade, M.J., and N.K. Luba. 1987. Serum triiodothyronine and thyroxine concentrations in weanling horses fed carbohydrate by direct gastric infusion. Amer. J. Vet. Res. 48:587.

Gibbs, P.G., G.D. Potter, R.W. Blake, and W.C. McMullan. 1982. Milk production of Quarter Horse mares during 150 days of lactation. J. Anim. Sci. 54:496-499.

Hay, W.W., Jr. 1995. Regulation of placental metabolism by glucose supply. Reprod. Fertil. Dev. 7:365-375.

Hintz, H.F., R.L. Hintz, and L.D. Van Vleck. 1978. Estimation of heritabilities for weight, height and cannon bone circumference of Thoroughbreds. J. Anim. Sci. 47:1243-1245.

Hoffman, R.M., D.S. Kronfeld, J.H. Herbein, W.S. Swecker, W.L. Cooper, and P.A. Harris. 1998. Dietary carbohydrates and fat influence milk composition and fatty acid profile of mare's milk. J. Nutr. 128:2708-2711.

Hoffman R.M., L.A. Lawrence, D.S. Kronfeld, W.L. Cooper, D.J. Sklan, J.J.Dascanio and P.A. Harris. 1999a. Dietary carbohydrates and fat influence radiographic bone mineral content of growing foals. J. Anim. Sci. 77: 3330-3338.

Hoffman, R.M., K.L. Morgan, M.P. Lynch, S.A. Zinn, C. Faustman, and P.A. Harris. 1999b. Dietary vitamin E supplemented in the preparturient period influences immunoglobulins in equine colostrum and passive transfer in foals. In: Proc. Equine Nutr. Physiol. Soc. 96-97.

Kronfeld, D.S., K.H. Treiber, T.M. Hess, and R.C. Boston. 2005. Insulin resistance in the horse: Definition, detection, and dietetics. J. Anim. Sci Suppl. 83:E22-E31.

Kruglik, V.L., J.M. Kouba, C.M. Hill, K.A. Skjolaas-Wilson, C. Armendariz, J.E. Minton, and S.K. Webel. 2005. Effect of feeding protected n-3 polyunsaturated fatty acids on plasma and milk fatty acid levels and IgG concentrations in mares and foals. In: Proc. Equine Sci. Soc. 135-136.

Martin, T.J., K.W. Ng, and T. Suda. 1989. Bone cell physiology. Endocr. Metab. Clin. North Am. 18: 833-859.

Pagan, J.D., and H.F. Hintz. 1986. Equine energetics I: Relationship between body weight and energy requirements in horses. J. Anim. Sci. 63:815-821.

Pagan, J.D., and S.G. Jackson. 1996. The incidence of developmental orthopedic disease on a Kentucky Thoroughbred farm. Pferdeheilunde 12:351-354.

Pagan, J.D., R.J. Geor, S.E. Caddel, P.B. Pryor, and K.E. Hoekstra. 2001. The relationship between glycemic response and the incidence of OCD in Thoroughbred weanlings: A field study. In: Proc. Amer. Assoc. Equine Prac. 47:322-325.

Pool-Anderson, R.H. Raub, and J.A. Warren. 1994. Maternal influences on growth and development of full-sibling foals. J. Anim. Sci.72:1661-1666.

Ralston, S.L. 1996. Hyperglycemia/hyperinsulinemia after feeding a meal of grain to young horses with osteochondritis dissecans (OCD) lesions. Pferdeheilkunde 12:320-322.

Ropp, J.K., R.H. Raub, and J.E. Minton. 2003. The effect of dietary energy source on serum concentration of insulin-like growth factor-I growth hormone, insulin, glucose and fat metabolites in weanling horses. J. Anim. Sci. 81:1581-1589.

Savage, C.J., R.N. McCarthy, and L.B. Jeffcott. 1993. Effects of dietary energy and protein on induction of dyschondroplasia in foals. Equine Vet. J. Supp 16:74-79.

Staniar, W. B. 2002. Growth and the somatotropic axis in young Thoroughbreds. Ph.D. Dissertation. Virginia Polytechnic and State University.

Staniar, W.B., D.S. Kronfeld, R.M. Akers, and J.R. Burk. 2002. Feeding-fasting cycle in meal fed yearling horses. J. Anim. Sci. Suppl: 80:156 (abstract).

Treiber, K.H., R.C. Boston, D.S. Kronfeld, R.M. Hoffman, W.B. Staniar, and P.A. Harris. 2004. Insulin resistance in growing Thoroughbreds is affected by diet. J. Anim. Sci. Vol 82, Suppl: 1:96 (abstract).

Treiber K.H., R.C. Boston, D.S. Kronfeld, W.B. Stanier, and P.A. Harris. 2005. Insulin resistance and a compensation in Thoroughbred weanlings adapted to high-glycemic meals. J. Anim. Sci. 83:2357-2364.

Williams, C.A., D.S. Kronfeld, W.B. Staniar, and P. A. Harris. 2001. Plasma glucose and insulin responses of Thoroughbred mares fed a meal high in starch and sugar of fat and fiber. J. Anim. Sci. 79:2196-2201.

NUTRITION AND MANAGEMENT OF THE GROWING HORSE

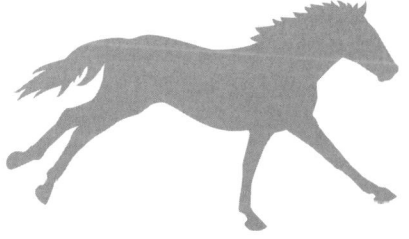

the study. In a subsequent study, 10 untrained Quarter Horse geldings were put into race training and were fed a diet balanced to meet NRC recommendations to further investigate the influence of early training on bone metabolism (Nielsen et al., 1998a). A similar decrease in the mineral content of the third metacarpal was observed during the first two months of the project. A follow-up study suggested that the NRC calcium recommendation was too low for young horses entering intense training (Nielsen et al., 1998b).

Kentucky Equine Research tracked bone density and morphology in a group of 15 Thoroughbred yearlings as they entered race training. Dorsopalmar radiographs of the third metacarpal bone (McIII) were taken on a monthly basis. An aluminum step wedge exposed simultaneously with the McIII was used as a reference standard. The radiographs were scanned into an image software program and a calibration curve was developed using the 11-step aluminum step wedge exposed with each film. Radiographic bone aluminum equivalencies (RBAE) were recorded at three sites: lateral and medial sites with peak densities and a central site of least density in the medullary cavity. Total RBAE was also calculated as the RBAE area under the curve for the entire bone cross section. The bone mineral content in grams per 2-cm cross section of bone was estimated using regression equations derived by Ott et al. (1987). Bone morphological measurements (bone width, medullary width, lateral, medial, dorsal, and palmar cortical width) were also measured from radiographs. Additionally, plasma concentrations of calcium, phosphorus, and calcitonin were measured monthly.

The yearlings entered training (day 0) in late November on a central Kentucky farm where regular turnout paddocks were available. The horses were confined in stalls for approximately 6 hours per day. The training intensity at this time was low, consisting of 15-20 minutes per day jogging in a paddock.

In late December (day 28) the horses were moved to a training center in central Kentucky where little or no turnout was available. For the remainder of the study the horses were confined in stalls for approximately 23 hours per day. In January and February (day 28-84), the horses (now 2-year-olds) were lightly exercised, mostly in an indoor arena since weather conditions prohibited training on the outside track. In March (day 84-112), weather conditions improved and training intensity increased. From this time period onwards, horses were kept at an intense level of training.

Bone mineral content (BMC) dropped from day 28 until day 84 when the horses were confined to stalls with only light exercise (Table 2 and Figure 1). By day 84, BMC was significantly lower than day 0. When training intensity increased in the spring, BMC increased to levels that were not different from pre-training.

Osteocalcin is a protein produced by the osteoblasts in bone and is an accepted marker of bone formation (McIlwraith, 2005). Plasma osteocalcin levels dropped slightly from day 0-84 when the horses were confined and in light training (Table 3 and Figure 2). Levels increased from day 84-112 when the horses began intense exercise, suggesting an increase in bone formation.

Table 2. Cannon bone density and morphology during early training.

Day	BMC (g/2-cm)	Bone Width (mm)	Medullary Width (mm)	Medial Cortical Width (mm)	Lateral Cortical Width (mm)
0	20.6 ± 0.7	40.5 ± 1.2	20.9 ± 1.8	11.0 ± 1.0	8.6 ± 0.7
28	21.0 ± 0.2	38.6 ± 0.7	18.2 ± 0.5*	11.2 ± 0.5	9.1 ± 0.4
56	20.5 ± 0.4	37.4 ± 0.7*	18.4 ± 0.5*	9.7 ± 0.4	9.3 ± 0.3
84	19.3 ± 0.3*	37.3 ± 0.8*	17.9 ± 0.5*	11.0 ± 0.7	8.4 ± 0.5
112	19.7 ± 0.3	37.1 ± 0.7*	18.0 ± 0.6*	10.7 ± 0.6	8.4 ± 0.3
140	21.1 ± 0.4	39.3 ± 0.8	18.1 ± 0.5*	12.0 ± 0.7	9.2 ± 0.5
168	21.5 ± 0.8	37.0 ± 1.3*	17.4 ± 0.5*	11.4 ± 0.8	8.2 ± 0.4
196	19.8 ± 0.2	38.6 ± 0.8	18.9 ± 0.4	10.7 ± 0.4	9.0 ± 0.5

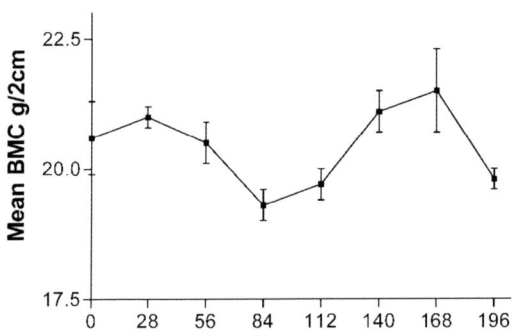

Figure 1. Bone mineral content (BMC) of the third metacarpal bone of young horses entering training.

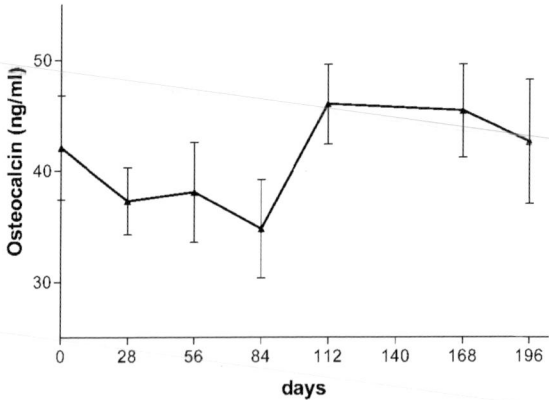

Figure 2. Plasma osteocalcin (ng/ml) in young horses entering training.

Plasma calcium also dropped significantly from day 28 to 84 (Table 3 and Figure 3). There was a large increase in plasma calcium levels when training intensity increased. Plasma phosphorus followed a similar pattern of change with exercise (Table 3 and Figure 4). These data illustrate how confinement and changes in exercise intensity can affect bone mineralization. These horses were consuming a commercial fortified feed and grass throughout the study. It is not known if additional nutrient supplementation could alter the pattern of skeletal changes that occurred. More research is needed in this area.

Table 3. Plasma osteocalcin, calcium and phosphorus during early training.

Day	Osteocalcin (ng/ml)	Calcium (mg/dl)	Phosphorus (mg/dl)
0	42.1 ± 4.7	12.7 ± 0.1	5.5 ± 0.1
28	37.3 ± 3.0	12.9 ± 0.1	5.3 ± 0.2
56	38.1 ± 4.5	12.3 ± 0.1*	4.6 ± 0.1*
84	34.8 ± 4.4	12.2 ± 0.1*	3.8 ± 0.1*
112	46.0 ± 3.6	13.6 ± 0.2*	5.1 ± 0.2
168	45.4 ± 4.2	12.9 ± 0.2	4.9 ± 0.3*
196	42.6 ± 5.6	12.5 ± 0.1	4.6 ± 0.2*

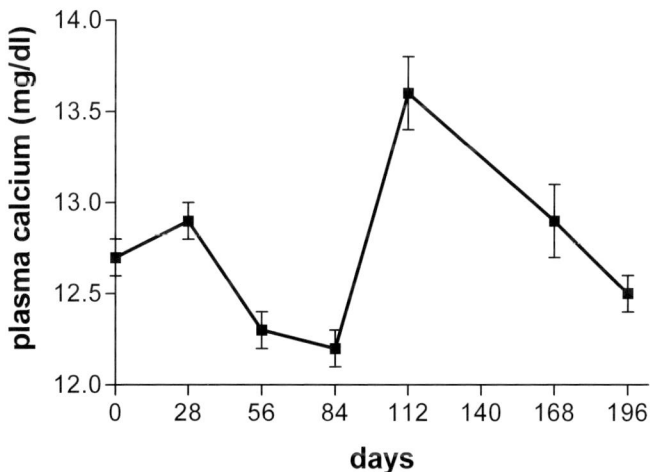

Figure 3. Plasma calcium (mg/dl) in young horses entering training.

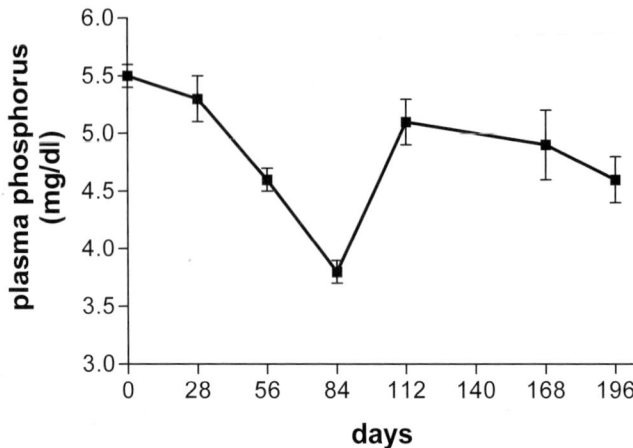

Figure 4. Plasma phosphorus (mg/dl) in young horses entering training.

BUCKED SHINS

Bucked shins and dorsal metacarpal disease are terms used to describe a condition of the third metacarpal bone which is related to bone fatigue and/or stress fractures. Bucked shins is a very common condition in young racehorses, normally occuring during the first year of training. The initial signs of the problem are heat and swelling over the dorsal aspect of the cannon bone. If work continues, horses can become extremely lame, resulting in long periods of inactivity (Nunamaker et al., 1990). A survey of veterinarians and trainers estimated that 80% of two-year-olds in Australia (Buckingham and Jeffcott, 1990) and 70% in the United States (Norwood, 1978) were affected by bucked shins. In a survey conducted by the Japanese Racing Association (JRA), a 66% incidence of bucked shin complex was recorded in horses during their first 8 months of training (Japan Racing Association, 1999).

In humans, inadequate calcium intake has been reported to play a significant role in skeletal injuries. In a study examining factors associated with shin soreness in human athletes (Myburgh et al., 1998), only 3 out of 25 athletes that developed shin soreness consumed the recommended dietary allowance of calcium in contrast to 15 of 25 control athletes who met their daily Ca requirement. Furthermore, only 2 of the control athletes consumed under half the recommended daily allowance compared to 10 of the injured athletes. No research has been conducted in horses to investigate the relationship between mineral intake and bucked shins.

Kentucky Equine Research studied the relationship between bucked shins, blood parameters, and cannon bone measurements in 30 two-year-olds as they were prepared for two-year-old in training (breeze-up) sales which took place in late winter or early spring. The horses were all trained by the same individual, but were housed at 3 different training facilities which were within a 2-mile radius of each other in South

Carolina. The study began in late December when the horses were already in moderate to intense training and lasted 56 days. Typically, each horse galloped four days, breezed once, and either lightly jogged or rested two days each week. Dorsopalmar and lateral radiographs of the third metacarpal bone (McIII) were taken on a monthly basis. An aluminum step wedge exposed simultaneously with the McIII was used as a reference standard. Bone density and morphology measurements were made using the same methods described earlier in this paper. Plasma concentrations of calcium, phosphorus, and calcitonin were also measured.

During the study, 5 of the 30 two-years-displayed clinical signs of shin bucking following breezing. These signs included swelling, heat, and soreness of the dorsal aspect of the cannon bone. Table 4 compares bone density and morphological measurements calculated from the dorsopalmar view radiograph in the bucked shin group (bucked) and the horses that did not buck their shins (normal). At the beginning of the study, the two groups' BMC, mean RBAE, total RBAE, and bone width were not significantly different. There was a trend towards greater medial and lateral cortical thickness in the normal group ($p<.10$). There was a significant increase in all dorsopalmar measurements in the normal horses over the 56-day training period ($p<.05$). In the bucked group BMC, mean RBAE, total RBAE, and bone width did not change significantly over the 56-day period ($p>.05$). In this group, lateral and medial cortical thickness increased ($p<.05$). At 56 days, there was a trend ($p<.10$) towards greater BMC and mean RBAE in the normal horses and normal horses had significantly greater lateral cortical width, bone width, and total RBAE ($p<.05$).

Table 4. Bone optical density and morphology of the third metacarpal bone (dorsopalmar view).

		Mean BMC (8/2-cm)	Mean RBAE (mm Al)	Total RBAE (mm Al)	Medial Cortical Width (mm)	Lateral Cortical Width (mm)	Dorsopalmar Bone Width (mm)
0 days	Bucked n =5	19.0 ± 0.5	23.0 ± 0.6	7870.4 ± 189.5	7.0 ± 0.4	5.3 ± 0.3	29.7 ± 1.2
	Normal n =25	18.5 ± 0.2	22.4 ± 0.2	8020.2 ± 211.0	8.6 ± 0.5	6.1±0.3	31.1 ± 0.8
56 days	Bucked n =5	18.60 ± 0.9	22.6 ± 1.0	8275.8 ± 456.7	9.7 ± 0.3	6.2 ± 0.2	31.8 ± 0.8
	Normal n =25	19.70 ± 0.3	23.7 ± 0.3	9411.5 ± 266.5	10.7 ± 0.4	7.5 ± 0.2	34.7 ± 0.6

There were no differences in the 0-day measurements taken from the lateral view with the exception of palmar cortical thickness which was significantly greater ($p<.05$) in the normal horses (Table 5). At 56 days, dorsal cortical width, total bone width, and mean and total RBAE had significantly increased ($p<.05$) in both groups. Palmar cortical width was unchanged in both groups, but remained greater in the normal group of horses ($p<.05$). There was a trend ($p<.10$) towards dorsal cortical thickness being greater in the bucked group.

168 Nutrition of the Young Equine Athlete

Table 5. Bone optical density and morphology of the third metacarpal bone (lateral view).

		Mean RBAE (mm AI)	Total RBAE (mm AI)	Dorsal Cortical Width (mm)	Palmar Cortical Width (mm)	Bone Width (mm)
0 days	Bucked n =5	17.3 ± 0.4	5206.4 ± 193.3	9.1 ± 0.5	5.1 ± 0.4	26.3 ± 0.6
	Normal n =25	17.3 ± 0.2	5361.2 ± 130.9	9.5 ± 0.2	6.5 ± 0.3	27.3 ± 0.5
56 days	Bucked n =5	17.8 ± 0.4	6029.5 ± 209.0	11.8 ± 0.3	5.4 ± 0.3	29.2 ± 0.7
	Normal n =25	17.7 ± 0.2	5833.3 ± 102.6	11.1 ± 0.2	6.2 ± 0.2	29.0 ± 0.3

Plasma calcium, phosphorus and osteocalcin dropped significantly in both groups from 0 to 56 days ($p<.05$)(Table 6). Calcium and phosphorus were not different between groups at either 0 or 56 days, but osteocalcin was significantly higher in the bucked group during both times ($p<.05$).

Table 6. Plasma calcium, phosphorus and osteocalcin.

	Sample Time (days)	0	56
Calcium (mg/dl)	Bucked n = 5	13.7 ± 0.1	13.1 ± 0.2
	Normal n = 25	13.5 ± 0.1	13.2 ± 0.1
Phosphorus (mg/dl)	Bucked n = 5	5.3 ± 0.2	4.5 ± 0.2
	Normal n = 25	5.0 ± 0.1	4.7 ± 0.1
Osteocalcin (ng/ml)	Bucked n = 5	42.1 ± 4.7	33.1 ± 2.4
	Normal n = 25	31.5 ± 1.3	28.0 ± 1.0

These data suggest that two-years-olds that buck shins do not produce as much McIII bone as unaffected horses. In spite of increased osteocalcin, bone width and total bone mineral deposition are reduced. The reason for this difference is not apparent since all the horses in the study were managed similarly.

Feeding Programs for Two-Year-Olds

A real concern for trainers is how differently to feed two-year-olds compared to older horses in the stable. Table 7 contains a typical feeding program for an adult

Thoroughbred in race training along with a feeding program for a two-year-old in moderate work using the same hay and grain mix. Both horses are fed 6 kg of timothy hay and a 12.0% protein grain mix that supplies 3.1 Mcal DE/kg. The adult racehorse would require 6.5 kg of grain to meet its energy requirement, while the two-year-old requires 5.25 kg/day.

Table 7. Feeding programs for adult racehorses and two-year-olds in training.

	Timothy Hay	Grain Mix Composition	Adult racehorse Timothy Hay	Grain Mix Daily Intake	Two-year-old Timothy Hay	Grain Mix Daily Intake
DM	93.8 %	88.0%	6.0 kg	6.5 kg	6.0 kg	5.25 kg
DE	2.1 Mcal/kg	3.1 Mcal/kg	12.5 Mcal	20.3 Mcal	12.5 Mcal	16.4 Mcal
CP	8.0%	12.0%	480 g	785 g	480 g	634 g
Lysine	0.24%	0.65%	14.4 g	42.2 g	14.4 g	34.1 g
Calcium	0.34%	0.60%	20.4 g	39.0 g	20.4 g	31.7 g
Phosphorus	0.21%	0.52%	12.6 g	33.8 g	12.6 g	27.5 g

Figures 5 and 6 show how well these rations meet the nutrient requirements of the two types of horses. Although the hay and grain are not excessively high in protein or minerals, the adult racehorse's ration supplies more protein, lysine, calcium, and phosphorus than needed because of the high level of intake required to meet the racehorse's energy requirement. A ration using the same hay and grain mix also meets the nutrient requirements of the two-year-old in moderate work. Again, a fairly high level of intake provides adequate nutrients from feedstuffs containing fairly low concentrations of protein and minerals. The bottom line from this comparison is that most rations fed to adult racehorses contain adequate protein, calcium, and phosphorus for two-year-olds. If caloric intake must be restricted in a two-year-old, higher levels of fortification may be needed.

In conclusion, the nutrient requirements of the two-year-old are intermediate between the growing foal and the adult performance horse. If the two-year-old is in training, it can be fed feeds that are typically formulated for adult performance horses because the elevated level of feed intake required to meet the energy required for exercise will provide the extra protein and minerals needed for growth. More research is needed to determine if nutrition can play a role in attenuating the loss in bone density that yearlings experience as they enter training or if nutritional manipulation can affect bone deposition in two-year-olds that are susceptible to bucked shins.

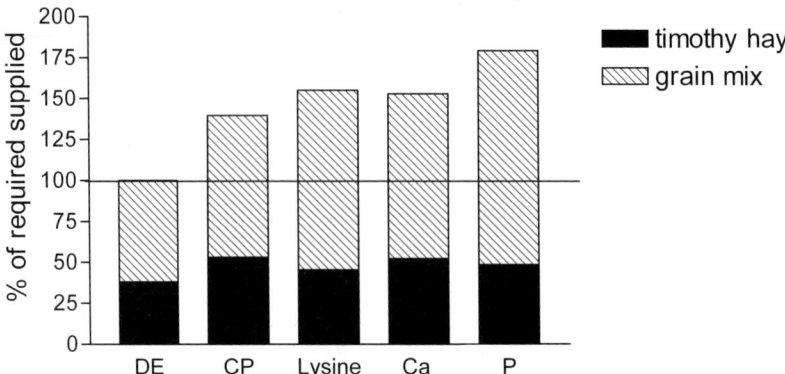

Figure 5. Nutrients supplied from a ration consisting of timothy hay and grain mix for an adult racehorse.

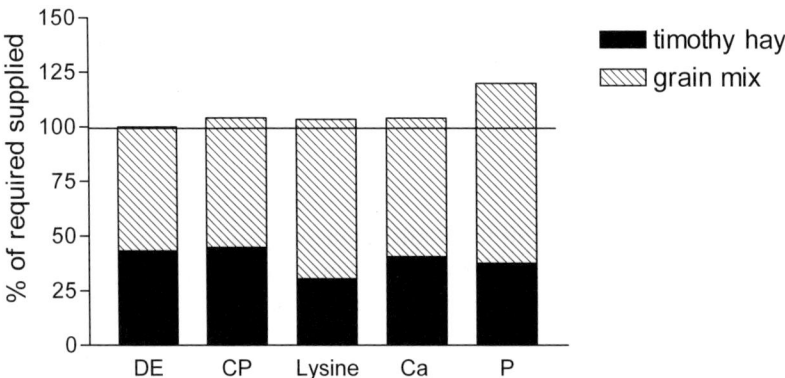

Figure 6. Nutrients supplied from a ration consisting of timothy hay and grain mix for a two-year-old in moderate work.

References

Buckingham S.H.W., and L.B Jeffcott. 1990. Shin soreness: A survey of Thoroughbred trainers and racetrack veterinarians. Aust. Equine Vet. 8:148-153.

Japan Racing Association. 1999. Annual Report on Racehorse Hygiene. Number of new patients. p. 24-44.

McIlwraith, C.W. 2005. Advanced techniques in the diagnosis of bone disease. In: J.D. Pagan (ed.) Advances in Equine Nutrition III. Nottingham University Press, Nottingham, U.K. p. 373-381.

Myburgh, K.H., N. Grobler, and T.D. Noakes. 1988. Factors associated with shin soreness in athletes. Phys. Sports Med. 16(4):129.

National Research Council. 1989. Nutrient requirements of horses, 5th edition. National Academic Press, Washington, D. C.

Nielsen B.D., G.D. Potter, L.W. Greene, E.L. Morris, M. Murray-Gerzik, W.B. Smith and M.T. Martin. 1998a. Characterization of changes related to mineral balance and bone metabolism in the young racing quarter horse. J. Equine Vet. Sci. 18:190-200.

Nielsen, B.D., G.D. Potter, L.W. Greene, E.L. Morris, M. Murray-Gerzik, W.B. Smith, and M.T. Martin. 1998b. Responses of young horses in training to varying concentrations of dietary Ca and P. J. Equine Vet. Sci. 18:397.

Nielsen, B.D., G.D. Potter, and L.W. Greene. 1997. An increased need for calcium in young racehorses beginning training. In: Proc. 15th Equine Nutr. Phys. Symp. p. 153-159.

Norwood, G.L. 1978. The bucked shin complex in Thoroughbreds. In: Proc. 24th Annu. Conv. Am. Assoc. Equine Pract. p. 319-336.

Nunamaker, D.M., D.M. Butterweck, and M.T. Provost. 1990. Fatigue fractures in Thoroughbred racehorses: Relationship with age, peak bone strain, and training. J. Orthop. Res. 8:604.

Ott, E.A., L.A. Lawrence, and C. Ice. 1987. Use of the image analyzer for radiographic photometric estimation of bone mineral content. In: Proc. 10th Equine Nutr. and Physiol. Symp., Ft. Collins, CO. p. 527.

DEVELOPMENT OF THE EQUINE GASTROINTESTINAL TRACT

LARRY A. LAWRENCE AND THERESA J. LAWRENCE
Kentucky Equine Research, Versailles, Kentucky

Introduction

Foals have a long gestational period (about 335 days) and are precocious at birth, standing and nursing within 20 minutes to 1 hour after birth. The transition from placental nutrition to enteral nutrition results in anatomic growth and differentiation of the gastrointestinal tract, gastric and pancreatic secretory development, and functional absorptive adaptations.

Development and maturation of the gastrointestinal tract begin in utero and continue through adulthood in the horse. The gastrointestinal tract and accessory glands must effectively secrete saliva, gastric acid, proteolytic enzymes, glycolytic enzymes, and bile. The gastric and intestinal mucosa must perform protective and absorptive functions.

Successful feeding of the equine neonate is dependent on optimal nutrition of the mare (Lawrence, 2006) and absorption of colostrum that contains specific nutrients, growth factors, and immunoglobulins. Changes in the gut and pancreas within 24 hours of birth increase the digestion and absorption of the nutrients found in mare's milk (Table 1).

Table 1. Composition of mare's milk.

Time After Foaling	Total Solids (%)	Energy (kcal/100 g)	Protein (%)	Fat (%)	Lactose (%)
1-4 weeks	10.7	58	2.7	1.8	6.2
5-8 weeks	10.5	52	2.2	1.7	6.4
9-21 weeks	10.0	50	1.8	1.4	6.5

Adapted from NRC, 2007.

Early Development of the Gastrointestinal Tract

The rate and extent of maturation of the equine gastrointestinal tract at any point in time is determined by genetics, a developmental biological clock, endogenous regulatory mechanisms, and environmental effects (Lebenthal and Lebenthal, 1999). As parturition approaches, systemic adrenocortical hormones are responsible for the final stages of tissue and system development. The equine gastrointestinal tract is affected by cortisol. Developmental changes influenced by glucocorticoids include structural, cellular, and functional differentiation. Prenatal development of gastric acid, gastrin secretion, and hydrolase activities including chymosin, pepsin, amylase, lactase, and aminopeptidases are all influenced by cortisol (Trahair and Sangild, 1997). Additionally, growth factors, hormones, and nutrients from swallowed amniotic fluid and colostrum may influence gastrointestinal tract development. Fetal fluid ingestion has been shown to modulate tissue growth, macromolecule and immunoglobulin absorption, enterocyte differentiation, cell turnover, and activity of brush-border hydrolases (Trahair and Sangild, 1997).

The structural and functional adaptations of the gastrointestinal tract in the fetus and neonate that are designed to provide passive transfer of antibodies, including low luminal proteolysis and macromolecule transport in the neonate, are thought to be controlled by growth factors derived from the lining of the gastrointestinal tract. One role of cortisol is to alter partitioning of uterine glucose uptake to favor uteroplacental tissues, which may limit uteroplacental prostaglandin production (Fowden et al., 1991). This alteration enhances the glucogenic capacity of the fetus in late gestation (Fowden et al., 2002). Cortisol is a critical signal in the maturation of the gastrointestinal tract's endocrine system. In the horse, fetal cortisol levels increase later in gestation than other species. The fetal hypothalamic-pituitary-adrenal axis of foals only increases activity during the final few weeks of gestation (Fowden et al., 1991). This may explain the frequency of premature births and neonatal hypoglycemia in horses.

A significant rise in cortisol takes place 2 to 3 days before parturition (Silver and Fowden, 1994). Cortisol is important for maturation of pancreatic b-cells in the fetal horse. Fowden et al. (1991) reported that concentrations of hepatic glycogen and glucose-6-phosphatase, the enzyme responsible for mobilization of glycogen, increase substantially between late gestation and after birth concurrent with the rise in fetal cortisol. Fetal cortisol correlates positively with the prepartum rise in glucose stimulated by a rise in fetal insulin.

Ousey et al. (1991) used respiratory quotients (RQ) to determine what energy sources are used by foals during the first 24 hours of life. They reported that the foal uses endogenous carbohydrate and fat until it establishes mare's milk as the primary source of nutrition. Initially, the newborn foal uses carbohydrate that is stored in the liver and glycogen from skeletal muscle. The authors estimate liver glycogen stores would provide energy for less than 1 hour. By 2 to 4 hours of age, the RQ indicates stored body fat is the primary energy source. In well-nourished foals, this energy could last over 24 hours (Meyer and Ahlswede, 1976). Beyond 2 to 4 hours, the RQ stabilizes at about 0.82, indicating energy is being supplied by a combination of carbohydrate and fat that reflects the nutrient composition of colostrum and milk.

Aside from essential nutrients, mare's milk and colostrum contain growth factors.

The gastrointestinal tract increases in length and diameter in response to mare's milk. Increased villi height, density, and width; crypt density and depth; and enterocyte differentiation are all associated with local luminal factors and systemic signals. Mare's milk and colostrum contain trophic hormones, growth factors, enzymes, and bioactive factors. Cortisol, insulin, thyroid hormones, insulin-like growth factors (IGF), epidermal growth factor (EGF), lysozyme, and lactoferrin are important in maturation of gut enterocytes and provide protective mechanisms for infection, disease, and gastric ulceration (Ousey et al., 1995).

Feeding stimulates gastrin production of the stomach. Gastrin causes the release of pepsinogen and hydrochloric acid (HCl) for protein digestion. Pancreatic polypeptide stimulates gastric emptying and inhibits pancreatic exocrine secretions. Gastrin increases in fed foals from 1 day of age to 30 days of age, resulting in increased gastric acid and lower stomach pH.

Gastrointestinal tract hormone response is different between the first feeding and subsequent meals (Ousey et al., 1995). Gastric pH of newborn foals is higher (4.1) than in older foals (2.6) (Baker and Gerring, 1993; Murray and Grodinsky, 1989). The first colostrum feeding does not stimulate high gastrin production and therefore HCl and pepsinogen secretion are limited. Plasma polypeptide is higher after the first feeding. Rapid gastric emptying reduces gastric acid and pepsinogen, resulting in rapid transfer of immunoglobulins through the stomach where they can be absorbed intact in the small intestine.

Development of Hydrolytic Enzyme Systems

Roberts et al. (1973) reported significant changes in the development of lactase enzymes from fetus to maturity in the horse. Neutral-ß-galactosidase can be isolated from the mucosal lining of the gastrointestinal tract in the fetus. This enzyme hydrolyzes lactose into the readily-absorbed monosaccharides glucose and galactose. The enzyme is located in the brush border of the enterocytes of the small intestinal mucosa. Neutral-ß-galactosidase has an optimum pH of 5.5 to 6.0 (Asp and Dahlquist, 1968). Acid-b-galactosidase is present at birth in the jejunal and ileal mucosa and has an optimal pH of 3.4. This enzyme has a maximal production (6.29 units) at 2 days portpartum. Neutral-ß- galactosidase (14.6 units) and ß-glucosidase (cellobiase) (3 units) peak at birth and decrease steadily for 3 years (Figure 1). These enzymes are virtually undetectable in adult horses.

Lactase is the primary hydrolase until 3 months of age, at which time maltase activity that had been relatively low begins to increase. Between 3 and 6 months of age, maltase and amylase reach adult levels in the gastrointestinal tract.

176 Development of the Equine Gastrointestinal Tract

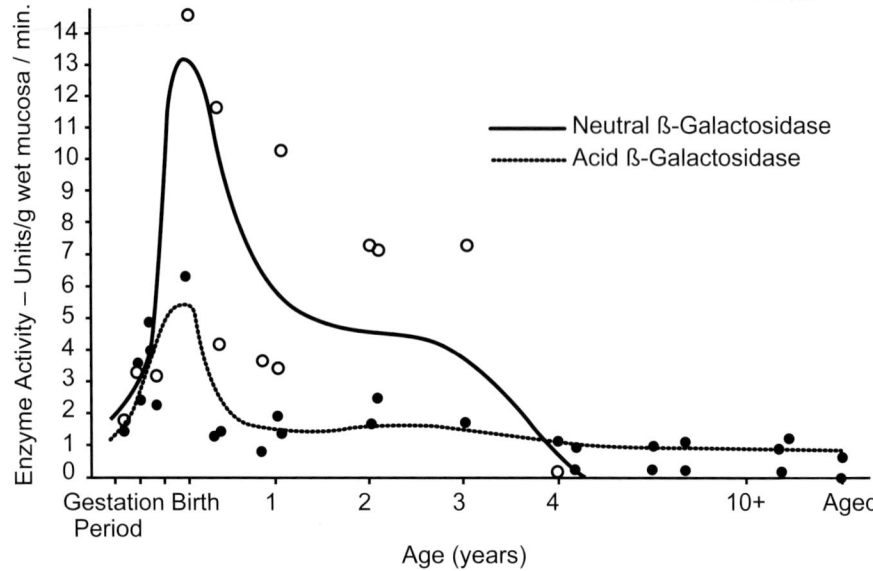

Figure 1. Development of ß-galactosidase activities in the horse (Roberts et al., 1973).

Physical Development of the Gastrointestinal Tract

Functional changes in the equine gastrointestinal tract are reflected in increases in length of the various segments including the initiation of hindgut fermentation. Smyth (1988) measured the length of the small intestine, cecum, ascending colon, and descending colon of fetuses, foals, growing horses, and adult horses (Figures 2 and 3). The horses ranged in age from 150 days of gestation to 35 years. Data was collected on 130 horses of multiple breeds. For analysis, he expressed the proportion of the various segments as a percentage of total length.

The total tract length increases from midgestation to one year of age. The total length ranged from 2.5 meters in a 150-day-old fetus to 29.7 meters in a 16-year-old adult horse. The proportional length of the small intestine increases during gestation and the early postnatal period. The greatest increase occurred between 1 and 4 weeks after birth (Smyth, 1988). The proportion of the small intestine was significantly greater from birth to 16 days of age when compared to fetuses and adult horses. Between 2 and 6 months of age, the proportional length of the small intestine decreased in comparison to changes in the large intestine.

The cecum ranged in length from 0.08 meters in a 150-day-old fetus to 1.1 meters in an 18-year-old adult horse. The greatest increase was between 1 and 6 months of age. The cecum continued to increase in length until 1 year of age.

The length of the ascending colon ranged from 0.2 meters in a 160-day-old fetus to 3.8 meters in an 18-year-old horse. The ascending colon was the major contributor

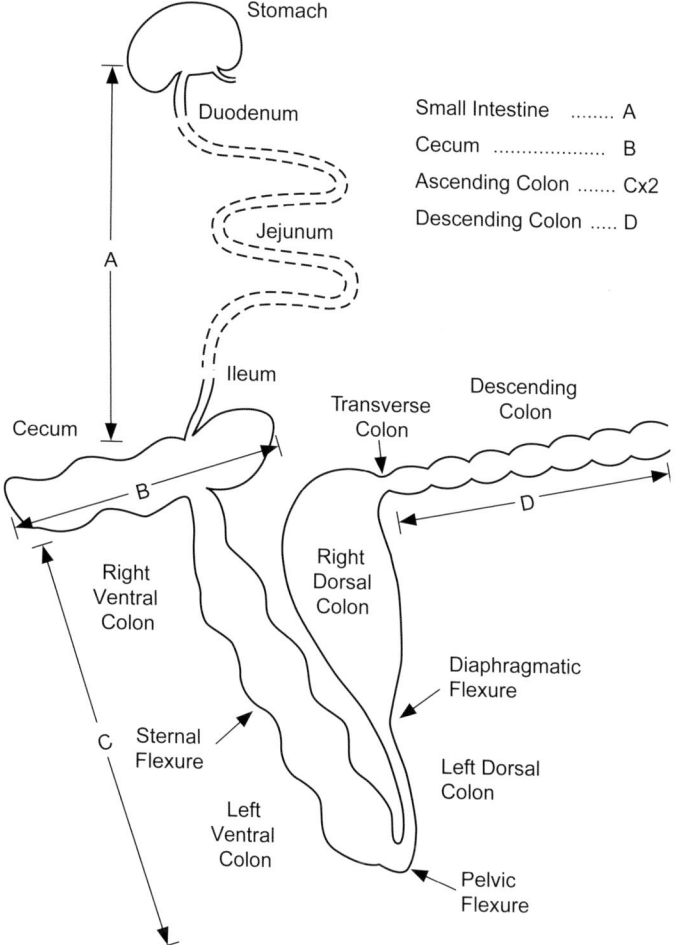

Figure 2. Diagram of the horse intestine showing points of reference used to measure lengths of the small intestine (A), cecum (B), ascending colon (Cx2), and descending colon (D) (Smyth, 1988).

to the increase in total intestinal length between 1 and 6 months after birth. It also was the most significant contributor to the increase in intestinal length between 1 and 2 years, and 10 and 20 years.

The length of the descending colon ranged from 0.32 meters in a 160-day fetus to 3.3 meters in an 11-year-old horse. The two most rapid periods of development of the descending colon were between 1 and 4 weeks of age and from 1 to 6 months of age. The percentage of gut length contributed by the descending colon was significantly greater in foals between 1 and 16 days and between 17 and 175 days. The period of

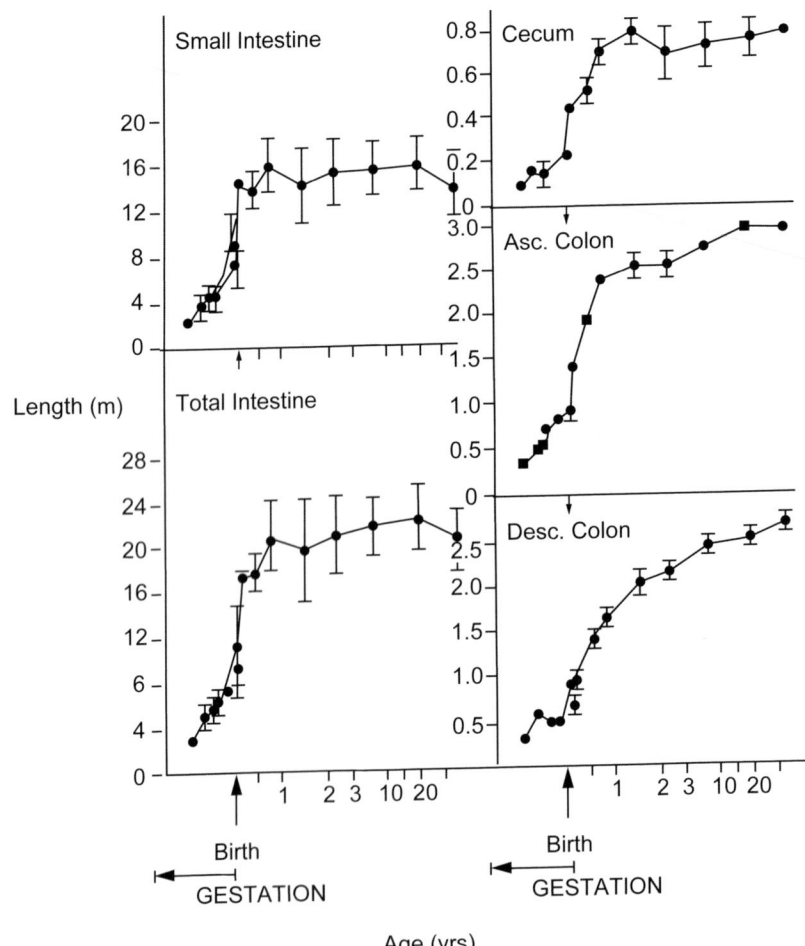

Figure 3. Lengths of the small intestine, cecum, ascending colon (ASC), descending colon (DESC), and total intestine in horses of different ages. Values represent mean ± SEM (Smyth, 1988).

greatest increase in intestinal length after birth was the increase in the length of the small intestine from 1 to 4 weeks postpartum. This corresponds to the period of most rapid growth in the foal (Hintz et al., 1979; Pagan et al., 1996).

The rapid increase in small intestinal length is in response to increased milk consumption. Intestinal growth in length is coordinated with increases in diameter. These morphological changes are also accompanied with structural changes including development of villi, crypts, blood vessels, and nerves (Trahair and Sangild, 1997). From 2 to 6 months of age, there were greater relative increases in lengths in the cecum, ascending colon, and descending colon. After one year of age, only the ascending and descending colons increase in relative length. Increases in length of the segments of the colon continue to a lesser degree through adulthood.

Foals forage very little when they are less than one month of age. As they mature, the amount of time spent foraging increases from 20 to almost 50% of the day from 1 to 5 months of age. By 10 months of age, growing horses are spending 60% of each day grazing (Boy and Duncan, 1979). Increased length of the hindgut corresponds to developmental age and changing diet (Smyth, 1988). The largest proportional change in length of hindgut segments is from 1 to 6 months of age. Foals increase forage intake dramatically during this time, suggesting that a functional hindgut is important during the dietary transition from milk and the soluble carbohydrates in grain to the structural carbohydrates of forage at weaning.

Development of Microbial Fermentation

The fetus develops in a sterile environment. Consequently, the gastrointestinal tract of the fetus is also devoid of microorganisms until parturition. The physical process of parturition exposes the newborn to environmental bacteria from the dam's vagina, feces, and saliva. In human infants bifidobacteria are the predominant lactic acid bacteria, whereas lactobacilli are the primary lactic acid bacteria colonizing the gastrointestinal tract of newborn farm animals (Eadie and Mann, 1970).

In 2000, Norikatsu et al. found a layer of lactobacilli lining the nonsecretory area of horse stomachs. Such bacterial layers were observed in animals from 1 to 23 years old. Their research indicated that this lactobacillus flora becomes established soon after birth and adheres to the stomach epithelium throughout the life of the horse. This host-microbe interaction demonstrates one mechanism of prevention of pathogenic microorganisms from inhabiting and colonizing the mucosal layers of the stomach as well as the subsequent small and large intestines.

Many organisms enter the gastrointestinal system only transiently and due to either internal or external factors are not able to colonize. Yukikiko and coworkers (1999) determined that the majority of the coliform bacteria identified in young foals at 3, 7, 14, 30, and 60 days of age were *Escherichia coli*. However, the α-toxin-producing bacterium *Clostridium perfringens*, suggested to be related to equine diarrhea, was detected at high levels in all specimens sampled at 3 and 7 days of age but was undetectable in any specimens obtained at 60 days of age, indicating that this organism only colonizes the gut transiently immediately after birth (Yukikiko et al., 1999).

The development of the large intestine (cecum, ascending colon, and descending colon) coincides with the development of the microbial ecology and microbial digestion. The succession of microbial colonization is most marked in the early stages of life. From suckling to weaning, the dramatic shifts in host-produced enzymatic digestion to anaerobic fermentation are directly associated with the changes in the type and quantity of feedstuffs ingested by the growing foal. Dynamic balances exist between the gastrointestinal microbiota, host physiology, and diet that directly influence the initial acquisition, developmental succession, and eventual stability of the gut ecosystem (Mackie et al., 1999).

Microbial succession during the first few weeks of life in the alimentary tracts of humans and farm animal species is remarkably similar even though neonatal animals are exposed to greater numbers of fecal and environmental bacteria than are human neonates (Smith, 1965). Within a few days of birth, coliforms and streptococci dominate the microbial environment in many mammalian species (Mackie et al., 1999). Obligate anaerobes appear later in the developmental process. Clostridia and lactobacilli species may also be present in most hosts within a short period of time.

After birth newborns are continually exposed to new microbes that enter the gastrointestinal tract via food intake. This process begins with the ingestion of milk, which contains up to 10^9 microbes/L (Moughan et al., 1992). The most abundant organisms cultured in mammalian milk secretions include staphylococci, streptococci, corynebacteria, lactobacilli, propionibacteria, and bifidobacteria. These commensal organisms originate from the nipple and surrounding skin as well as the milk duct within the mammary gland (Mackie et al., 1999).

Both adults and newborns are continually exposed to microorganisms that enter the alimentary system with food, but the two groups are affected differently. The microorganisms entering newborns via milk consumption are more likely to colonize than are those entering healthy adults with stabilized populations. Opportunities arise, both internal and external, in which colonization of ingested microbes is favored in newborn and developing foals.

External factors that affect microbial colonization and succession in the gastrointestinal tract include the microbial load of the immediate environment, food and feeding habits, and composition of the maternal microbiota. As previously described, the feeding habits of foals change drastically during the first 5 months of life as they spend less time nursing and more time grazing (Boy and Duncan, 1979). As this shift in feeding occurs, so too do the profile and population of the gastrointestinal microorganisms.

The increased intake of feeds high in complex carbohydrates such as cellulose and hemicellulose requires the establishment of colonies of bacteria that can ferment such compounds in an anaerobic environment. Examples of anaerobic, cellulolytic organisms include *Ruminococcus albus*, *Fibrobacter succinogenes*, and *Butyrivibrio fibrisolvens*. Young foals are frequently observed consuming their dam's feces, and this serves as a direct inoculation of these vital gastrointestinal organisms. Due to the increased time required for bacterial digestion, the rate of passage through the large intestine greatly increases, particularly after weaning. In the young suckling foal, the stomach empties more slowly after a meal allowing more time for milk digestion by the acids and enzymes in the stomach and small intestine. After weaning, however, the stomach empties rapidly and the ingesta spends the majority of its time in the large intestine, where the relatively slow process of microbial digestion occurs, along with reabsorption of the large volumes of digestive secretions (Findlay, 1998). Internal or host-related factors affecting microbial succession include intestinal pH, microbial interactions, environmental temperature (within the host animal), physiologic factors, peristalsis, bile acids, host secretions, immune responses, drug therapy, and bacterial mucosal receptors (Conway, 1997).

As the foal matures and ingests a greater variety of feedstuffs, its microbiota also multiplies and develops in much the same way an organ would. The function and development of the equine hindgut and its microbial inhabitants are markedly similar to that of the rumen of the growing calf (Hungate, 1966). For this reason, much of the research performed on calf rumens is highly correlated with the processes that occur in the hindgut of the foal. Researchers in the mid-1950s evaluated the functionality of the rumen and its dynamic microflora. The scientists determined that in vitro cellulose digestion by rumen contents was 25 to 40% by 1 week of age and had essentially doubled by 15 weeks (McCarthy and Kesler, 1956). Ruminal volatile fatty acid (VFA) production, the end products of fermentation transformed to energy sources in the liver of the bovine and equine, peaked at 7 weeks and then leveled off. The researchers concluded that although the rumen continues to increase in size and volume, rumen function in the calf can be considered qualitatively similar to that of an adult by six weeks of age. Several other reports have confirmed that rumen concentration of VFA from calves on solid feeds reaches adult proportions between the sixth and eighth week of life (Huber, 1968). Cellulolytic activity of rumen microorganisms approached adult levels by six weeks of age (Huber, 1968).

It is important to clarify that efficiency, activity, and VFA concentrations that are similar to adult levels do not imply that volumes or population sizes are comparable. The proportional growth of the large intestine and the distention of the cecum due to significant quantities of forage ingestion are some necessary components for increasing the quantity of the microbial population and volumes of VFA. The cyclic and dynamic processes that stimulate cecal growth and function are all directly related to the ingestion of diverse nutrients, plant constituents, and environmental inoculum, and help in establishing each horse's hindgut ecology. A consistent diet including quality forages will help develop the neonate's hindgut microbial population into an efficient organ of plant and forage digestion that will play an essential role in the nutrition of the horse throughout its lifetime.

References

Asp, N.G., and A. Dahlquist. 1968. Rat small intestinal ß-galactosidases: Separation by ion-exchange chromatography and gel filtration. Biochem. J. 106:841-845.

Baker, S.J., and E.L. Gerring. 1993. Gastric pH monitoring in healthy, suckling pony foals. Amer. J. Vet. Res. 54:959-964.

Boy, V., and P. Duncan. 1979. Time budgets of Camargue horses. 1. Developmental changes in the timebudgets of foals. Behavior. 21:187-201.

Conway, P. 1997. Development of intestinal microbiota. In: R.I. Mackie, B.A. White, and R.E. Isaacson (Eds.) Gastrointestinal microbiology. Vol. II. p. 3-38. Chapman and Hall. New York.

Eadie, J.M., and S.O. Mann. 1970. Development of the rumen microbial population: High starch diets and instability. Physiol. Digest. Metabo. Rumin. 335-347.

Findlay, A.L.R. 1998. The developing gastrointestinal system. www.chu.com.ac.uk.

Fowden, A.L., L. Mundy, J.C. Ousey, A. McGladdery, and M. Silver. 1991. Tissue glycogen and glucose 6-phosphatase levels in fetal and newborn foals. J. Reprod. Fertil. Suppl. 44:537-542.

Fowden, A.L., A.J. Forhead, K.L. White, and P.M. Taylor. 2002. Equine uteroplacental metabolisms at mid and late gestation. Exp. Physiol. 85:539-545.

Fowden, A.L., J.C. Ousey, and A.J. Forhead. 2001. Comparative aspects of prepartum maturation; provision of nutrients. Pferdeheilkunde 17:653-658.

Hintz, H.F., R.L Hintz, and L.D. Van Vleck. 1979. Growth rate of Thoroughbreds: Effect of age of dam, year and month of birth, and sex of foal. J. Ani. Sci. 48:480-487.

Huber, J.T. 1968. Development of the digestive and metabolic apparatus of the calf. In: Symposium: Calf nutrition and rearing. 63rd Annual Meeting of the American Dairy Science Association, The Ohio State University, Columbus, Ohio.

Hungate, R.E. 1966. The rumen and its microbes. Academic Press. New York, New York.

Lawrence, L.A. 2006. Nutrition of the dam influences growth and development of the foal. In: Proc. Kentucky Equine Research Nutr. Conf. 17:89-98.

Lebenthal, A., and E. Lebenthal. 1999. The ontogeny of the small intestinal epithelium. J. Parenteral Enteral Nutr. Suppl. 23:S3-6.

Mackie, R.J., S. Abdelghani, and H.R. Gaskins. 1999. Developmental microbial ecology of the neonatal gastrointestinal tract. Amer. J. Clin. Nutr. Suppl. 69:1035S-1045S.

McCarthy, R.D., and E.M. Kesler. 1956. Relation between age of calf, blood glucose, blood and rumen levels of volatile fatty acids and in vitro cellulose digestion. J. Dairy Sci. 39:1280.

Meyer, H., and L. Ahlsede. 1976. Uber das intrauterine wachstum und die korperzusammentragender stuten. Ubersicht. Tierernahr. 4:263-292.

Moughan, P.J., M.J. Birties, P.D. Cranwell, W.C. Smith, and M. Pedraza. 1992. The piglet as a model animal for studying aspects of digestion and absorption in milk-fed human infants. In: A.P. Simopoulos (Ed.). Nutritional triggers for health and in disease. p. 4-113. Karger. Basel, Switzerland.

Murray, M.J., and C. Grodinsky. 1989. Regional gastric pH measurement in horses and foals. Equine Vet. J. Suppl. 7:73-76.

NRC. 2007. Nutrient Requirements of Horses, Sixth Revised Edition. National Academy Press, Washington, D.C.

Norikatsu, Y., T. Shimazaki, A. Kushiro, K. Watanabe, K. Uchida, T. Yuyama, and M. Morotomi. 2000. Colonization of the stratified squamous epithelium of the nonsecreting area of horse stomach by lactobacilli. Appl. Environ. Microb. 11:5030-5034.

Ousey, J.C., M. Ghatei, P.D. Rossdale, and S.R. Bloom. 1995. Gut hormone responses to feeding in healthy pony foals aged 0 to 7 days. Biol. Reprod. Mono. 11:87-96.

Ousey, J.C., A.J. McArthus, and P.D. Rossdale. 1991. Metabolic changes in Thoroughbred and pony foals during the first 24 h post partum. J. Reprod. Fertil. Suppl. 44:561-570.

Pagan, J.D., S.G. Jackson, and S. Caddel. 1996. A summary of growth rates of Thoroughbreds in Kentucky. Pferdeheilkunde. 12:285-289.

Roberts, M.C., D.E. Kidder, and F.W.G. Hill. 1973. Small intestinal beta-galactosidase activity in the horse. Gut. 14:535-540.

Silver, M., and A.L. Fowden. 1994. Prepartum adrenocortical maturation in the fetal foal: Responses to ACTH. J. Endocrinol. 142:417-425.

Smith, H.W. 1965. Development of the flora of the alimentary tract in young animals. J. Pathol. Bacteriol. 90:495-513.

Smyth, G.B. 1988. Effects of age, sex and post mortem interval on intestinal lengths of horses during development. Equine Vet. J. 20:104-108.

Trahair, J.F., and P.T. Sangild. 1997. Systemic and luminal influences on the perinatal development of the gut. Equine Vet. J. Suppl. 24:40-50.

Yukikiko, S., N. Yuki, F. Nakajima, S. Hakanishi, H, Tanaka, R. Tanaka, and M. Morotomi. 1999. Colonization of intestinal microflora in newborn foals. J. Int. Microb. 13:9-14.

SKELETAL ADAPTATION DURING GROWTH AND DEVELOPMENT: A GLOBAL RESEARCH ALLIANCE

CHRIS E. KAWCAK
Colorado State University, Fort Collins, Colorado

Acknowledgements: The Global Equine Research Alliance designed and carried out the following work. It is comprised of researchers from Massey University, NZ (Elwyn Firth and Chris Rogers); Colorado State University, US (C.W. McIlwraith and Chris Kawcak); Royal Veterinary College, UK (Allen Goodship and Roger Smith); and University of Utrecht, Netherlands (Ab Barneveld and Rene van Weeren). Funding for this study came from several sources, namely Arthritis Foundation, Marilyn M. Simpson Trust, NASA, NIH, NSF, pre-doctoral fellowship from Whitaker Foundation, The New Zealand Equine Research Foundation, Palmerston North, New Zealand, New Zealand Racing Board, and the Grayson Jockey Club Research Foundation.

Introduction

Musculoskeletal diseases in racehorses are common and can lead to catastrophic injuries requiring euthanasia of the horse. Consequently, results of intensive studies concerning the pathogenesis of these injuries have revealed that many of these problems are due to chronic fatigue damage in the tissues from repetitive stress of racing and training (Kawcak et al., 2001). A horse's predisposition to tissue damage may be due to high mechanical loads imposed on a particular tissue, relatively poor material properties of a specific tissue, or both. Abnormal mechanical loading on a particular tissue can be due to a number of factors, including neurologic dysfunction and remote pain leading to overload of an opposing limb. In addition, we know clinically that conformation can greatly influence the forces on a specific joint, tendon, or ligament, often leading to clinically detectable diseases. Recent evidence is also starting to show that certain joints may be predisposed to high mechanical loads due to subtle geometric differences within the joint tissues (Muller-Gerbl, 1998). The material properties of a tissue, whether it is bone, articular cartilage, ligament, tendon, or muscle, are dictated by its collagenous and noncollagenous protein characteristics. For bone, the material properties are also dictated by the quantity and quality of mineral (Kawcak et al., 2001). Therefore, aberrant characteristics in any of these matrix components can lead to reduction in strength of the tissues.

Matrix components within tissues can be influenced by things such as genetics, nutrition, and physical loading history. As an example, in humans, there is considerable evidence that genetics is a strong factor in dictating the presence of osteoporosis (Runyan et al., 2003; Seeman et al., 1996). Nutrition is also a factor, which is suggested in horses as well (Runyan et al., 2003). Recently, exercise has been shown to strongly influence tissue material properties. In humans, it has been shown that, regardless of genetic and nutritional influences, people with a long history of moderate levels of exercise have a protective effect for osteoporosis (Runyan et al., 2003; Daly and Bass, 2006; Micklesfield et al., 2005). To further those investigations, it appears that when exercise was imposed during the greatest growth period, bone strength was maximized later in life, providing a protective factor from osteoporosis (Cooper et al., 1995; Janz, 2002; McKay et al., 2005; Wang et al., 2005; MacDonald, et al., 2006). In addition to these clinical results, experimental studies in several different species show, in general, that there is a threshold of exercise beyond which tissues are strengthened, but as importantly, a threshold above that which can be damaging (Kawcak et al., 2000; Kawcak et al., 2001).

The problem with these findings is that usually only one tissue such as bone is studied, and there are no conclusions as to the effects of a particular exercise level on all tissues.

Exercise studies in horses have shown that beyond a certain level, tissue damage can occur to certain tissues (Kawcak et al., 2000; Kawcak et al., 2001). In addition, limited exercise or nonweight-bearing events, such as casting, can also cause tissue damage (Richardson and Clark, 1993; van Harreveld et al., 2002a; van Harreveld et al., 2002b). Therefore, it appears that the results for horses are similar to other species. However, in order to use physical loading to positively affect tissue material properties, guidelines are needed to show whether loading during growth will be protective of all tissues.

The goal of the current study was to determine the effects of exercise at an early age on musculoskeletal tissues in the horse. Our hypothesis was that early imposed exercise would strengthen all tissues, thus preventing tissue damage later in life.

Materials and Methods

Thirty-three Thoroughbred foals were divided into two groups and subjected to different exercise regimens. In phase 1 (Figure 1), from birth until 18 months of age, the conditioned group was raised on pasture as well as subjected to a conditioning program (1020 meters) of increasing exercise level from approximately 10 days of age. The control group exercised spontaneously at pasture. At 18 months of age, 6 random foals from each group were euthanized for postmortem analysis. The remaining 21 foals entered phase 2, during which they were trained for two-year-old racing.

Horses were observed daily for general health, and clinical examination was carried out by a veterinarian at approximately four days of age and monthly thereafter in phase 1. This examination consisted of a general physical and lameness examination. At the end of phase 1, horses underwent clinical examinations, together with full radiographic, scintigraphic, and ultrasononographic examinations at the Massey University Equine Hospital. The behavior and plasma cortisol levels of the foals between average ages of three and five months were quantified (Crowell-Davis, 1986; Crowell-Davis and

Houpt, 1986). The following detailed evaluations have been completed on the tissues acquired at 18 months.

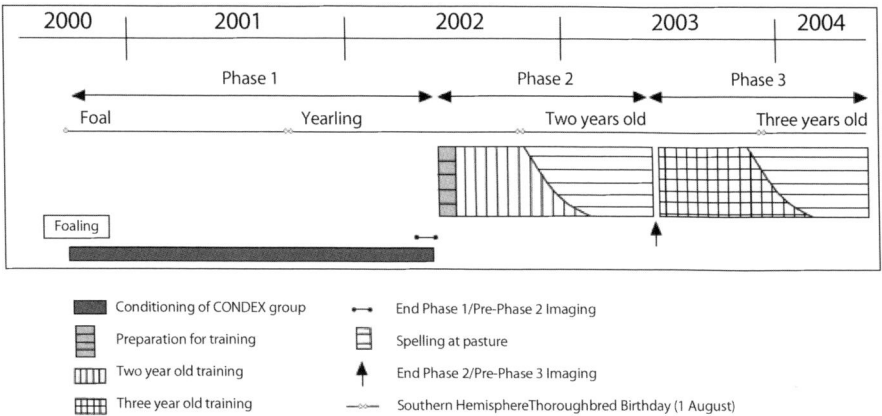

Figure 1. Timeline showing the three phases of the project (Rogers et al., 2006).

EFFECTS OF EARLY EXERCISE ON ARTICULAR CARTILAGE VIABILITY

In order to determine the effects of early exercise on articular cartilage and subchondral bone in specific sites of the metacarpophalangeal and metatarsophalangeal joints of young Thoroughbred horses, articular cartilage samples from four sites of the distal third metacarpal/metatarsal bones were stained with calcein-AM and propidium iodide. Confocal laser scanning microscopy was used to count live and dead cells. Proteoglycan scoring and modified Mankin scoring were also determined. The subchondral epiphyseal bone mineral density at the sites was measured using computed tomography (Dykgraaf et al., 2006).

EFFECTS OF EARLY EXERCISE ON MECHANICAL PROPERTIES OF ARTICULAR CARTILAGE

The objectives of the study were to determine (1) the site-associated response of articular cartilage of the equine distal metacarpal condyle to training at a young age as assessed by changes in indentation stiffness and alterations in cartilage structure and composition, and (2) relationships between indentation stiffness and indices of cartilage structure and composition. Four osteochondral samples were harvested per metacarpal condyle from dorsal-medial, dorsal-lateral, palmar-medial, and palmar-lateral aspects. Cartilage was analyzed for India ink staining (quantified as reflectance score), short-term indentation stiffness (sphere-ended, 0.4 mm diameter), thickness, and biochemical composition (Nugent et al., 2004).

EFFECTS OF EARLY EXERCISE ON SUBCHONDRAL MINERALIZATION PATTERN IN THE THIRD METACARPAL CONDYLES

Metacarpophalangeal joints were scanned using a conventional computed tomographic scanner and the files were exported to a custom-designed program for three-dimensional analysis of the joint. In the computer program, the third metacarpal condyles were disarticulated and analyzed. The bones were further cut into slices at 20, 30, and 40 degrees palmar from the mid-frontal plane. This allowed analysis of bone density and density pattern in the area most susceptible to injury.

EFFECTS OF EARLY EXERCISE ON OSTEOCHONDRAL TISSUES

Articular cartilage was harvested for analysis of glycosaminoglycan content and synthesis. In addition, synovial membrane, articular cartilage, and osteochondral samples were collected for histologic analyses using published techniques. All data were analyzed to determine the effects of exercise and site within the joint on dependent variables.

Results

Ten colts and 23 fillies were born with an average birth weight of 56.4 ± 5.54 kg. Foals were weaned at a mean age of 133 ± 9.51 days. No significant differences in behavior, plasma cortisol levels, or body weights existed between groups. Control foals had significantly higher condition scores compared to conditioned foals at 3 and 4 months.

The analysis of these clinical data indicated that conditioning increased the risk of joint effusion in the metacarpophalangeal, intercarpal, and radial carpal joints, and was protective for tarsocrural effusion. Significant differences in physitis scores for the distal radius between the conditioned and control groups were observed in months 2, 3, 4, 6, and 10. Analysis of the third metacarpal scores identified significant differences between the control and exercise groups at 2, 4, 6, 7, and 8 months of age ($p<0.05$).

EFFECTS OF EARLY EXERCISE ON ARTICULAR CARTILAGE VIABILITY

The mean number of viable chondrocytes was 14% more in the exercised horses than non-exercised horses ($88\% \pm 1.3$ vs. $74\% \pm 1.3$, $p=0.001$), and 34% greater at the dorsal sites of the exercised horses than dorsal sites of non-exercised horses ($87\% \pm 1.2$ vs. $53\% \pm 2.1$, $p=0.001$). The exercised group had a greater overall proteoglycan staining score than the non-exercised group (2.0 ± 0.1 vs 1.2 ± 0.1, $p=0.001$).

EFFECTS OF EARLY EXERCISE ON MECHANICAL PROPERTIES OF ARTICULAR CARTILAGE

Cartilage structural, biochemical, and biomechanical properties varied markedly with site in the joint. Sites just medial and just lateral to the saggital ridge showed signs of early degeneration, with relatively low reflectance score, indentation stiffness, and collagen content, and relatively high water content. Effects of exercise and side (left vs. right) were not detected for any measure. Overall, indentation stiffness correlated positively with reflectance score and collagen content, and inversely with thickness and water content.

EFFECTS OF EARLY EXERCISE ON SUBCHONDRAL MINERALIZATION PATTERN IN THE THIRD METACARPAL CONDYLES

Results showed that there was a modest increase in bone density in the fetlock joints of horses that were exercised from an early age. In addition, there appeared to be a density pattern that might predispose some horses to condylar fracture. There was no effect of exercise on this pattern, but it was concerning that some horses showed a significant density gradient in the parasaggital groove of the third metacarpal condyle–the area where condylar fractures occur.

There were no significant effects of exercise on synovial membrane or articular cartilage histologic parameters. There was a trend for articular cartilage glycosaminoglycan content to be higher in exercised horses, although a trend existed for articular cartilage glycosaminoglycan synthesis to be higher in control horses. Analysis of subchondral bone parameters showed minimal effect of exercise on differences in bone fraction in each area, and significant increase in bone formation in the subchondral bone areas of the lateral and medial aspects of the third metacarpal condyles.

Discussion

Exercise beginning at 10 days of age did not have a detrimental effect on clinical, histologic, and biochemical parameters of musculoskeletal tissues. However, only osteochondral tissues were evaluated in this report, and results of tendon and ligament analyses are pending. One concern during development of this protocol was that early exercise might be detrimental to tissues. However, the level of exercise used in this study did not adversely affect tissues, but also had only a mild effect on positive tissue characteristics. Therefore, exercise levels beyond that used in this study would be recommended for future studies.

Early exercise had a beneficial effect on cellular and matrix features of the articular cartilage. The sequence of events leading to articular cartilage change appeared to be unrelated to SCB sclerosis. These findings may have implications for the use of exercise to condition developing mammalian articular cartilage. Increased chondrocyte viability and matrix quality could improve resilience of the articular cartilage to injury (Dykgraaf et al., 2006). However, exercise-imposed mechanical stimulation did not markedly affect articular cartilage function or structure. The marked site-associated variation suggests that biomechanical environment can initiate degenerative changes in immature cartilage during joint growth and maturation (Nugent et al., 2004).

Early exercise did induce significant increase in bone formation rate when the bone labels were given at 8 months of age. However, the overall effect on bone fraction at the end of the study (18 months) was minimal. Therefore, it appears that control horses may have regulated bone content with normal pasture exercise and growth. There were modest increases in bone density in certain areas of the metacarpal condyles; therefore, some protective effect may have occurred due to early exercise.

References

Cooper, C., M. Cawley, A. Bhalla, et al. 1995. Childhood growth, physical activity, and peak bone mass in women. J. Bone Miner. Res. 10:940-947.

Crowell-Davis, S.L. 1986. Developmental behavior. Vet. Clin. North Amer. Equine Pract. 2:573-590.

Crowell-Davis, S.L., and K.A. Houpt. 1986. Techniques for taking a behavioral history. Vet Clin. North Amer. Equine Pract. 2:507-518.

Daly, R.M., and S.L. Bass. 2006. Lifetime sport and leisure activity participation is associated with greater bone size, quality and strength in older men. Osteoporos. Int. 17:1258-1267.

Dykgraaf, S., E.C. Firth, C.W. Rogers, et al. 2006. Effect of exercise on chondrocyte viability and subchondral bone sclerosis of the distal third metacarpal and metatarsal bones of young horses. Amer. J. Vet. Res. In preparation.

Janz, K. 2002. Physical activity and bone development during childhood and adolescence: Implications for the prevention of osteoporosis. Minerva Pediatr. 54:93-104.

Kawcak, C.E., C.W. McIlwraith, R.W. Norrdin, et al. 2000. Clinical effects of exercise on subchondral bone of carpal and metacarpophalangeal joints in horses. Amer. J. Vet. Res. 61:1252-1258.

Kawcak, C.E., C.W. McIlwraith, R.W. Norrdin, et al. 2001. The role of subchondral bone in joint disease: A review. Equine Vet. J. 33:120-126.

MacDonald, H., S. Kontulainen, M. Petit, et al. 2006. Bone strength and its determinants in pre- and early pubertal boys and girls. Bone 39:598-608.

McKay, H.A., L. MacLean, M. Petit, et al. 2005. "Bounce at the Bell:" A novel program of short bouts of exercise improves proximal femur bone mass in early pubertal children. Br. J. Sports Med. 39:521-526.

Micklesfield, L.K., L. van der Merwe, and E.V. Lambert. 2005. Lifestyle questionnaire to evaluate risk for reduced bone mineral density in women. Clin. J. Sports Med. 15:340-348.

Muller-Gerbl, M. 1998. The SCB Plate. Advances in Anatomy, Embryology and Cell Biology.

Nugent, G.E., A.W. Law, E.G. Wong, et al. 2004. Site- and exercise-related variation in structure and function of cartilage from equine distal metacarpal condyle. Osteoarthritis Cartilage 12:826-833.

Richardson, D.W., and C.C. Clark. 1993. Effects of short-term cast immobilization on equine articular cartilage. Amer. J. Vet. Res. 54:449-453.

Rogers, C., R. van Weeren, A. Barneveld, et al. 2006. Evaluation of a new strategy to modulate skeletal development in the equine athlete by imposing track-based exercise during growth. In preparation.

Runyan, S.M., D.D. Stadler, C.N. Bainbridge, et al. 2003. Familial resemblance of bone mineralization, calcium intake, and physical activity in early-adolescent daughters, their mothers, and maternal grandmothers. J. Amer. Diet. Assoc.103:1320-1325.

Seeman, E., J.L. Hopper, N.R. Young, et al. 1996. Do genetic factors explain associations between muscle strength, lean mass, and bone density? A twin study. Amer. J. Physiol. 270:E320-327.

van Harreveld, P.D., J.D. Lillich, C.E. Kawcak, et al. 2002a. Clinical evaluation of the effects of immobilization followed by remobilization and exercise on the metacarpophalangeal joint in horses. Amer. J. Vet. Res. 63:282-288.

van Harreveld, P.D., J.D. Lillich, C.E. Kawcak, et al. 2002b. Effects of immobilization followed by remobilization on mineral density, histomorphometric features, and formation of the bones of the metacarpophalangeal joint in horses. Amer. J. Vet. Res. 63:276-281.

Wang, Q.J., H. Suominen, P.H. Nicholson, et al. 2005. Influence of physical activity and maturation status on bone mass and geometry in early pubertal girls. Scand. J. Med. Sci. Sports 15:100-106.

MUSCLE ADAPTATIONS DURING GROWTH AND EARLY TRAINING

STEPHANIE J. VALBERG AND LISA BORGIA
University of Minnesota, St. Paul, Minnesota

Introduction

It is well documented that mammalian muscle, while influenced by heredity, is highly plastic tissue that is capable of changing dramatically in response to growth, exercise, hormonal influences, disease, and dietary deficiencies. The increased demand for performance capacity in young racehorses has prompted investigations to determine if instituting training at a young age can have a major impact on muscle development, thereby promoting long-term benefits to equine performance. The purpose of this review is to highlight the changes that occur in foals and weanlings with growth as well as to review the findings from studies where training has been introduced to foals in the weanling or yearling stage.

Much of our knowledge of skeletal muscle in horses has been gained through the study of muscle biopsies. A muscle biopsy technique for horses was developed in the 1970s (Lindholm and Piehl, 1974; Snow and Guy, 1980). The technique involves insertion of a 6-mm diameter needle into the muscle through a 10-mm skin incision and removal of approximately 400 mg of tissue from a standardized depth. A battery of tinctorial and histochemical stains are applied to specially frozen muscle to identify muscle fiber sizes, shapes, and contractile and metabolic properties, as well as neuromuscular junctions, nerve branches, connective tissue, and blood vessels. Biochemical evaluation of skeletal muscle samples provides quantitative information regarding the activity of various metabolic enzymes and substrate and metabolite concentrations. Muscle biopsy has greatly expanded our understanding of normal muscle structure and function, as well as disease processes.

Contractile Fiber Types

Skeletal muscle comprises approximately 50% of the body's mass. It consists largely of long multinucleated spindle-shaped cells (myofibers) that are highly specialized by virtue of a structured array of muscle-specific contractile proteins that confer the ability to shorten rapidly and efficiently. Myosin, one of the main contractile proteins, possesses enzymatic properties that allow the hydrolysis of adenosine triphosphate (ATPase). The speed of contraction of individual muscle fibers differs depending on the type of myosin and the activity of the myosin ATPase. Contractile properties of muscle fibers can be differentiated using a histochemical staining technique that is based on the sensitivity of myosin ATPase activity to acid and alkaline pre-incubation. Slow twitch type I fibers stain darkly after acid and lightly after alkaline pre-incubation. In contrast, fast twitch type II myofibers stain lightly with acid and darkly with alkaline pre-incubation (Brooke and Kaiser, 1970). Some fibers do not reverse their staining properties in acid and alkaline media and are classified as type IIC or intermediate myofibers. This likely corresponds to fibers containing either slow and fast twitch myosin or embryonic myosin. Further, type IIA and type IIB myofibers may be differentiated if muscle sections are pre-incubated at pH 4.6 prior to ATPase staining.

Myosin also has structural properties that can be used to differentiate fiber types. Two identical myosin heavy chains (MHC) and two pairs of light chains form each myosin molecule. Different forms of MHC (termed isoforms) are expressed in individual muscle fibers. Immunohistochemical techniques recently have been developed to specifically identify fiber types based on antibodies directed against various MHC isoforms (Gorza, 1990). Embryonic and slow twitch myosin isoforms as well as type 2a, type 2b, and 2x (also called 2d) in skeletal muscle and type 2m fibers in the jaw muscles can be distinguished by this technique. Some hybrid fibers contain a mixture of these isoforms (i.e., type 2a/x). Fibers with type 2x myosin contract faster than fibers with type 2a myosin, which in turn contract faster than type 1 myosin.

Unfortunately, type IIB fibers distinguished by myosin ATPase activity do not correspond to type 2b fibers distinguished by immunohistochemical staining for MHC. Rather, type IIB fibers correspond more closely with type 2x fibers, and type 2b fibers correspond to a very rapidly contracting fiber type found in rodents and camelids (Gorza, 1990; Linnane et al., 1999). In the following sections, information derived from studies using histochemistry is designated by Roman numerals for fiber types (I, IIA, IIB), whereas studies using immunohistochemistry use types 1, 2a, and 2x.

Metabolic Fiber Types

Type 1 fibers generally have higher concentrations of triglycerides and myoglobin and are better suited to derive their energy by oxidative phosphorylation via the electron transport system following the oxidation of fatty acids and glucose via the Krebs cycle. The oxidative capacity of type 1 fibers can be demonstrated by dark histochemical staining for the activity of oxidative enzymes such as succinate dehydrogenase (SDH) and reduced nicotinamide adenine dinucleotide tetrazolium reductase (NADHTR) (Dubowitz et al., 1973).

In general, type II fibers are suited to derive energy for contraction by anaerobic glyco(geno)lysis. Fast twitch fibers, particularly type IIx and IIb fibers, tend to have higher concentrations of glycogen as well as higher activities of enzymes associated with glycogenolysis and glycolysis such as phosphofructokinase (PFK) and lactate dehydrogenase (LDH) activity. The oxidative staining of type II fibers can be variable with some fibers containing higher oxidative staining than others. In general type 2a fibers have higher oxidative staining than type 2b fibers. However, this is not always the case and may vary with age and training (Valberg et al., 1988). A further means to subtype fibers is by both their ATPase and oxidative staining for SDH or NADH. This fiber typing distinguishes slow twitch, fast twitch oxidative, and fast twitch glycolytic (or non-oxidative) fibers.

Measures of Metabolic Capacity

Aerobic pathways such as the citric acid cycle, ß oxidation of free fatty acids, and the electron transport chain are located within mitochondria and provide the bulk of ATP for the cell as long as oxygen is plentiful. The activity of key enzymes in the pathways can be used as an indicator of oxidative capacity. Citric acid cycle enzymes such as citrate synthase (CS) and succinate dehydrogenase (SDH) are often measured in snap frozen muscle biopsies as oxidative markers. Often used as a marker for the capacity for ß oxidation of free fatty acids is 3-hydroxy-acyl-CoA dehydrogenase (HAD). Anaerobic pathways such as glycolysis, creatine phosphate, and the purine nucleotide cycle are found within the cell cytoplasm. Markers for the capacity for anaerobic glycolysis that are commonly measured in frozen muscle include PFK and LDH enzyme activities.

The main fuels for aerobic muscular contraction are fatty acids and glucose, which are supplied by intramuscular (lipid droplets, ß glycogen particles) and extramuscular (liver and adipose tissue) depots during exercise. The rate-limiting factor in the supply of plasma free fatty acid (FFA) to muscle appears to be the rate of FFA release from adipose tissues (Bennard et al., 2005). The rate-limiting factor in the extramuscular supply of glucose to working muscle is glucose uptake by the myofibers under the influence of insulin. Muscle triglyceride levels can be estimated by Oil red O staining in muscle. Glycogen stores in muscle can be measured biochemically in snap frozen samples and estimated from periodic acid Schiff's stains of frozen sections.

Variation in Muscle Fiber Type Composition

The speed and force developed by a muscle during contraction differs qualitatively and quantitatively depending on its fast and slow twitch fiber type composition. Most muscles in horses contain a mixture of types 1, 2a, and 2x fibers (or I, IIA, and IIB, depending on the technique used for fiber typing). Locomotor muscles have a high proportion of type 2a and 2x fibers relative to type 1 fibers, whereas postural muscle have a higher proportion of type 1 fibers than most locomotor muscles. The proportion of muscle fiber types within a given muscle will also vary along its length and depth.

Generally, deeper muscles or portions of muscles have a higher percentage of type 1 muscle fibers. Due to this variation, when comparing the fiber type composition of different individuals, a standardized site within a muscle must be used. Fiber type composition of muscles on the left and right side of the body will be identical if samples are taken from the same site and depth. The gluteus muscle is often chosen for study in horses because it is a major propulsive muscle active in locomotion, is easily accessible, and shows adaptations to growth and training. Some studies have also evaluated the semimembranosus or tendinosus muscle.

When standardized techniques are used to assess muscle fiber composition, individual horses have been shown to have a wide variation in muscle fiber type composition. This phenomenon has been attributed to effects of genetic background, breed, sex, age, and state of training. Heritability is believed to have a strong influence on MHC isoforms in muscle and is estimated to be 13% (Rivero et al., 1996; Barrey et al., 1999). Breed differences have been extensively studied in horses (Snow and Valberg, 1994). In general, Quarter Horses and Thoroughbreds have the highest percentage of type II fibers in the gluteus medius, about 80-90%; Standardbreds and Andalusians have an intermediate number, about 75%; and donkeys have the lowest percentage of type II fibers in locomotor muscles. There are, however, wide variations between individuals of the same breed.

Stallions have a higher proportion of type IIA and lower proportion of type IIB fibers on average in their locomotor muscles than mares (Rivero et al., 1993a; Roneus, 1993). No differences in type I fibers or oxidative enzyme activities have been identified between age-matched Standardbred mares and stallions (Roneus, 1993). Andalusian mares have a higher percentage of type I fibers than stallions (Rivero et al., 1993a), a finding which has been inconsistently reported in Thoroughbreds (Snow and Guy, 1980; Roneus et al., 1991).

With growth and training, there is a change in the length and breadth of all fibers, and a change in the proportion of fiber types rather than an increase in the number of muscle fibers.

Effect of Growth on Metabolic and Contractile Properties

In the embryo, primitive muscle cells migrate to their position in the limb where their eventual fiber type is influenced by innate developmental directives, temporal and positional factors, neural enervation, and activation of specific signal transduction pathways. Fetal muscle cells initially express perinatal MHC, which is subsequently replaced by one of the fast or slow twitch MHC isoforms. Further development of subtypes of fast twitch fibers (2a, 2ax, or 2x) occurs in concert with the emergence of thyroid function (Emerson and Hauschka, 2004). Positional factors dictate that those portions of muscles that are primarily postural have a higher percentage of slow twitch type 1 muscle fibers. Eventual neural enervation dictates that all fibers supplied by the same nerve branch have the same muscle fiber type. These factors combine to produce a mosaic of fiber types with fiber type predominance programmed into certain muscles or portions of muscles. Muscle remains plastic well into adulthood, however, and contractile fiber types may be altered by growth and training.

The change in metabolic and contractile properties of the gluteus medius muscle with growth and development have been studied in Standardbreds, Quarter Horses,

Andalusians, Arabians, and Thoroughbreds (Essen-Gustavsson et al., 1983; Thornton and Taylor, 1983; Kline and Bechtel, 1990; Fowden et al., 1991; Roneus et al., 1991; Galisteo et al., 1992; Rivero et al., 1993a; Roneus, 1993; Yamano et al., 2005). A confounding factor in some of these studies is the degree of standardization of the biopsy site. Ideally, the same relative position within the muscle would be sampled as the animal grows. In studies where standardization was not accomplished, attributions of variation in both metabolic and contractile properties with growth may in fact reflect the sample depth-age relationship. In particular, if biopsy sample depth was not increased as foals aged, samples from older foals would underestimate any real increase in oxidative fiber types or oxidative capacity.

PERINATAL PERIOD

In utero, maternal glucose is the primary source of energy for equine muscle. During the third trimester of pregnancy, the equine fetus shows a clear insulin response to blood glucose, which serves to drive glucose into muscle and increase glycogen stores (Fowden et al., 1984; Fowden et al., 1991). Newborn foals continue their dependence on glucose as fuel via mare's milk, which is relatively high in sugar (59% DM) and low in lipid (13% DM) relative to other domestic animals (Rossdale, 1967). Muscle glycogen concentrations in newborn foals are relatively high (119-220 µmol/g wet weight) and similar to those found in yearling and two-year-old horses (Fowden et al., 1991; Valberg et al., 2001; de la Corte et al., 2002).

Few studies have addressed the metabolic characteristics of skeletal muscle of newborn foals. Kline (1990) found that Quarter Horses and Standardbreds followed from 1 to 100 days of age showed a significant increase in glycolytic enzymes (250% increase in LDH) and a decline in oxidative enzymes (37% decrease in HAD) in muscle. This corresponded to a tendency for fast twitch glycolytic fibers to increase and fast twitch oxidative fibers to decrease in these foals. The depth of the biopsy was not adjusted for growth in this study. We performed a study evaluating the activity of three enzymes involved in the ß oxidation of fat in gluteal muscle of Thoroughbred foals using a technique to standardize the depth of sampling. The activity of the enzyme crotonase decreased from 7.2 ± 1.6 µmol/g/min at 48 h of age to 4.4 ± 0.4 µmol/g/min at 1 month of age, whereas the activity of HAD and thiolase remained unchanged at 5.7 ± 2.2 to 4.1 ± 0.4 µmol/g/min and 1.1 ± 0.13 to 1.1 ± 0.3 µmol/g/min.

Mature fast and slow twitch MHC isoforms are expressed in newborn foal muscle. Fast twitch fibers in foals may coexpress perinatal MHC up to 10 weeks of age (Dingboom et al., 2002). In addition, many slow twitch fibers in foal muscle coexpress cardiac MHC isoforms up to 22 weeks of age.

BIRTH TO 1 YEAR OF AGE

The metabolic changes that occur in gluteal muscle with growth are not consistent across the studies available. Standardbred weanlings followed from 6 months to 1 year of age showed no change in CS or HAD activity and a decline in glycolytic capacity (LDH) (Essen-Gustavsson et al., 1983). In contrast, a study of Arabian and Thoroughbred crossbred foals showed a 23% decline in oxidative enzyme activity (SDH) and oxidative staining intensity of fast twitch fibers from 2 weeks to 8 months of age (Thornton et al., 1983). A 25% increase in glycolytic capacity (PFK activity) was also recorded. It is unclear what the depth of sampling was in these foals. This decline in oxidative fast twitch fibers was also documented in Arabian and Andalusian horses from birth to 1 year of age in a study where depth was not adjusted (Galisteo et al., 1992). A semi-quantitative study of SDH activity indicated an increase in activity in all fiber types with growth in Thoroughbred foals (Eto et al., 2003). We evaluated the activity of three enzymes involved in ß oxidation of fat in Thoroughbred foals using a biopsy technique that accounted for changes in muscle size with growth. The activity of the enzyme crotonase increased from 4.4 ± 0.4 µmol/g/min to 6.9 ± 0.9 µmol/g/min at 1 year of age, HAD increased from 4.1 ± 0.4 to 6.0 ± 1.2 µmol/g/min, and thiolase remained unchanged at 1.2 ± 0.1 µmol/g/min. Thus, it would appear that there might be a variable change in oxidative capacity during the first year of life and an increase in glycolytic capacity.

From 6 months to 1 year of age, Standardbred foals showed no change in the percentage of type 1 fibers, an increase in type IIA fibers and a decrease in type IIB fibers (Essen-Gustavsson et al., 1983). In a study of Arabian and Andalusian foals, the percentage of type I and IIA fibers increased, and type IIB decreased from 10 days to 1 year of age (Galisteo et al., 1992, Rivero et al., 1993a). Thoroughbred foal gluteal muscles showed no change in the percentage of type 1 fibers from birth to 1 year of age, an increase in the percentage of type 2a fibers, and a decrease in 2x fibers (Eto et al., 2003). In warmblood foals, the percentage of type 1 and type 2a fibers increased and the percentage of hybrid type 2a/2x and type 2x fibers decreased from birth to 1 year of age (Dingboom et al., 1999; Dingboom et al., 2002). Thus, there is a small increase in type 1 fibers and a consistent increase in fast twitch type 2a (IIA) fibers and a decrease in type 2x (IIB) in foals of a variety of breeds as they reach 1 year of age. Between 1 year and 2 years of age, these changes in fiber type proportions continue and appear to level off at about 3 1/2 years of age in those breeds that have been studied (Roneus et al., 1991).

Thus, glycolytic metabolism appears to be of prime importance in young foals with a gradual increase in the ratio of type IIA:IIB with development over the first year of life.

Adaptations to Training

BIRTH TO 1 YEAR OF AGE

A study of five Standardbred colts was conducted where weanlings between 7 and 8 months of age were started into training and continued until 17-18 months of age

(Essen-Gustavsson et al., 1983). Training consisted of walk for 5 min and trot for 1800 m with the distance gradually increasing over the next 4 months to 3600 meters. This exercise was performed 4-5 days/week. For the next 6 months, yearlings were trained with a sulky at a trot over 3000 meters 4-5 days/week at increasing tempo. During this period, 1 day of speed training (500 m/min or faster) over 1600 m was added. An age- and sex-matched control group remained untrained. The increase in type IIA:IIB ratio that occurred with growth was similar between trained and untrained groups. The activity of the oxidative enzyme CS increased significantly (18%) in the trained group but not the untrained group and glycolytic enzyme activities declined (LDH 33%) similarly with age in both trained and untrained weanlings.

Thoroughbreds. A training study of Thoroughbred foals began at 2 months of age and continued to 1 year of age with foals weaned at 5 months of age. An age-matched control group was untrained. Foals began treadmill exercise with 15 s of cantering interspersed with 4 min of trot and gradually increased their speed, reaching 3.3 m/s of trot and 11 m/s of cantering (Eto et al., 2003). There was no difference in fiber type composition between the control and training group; however, SDH activity was higher in type 2x fibers of trained foals than controls. Muscle fiber sizes were larger in the trained vs. untrained foals.

Warmbloods. A comparison of Dutch warmbloods that were either stall-rested, turned out on pasture, or chased in the paddock for repeated sprints from birth to 5 months of age showed little effect of exercise on contractile fiber types (Dingboom et al., 1999; Dingboom et al., 2002).

Training studies of two- to four-year-old Standardbred, Andalusian, and Thoroughbred horses show an increase in the type IIA:IIB or 2a:2x ratio and an increase in oxidative capacity (CS: 31% increase Andalusians, 50% increase Standardbreds; SDH: 37% increase Thoroughbreds) (Roneus et al., 1992; Serrano et al., 2000; Yamano et al., 2005). When training is imposed on young growing weanlings, it does not appear to have a major impact on muscle development over and above the changes which occur naturally with growth. Enhanced oxidative capacity of type 2b fibers may occur with training but this change is not permanent, as studies have shown that after 3 months of detraining, oxidative enzyme activity will revert to pre-training levels (Serrano et al., 2000).

Conclusion

In summary, the metabolic and contractile adaptations in skeletal muscle that are present at birth provide the means by which young foals stand within minutes of being born and develop the quick burst of speed and rapid glycolytic metabolism necessary to evade predators. Equine muscle contains high muscle glycogen content and glycolytic capacity from birth, and mare's milk provides a rich source of sugar for energy metabolism. During the first years of a horse's life, there is a shift in fiber type proportions in favor of type 2a fibers at the expense of type 2b fibers. Depending on the breed, there may be a gradual increase in the oxidative capacity of type 2 fibers in the first year of life, which progressively evolves over the next 2 years providing enhanced staying power and a slightly slower speed of muscle contraction (decreased type 2a:2x ratio). Initiating training at less than a year of age does not appear to hasten the changes that occur naturally with growth and its impact appears to be less in young growing horses than is seen when training is begun at 18 months to 3 years of age.

References

Barrey, E., J.P. Valette, M. Jouglin, C. Blouin, and B. Langlois 1999. Heritability of percentage of fast myosin heavy chains in skeletal muscles and relationship with performance. Equine Vet. J. Suppl. 30:289-92.

Bennard, P., P. Imbeault, and E. Doucet. 2005. Maximizing acute fat utilization: Effects of exercise, food, and individual characteristics. Can. J. Appl. Physiol. 30:475-499.

Brooke, M.H., and K.K. Kaiser. 1970. Muscle fiber types: How many and what kind? Arch. Neurol. 23:369-379.

de la Corte, F.D., S.J. Valberg, J.M. MacLeay, and J.R. Mickelson. 2002. Developmental onset of polysaccharide storage myopathy in 4 Quarter Horse foals. J. Vet. Intern. Med. 16:581-587.

Dingboom, E.G., G. Dijkstra, E. Enzerink, H.C. van Oudheusden, and W.A. Weijs. 1999. Postnatal muscle fibre composition of the gluteus medius muscle of Dutch Warmblood foals: Maturation and the influence of exercise. Equine Vet. J. Suppl. 31:95-100.

Dingboom, E.G., H. van Oudheusden, K. Eizema, and W.A. Weijs. 2002. Changes in fibre type composition of gluteus medius and semitendinosus muscles of Dutch Warmblood foals and the effect of exercise during the first year postpartum. Equine Vet. J. 34:177-183.

Dubowitz, V., M.H. Brooke, and H.E. Neville. 1973. Muscle biopsy: A modern approach. W. B. Saunders, London, Philadelphia. p. 475.

Emerson Jr, C.P., and A.D. Hauschka. 2004. Embryonic origins of skeletal muscles. In: Myology. McGraw-Hill Co. New York. A. Engel and C. Franzini-Armstrong, ed. pp. 3-44.

Essen-Gustavsson, B., D. Lindholm, S.G.B. Persson, and J. Thornton. 1983. Skeletal muscle characteristics of young Standardbreds in relation to growth and early training. In: Equine Exercise Physiology, Burlington Press, Cambridge. Snow et al., ed. pp. 200-210.

Eto, D., S. Yamano, Y. Kasashima, T. Sugiura, T. Nasu, M. Tokuriki, and H. Miyata. 2003. Effect of controlled exercise on middle gluteal muscle fibre composition in Thoroughbred foals. Equine Vet. J. 35:676-680.

Fowden, A.L., L. Mundy, J.C. Ousey, A. McGladdery, and M. Silver. 1991. Tissue glycogen and glucose 6-phosphatase levels in fetal and newborn foals. J. Reprod. Fertil. Suppl. 44:537-542.

Fowden, A.L., M. Silver, L. Ellis, J. Ousey, and P.D. Rossdale. 1984. Studies on equine prematurity 3: Insulin secretion in the foal during the perinatal period. Equine Vet. J. 16:286-291.

Galisteo, A.M., E. Aguera, J.G. Monterde, and F. Miro. 1992. Gluteus medius muscle fiber type composition in young Andalusian and Arabian horses. Equine Vet. Sci. 12:254-258.

Gorza, L. 1990. Identification of a novel type 2 fiber population in mammalian skeletal muscle by combined use of histochemical myosin ATPase and anti-myosin monoclonal antibodies. J. Histochem. Cytochem. 38:257-265.

Kline, K.H., and P.J. Bechtel. 1990. Changes in the metabolic profile of equine muscle from birth through 1 year of age. J. Appl. Physiol. 68:1399-1404.

Lindholm, A., and K. Piehl. 1974. Fibre composition, enzyme activity and concentrations of metabolites and electrolytes in muscles of Standardbred horses. Acta Vet. Scand. 15:287-309.

Linnane, L., A.L. Serrano, and J.L. Rivero. 1999. Distribution of fast myosin heavy chain-based muscle fibres in the gluteus medius of untrained horses: Mismatch between antigenic and ATPase determinants. J. Anat. 194:363-372.

Rivero, J.L., M. Valera, A.L. Serrano, and M. Vineuesa. 1996. Variability of muscle fibre type composition in a number of genealogical bloodlines in Arabian and Andalusian horses. Pferdeheilkunde 12:661-665.

Rivero, J.L., A.M. Galisteo, E. Aguera, and F. Miro. 1993a. Skeletal muscle histochemistry in male and female Andalusian and Arabian horses of different ages. Res. Vet. Sci. 54:160-169.

Rivero, J.L., A.L. Serrano, A.M. Diz, and J.L. Morales. 1993b. Changes in cross-sectional area and capillary supply of the muscle fiber population in equine gluteus medius muscle as a function of sampling depth. Am. J. Vet. Res. 54:32-37.

Roneus, M. 1993. Muscle characteristics in Standardbreds of different ages and sexes. Equine Vet. J. 25:143-146.

Roneus, M., B. Essen-Gustavsson, A. Lindholm, and S.G. Persson. 1992. Skeletal muscle characteristics in young trained and untrained Standardbred trotters. Equine Vet. J. 24:292-294.

Roneus, M., A. Lindholm, and A. Asheim. 1991. Muscle characteristics in Thoroughbreds of different ages and sexes. Equine Vet. J. 23:207-210.

Rossdale, P.D. 1967. Clinical studies on the newborn Thoroughbred foal. I. Perinatal behaviour. Br. Vet. J. 123:470-481.

Serrano, A.L., E. Quiroz-Rothe, and J.L. Rivero. 2000. Early and long-term changes of equine skeletal muscle in response to endurance training and detraining. Pflugers Arch. 441:263-274.

Snow, D.H., and P.S. Guy. 1980. Muscle fibre composition of a number of limb muscles in different types of horses. Res. Vet. Sci. 28:134-144.

Snow, D.H., and S.J. Valberg. 1994. Muscle anatomy: Adaptations to exercise and training. In: The Athletic Horse: Principles and Practice of Equine Sports Medicine, Sanders, New York. Rose et al. (eds.) pp 145-179.

Thornton, J.R., and A.W. Taylor. 1983. Skeletal muscle characteristics of foals at two and four weeks and eight months of age. In: Equine Exercise Physiology, Burlington Press, Cambridge. Snow et al. (eds.) pp. 218-224.

Valberg, S., B. Essen-Gustavsson, and H. Skoglund-Wallberg. 1988. Oxidative capacity of skeletal muscle fibres in racehorses: Histochemical versus biochemical analysis. Equine Vet. J. 20:291-295.

Valberg, S.J., J.R. Mickelson, E.M. Gallant, J.M. MacLeay, L. Lentz, and F. de la Corte. 1999. Exertional rhabdomyolysis in Quarter Horses and Thoroughbreds: One syndrome, multiple aetiologies. Equine Vet. J. Suppl. 30:533-538.

Valberg, S.J., T.L. Ward, B. Rush, H. Kinde, H. Hiraragi, D. Nahey, J. Fyfe, and J.R. Mickelson. 2001. Glycogen branching enzyme deficiency in Quarter Horse foals. J. Vet. Intern. Med. 15:572-580.

Yamano, S., D. Eto, Y. Kasashima, A. Hiraga, T. Sugiura, and H. Miyata. 2005. Evaluation of developmental changes in the coexpression of myosin heavy chains and metabolic properties of equine skeletal muscle fibers. Am. J. Vet. Res. 66:401-405.

THE BALANCING ACT OF GROWING A SOUND, ATHLETIC HORSE

CLARISSA G. BROWN-DOUGLAS
Kentucky Equine Research, Versailles, Kentucky

Introduction

The genetic makeup, or genotype, contributes to a horse's performance ability by determining ultimate size and influencing conformation and athletic potential. Growth rate is not predestined and is affected by factors such as the environment, nutrition, and management.

Latest research shows that "bigger is better," as heavy and tall Thoroughbreds sold for the highest prices at yearling sales and when raced had the most earnings, graded stakes wins and grade-1 stakes wins (Pagan et al., 2005; Brown-Douglas and Pagan, 2006). Horses are therefore grown to be as large as possible at a young age, despite not achieving their mature weight and height until around four or five years of age. Unlike meat-producing animals, achieving maximal size in the least amount of time is undesirable in the horse as there are many career-ending developmental conditions such as osteochondritis dissecans (OCD) that occur in rapidly growing horses. Growing a foal too slowly, however, can prevent the animal from ever reaching its mature size. Optimal growth rate results in a desirable body size with the least amount of developmental problems, making the art of raising a successful athlete a sensitive balancing act.

Kentucky Equine Research (KER) has studied Thoroughbred growth and development over the last 20 years. Body weight and height data have been collected from foals born and raised in the major Thoroughbred-producing countries of the world including the United States, England, Ireland, Australia, New Zealand, South Africa, and India. Using this database of over 15,000 Thoroughbred foals, KER has compiled detailed reference growth curves for breeders to use when monitoring their horses' growth. Using Gro-Trac, KER's innovative growth and ration management software, breeders can track and compare the growth rates of their horses to the average growth parameters of a chosen reference peer group. KER studies have also focused on the effects of nutrition and management on equine growth. This paper will review the major results of KER's growth and development research and discuss the various management factors that influence the growing horse from foal to athlete.

Gro-Trac and Percentiles

Traditionally, Gro-Trac has provided some indication of how a horse is growing by comparing it to a reference population and indicating the percentage of reference. This method is useful, but it does not take into account the spread of the data around the average. For example, there is a much wider range for a horse's body weight than for wither height at a particular age. Body weights can differ by as much as 110 pounds (50 kg), whereas differences in height will be only a few centimeters. A horse that is plus four percent of reference body weight is not that much heavier than the average, but if he is plus four percent of reference height then he is a lot taller! Percentiles deal with this spread issue and allow a more relative comparison with the entire population. Furthermore, this method allows horses to be compared regardless of gender and age. Using percentiles, breeders can assess if there are any abnormalities in the growth pattern and adjust nutritional and conditioning regimens as necessary. The use of percentiles is not a new concept in growth studies and is commonly used in pediatrics. However, this is the first time such a large equine data set has been acquired to create reference populations from which percentiles can be calculated for Thoroughbred horses.

Nature versus Nurture

Thoroughbreds share a fairly narrow genetic base, so geography has a significant influence on growth patterns in young Thoroughbreds. Body weight data collected from the major Thoroughbred breeding countries revealed that Australian and New Zealand Thoroughbreds tend to be larger than American Thoroughbreds, which in turn are larger than those reared in England (Brown-Douglas and Pagan, 2006). Indian Thoroughbreds are smaller than all other populations (Figure 1). Thoroughbreds in all countries except India showed seasonal changes in daily weight gain in winter and spring that coincided with changes in pasture quality and availability. English Thoroughbreds are as much as four percent below the American average and seven percent below the Australian reference. In percentile terms, English Thoroughbreds are in the 30th-40th (body weight) and 40th-45th (body weight) percentiles on average when compared with Australian and American Thoroughbreds, respectively. American Thoroughbreds average in the 40th-45th percentile for body weight when compared with Australian Thoroughbreds, but there is little difference in height between these two populations.

Indian Thoroughbreds are smaller than all other populations, averaging 7-11% below the reference curve of English and American Thoroughbreds and falling in the 5th-10th percentile for weight. The observed differences in weight and height between other populations of Thoroughbreds are probably due to the different environments in which they are reared as well as varying management factors during the growth and development period.

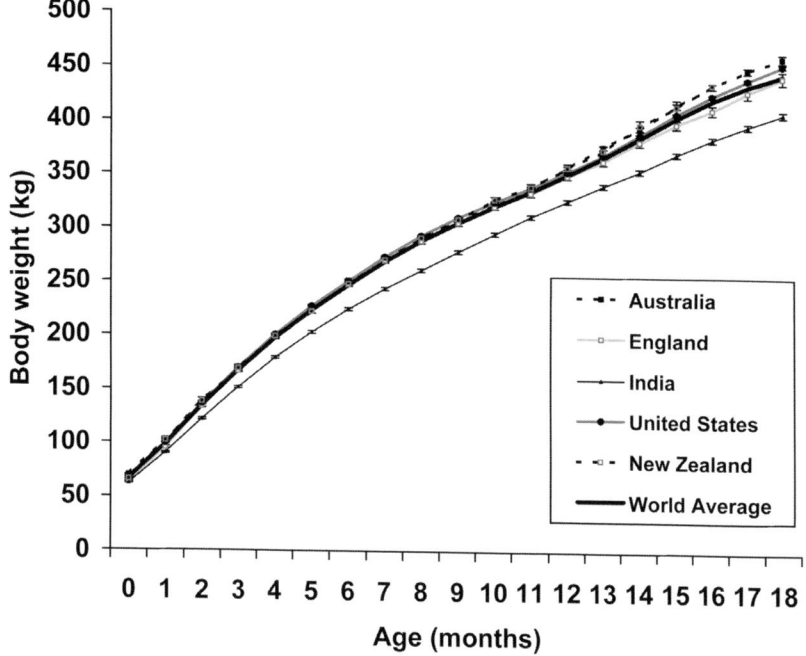

Figure 1. Body weight ± 95% confidence interval (kg) of Thoroughbreds reared in Australia, England, India, United States and New Zealand compared with the world average (Brown-Douglas and Pagan, 2006).

Is Growth Important to a Horse's Career?

Growth management of the young foal will vary depending on the commercial end point. A large, well-grown Thoroughbred yearling is desirable when offered for sale at public auction as selling price is influenced by body size. Yearlings that sold higher than the median of the session in which they were sold were heavier and taller, but not fatter, than yearlings which sold below the session median (Pagan et al., 2005). Sold yearlings were also heavier and taller than those listed as RNA (reserve not attained), and fewer lightweight yearlings (those in the lowest weight quartile) were sold compared with the heaviest yearlings (Brown-Douglas et al., 2007). Early rapid growth may not be favored in Thoroughbreds that are "bred to race" with no intention of being prepared for sale as weanlings or yearlings. Many breeders selling horses at public auction aim to produce early-born foals to maximize growing time before a July or September sale. This practice may not be that advantageous as foals born in the central Kentucky winter (January and February) were smaller at birth and grew slower during the first two months compared with spring-born foals (Figure 2), but compensated by growing faster later in lactation so that by 5 months of age there was no difference between body weights in any of the groups (Pagan et al., 2006).

April- and May-born yearlings at 16 months of age are also taller and heavier than winter-born yearlings (Brown-Douglas et al., 2006). September sale yearlings are between 16-20 months of age, so buyers may mistake January-born yearlings for the largest when in fact they are only the oldest.

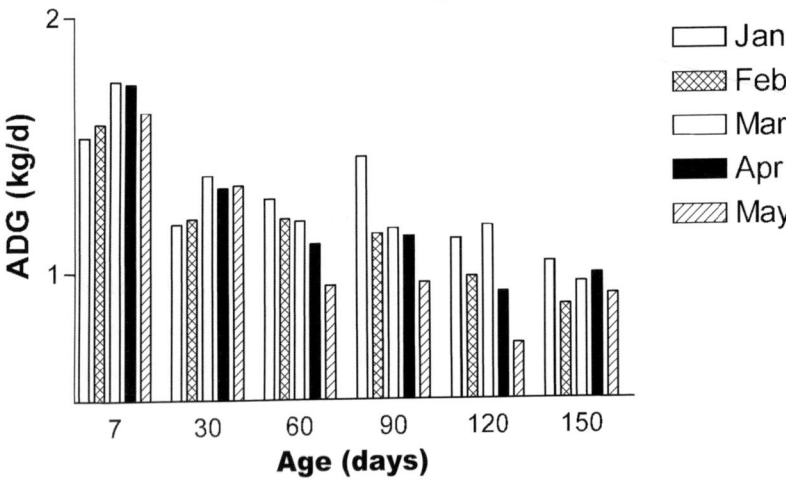

Figure 2. ADG (kg/d) of Kentucky foals separated by month of birth (Pagan et al., 2006).

Furthermore, recent research at KER has shown that yearling size does not necessarily predict athletic success (Brown-Douglas et al., 2006). KER recently analyzed the growth and racing performance records of nearly 4,000 American Thoroughbreds to determine if certain growth characteristics affect the odds of success as a racehorse. Findings suggest some significant trends between growth and racing success. Horses that started as two-year-olds were shorter and weighed less as foals and yearlings than those that did not, regardless of birth month. However, fewer May-born yearlings started as two-year-olds compared with earlier-born yearlings. It is generally accepted that faster-maturing, heavier horses are more likely to be raced as two-year-olds, but these results suggest just the opposite; smaller horses are more likely to run early. Furthermore, smaller horses had more career starts, suggesting that smaller horses are sounder.

Conversely, stakes winners, graded stakes winners, grade-1 stakes winners, and millionaires were heavier and taller than average as yearlings. Interestingly, the 21 millionaires in the study were, on average, taller than 79% of the population as yearlings. These results indicate different growth characteristics for different performance outcomes. If one wants an early-starting horse that races for longer, then a smaller horse is more desirable. If, however, one wishes a stakes winner and high earner, then bigger is better, although there is a greater risk of the horse not starting at all. Furthermore, a greater percentage of two-year-old starters were born in March and April and a greater percentage of stakes winners were born in March.

To further evaluate the relationship between size and racing performance, the yearlings were divided into four groups (quartiles) based on weight and height so that the lightest or shortest yearlings were in the lowest quartile, and the heaviest and tallest in the highest quartile. This method allowed comparison among all horses regardless of age or gender and ranks the relative position of an individual in a population by indicating what percent of the reference population that individual will equal or exceed for each measurement. Yearlings in the lowest weight quartile (those that weighed less than 75% of the population) had lower sales prices, and went on to have lower earnings, fewer stakes wins, and a lower sire index than the rest of the population (Table 1 and Figures 3 and 4). Sire index was examined to account for genetic variation and indicates the average racing class of foals sired by a stallion. However, yearlings below the 50th weight and height percentiles were more likely to start as two-year-olds and had more career starts than those above the 50th percentile.

Table 1. Median sale price of yearlings compared with average sire index, percent stakes winners, and average and median career earnings; letters indicate significant differences within factor (P<0.05) (Brown-Douglas et al., 2007).

Yearling weight quartile	1 (percentiles 0-25)	2 (percentiles 26-50)	3 (percentiles 51-75)	4 (percentiles 76-100)
Median sale price (USD)	$21,500	$30,000	$40,000	$50,000
Sire index	2.09 ± 0.03^a	2.16 ± 0.03^a	2.33 ± 0.03^b	2.45 ± 0.03^c
Stakes winners (%)	4.64^a	8.68^b	8.44^b	8.26^b
Average career earnings (USD)	$51,226 \pm 4480^a$	$86,443 \pm 4964^b$	$69,339 \pm 5236^c$	$72,606 \pm 2221^{b,c}$
Median earnings (USD)	$13,795	$17,058	$19,050	$18,081

Yearlings that weighed less than half the population had lower sire indexes than those in the heavier quartiles, indicating that successful sires tend to produce larger yearlings. Interestingly, foals in the second quartile (between the 25th and 50th weight percentiles) had as many stakes wins and greater earnings than the larger yearlings even though they were by sires with significantly lower sire indexes. This suggests that these moderately lighter yearlings outperformed their pedigrees.

These data provide insight into managing horses for different strategies. Smaller horses are more likely to start as two-year-olds and have more career starts; however, elite performers (graded stakes winners, grade-1 stakes winners, and millionaires) tend to be taller and heavier.

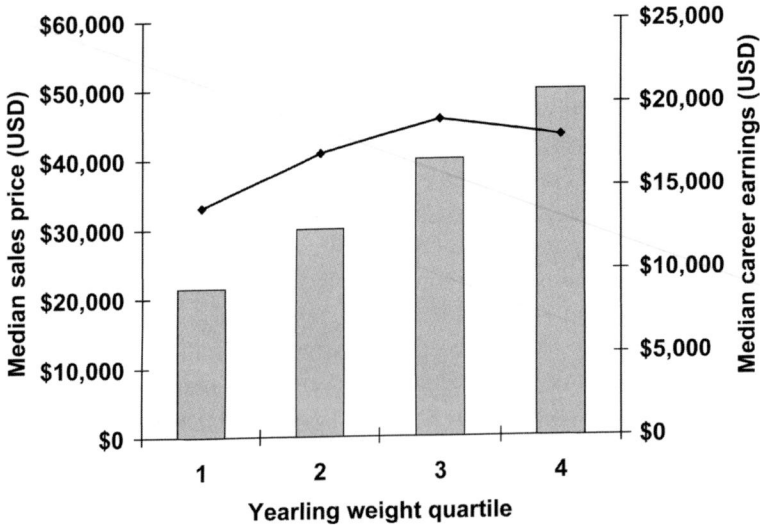

Figure 3. Median sales price (☐) and median career earnings (-◆-) in each weight quartile (Brown-Douglas et al., 2007).

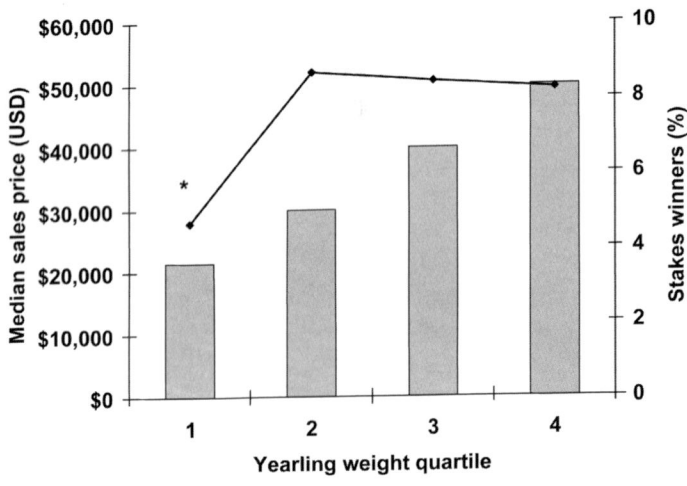

Figure 4. Median sales price (☐) and percent stakes winners (-◆-) in each weight quartile; *indicates point is significantly different from all others within factor (P<0.05) (Brown-Douglas et al., 2007).

Nutrition of the Young, Growing Horse

Because of the premium price paid for mass, young Thoroughbreds prepared for sale are grown rapidly to achieve maximal size. To fuel maximum growth, these young horses are often fed large amounts of grain. Extremely rapid growth by overfeeding energy has been implicated in developmental orthopedic disease (DOD). Periods of slow or decreased growth followed by growth spurts are also risky. Therefore, nutrition mistakes made during a foal's early growth can lead to developmental problems that limit performance later in life.

The best way to evaluate the success of a feeding and conditioning program of young horses is through assessment of body weight, height, and condition. Regular monitoring of weight allows farm managers to maintain a steady growth rate while preventing the animal from becoming too heavy.

During the first few months of life, foals grow rapidly, quadrupling their body weights by 5 months of age (Pagan et al., 1996; Lawrence, 2003; Brown-Douglas and Pagan, 2006). During this time, foals derive the energy, protein, and minerals necessary to support rapid growth from a combination of mare milk, pasture, supplemental grain, and mineral stores in the foal's liver. If the broodmare has received a correctly fortified feed during late pregnancy and is producing adequate milk, in most cases it is unnecessary to supplement the foal with grain until it reaches 90 days of age.

Proper nutrient intake is vital during the weanling stage as the skeleton is most vulnerable to disease. Most types of DOD are unlikely to form after 12 months of age. Lesions that become clinically relevant after this age have typically been formed at a younger age; nevertheless, correct nutrient balance is important in the growing yearling (Pagan, 2003).

The amount of supplementary grain required to maintain a desired growth rate varies, and it is important to feed each horse as an individual. "Easy-keeping" yearlings should be prevented from becoming fat by being fed a low-intake, low-calorie source of essential protein, vitamins, and minerals. On the other hand, yearlings that are large-framed with much growth potential can consume normal amounts of fortified concentrate.

Nutrition plays an important role in the pathogenesis of DOD in horses as deficiencies, excesses, and imbalances of nutrients affect the incidence and severity of physitis, angular limb deformity, wobbler syndrome, and osteochondritis dissecans (OCD) (Pagan, 2003). The most common feeding errors attributed to DOD are excessive grain intake, feeding an inappropriate grain for the forage being fed, and inadequate fortification of grain. These three scenarios are easily fixed by feeding an appropriate grain mix fortified for the young, growing horse and feeding it at the correct intake. Young horses already suffering from DOD should have their energy intakes reduced while maintaining correct levels of protein, vitamins, and minerals.

It is now commonly accepted that excessive energy intake can lead to rapid growth and increased body fat, which is thought to increase the incidence of certain types of DOD in Thoroughbred foals. Yearlings with OCD of the hock and stifle were large at birth, grew rapidly from 3 to 8 months of age, and were heavier than the average population as weanlings (Figure 5) (Pagan, 1998).

In addition to excessive energy, the source of calories for young horses may also be important. Foals that experience an exaggerated and sustained increase in circulating glucose or insulin in response to a carbohydrate (grain) meal may be predisposed to

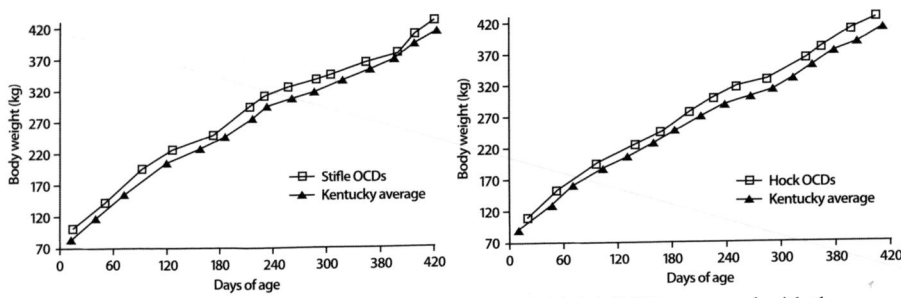

Figure 5. Body weights of foals with stifle (left) and hock (right) OCD compared with the Kentucky average (Pagan, 1998).

OCD. Research conducted by KER suggests that hyperinsulinemia may influence the incidence of OCD (surgically treated) in Thoroughbred weanlings (Pagan et al., 2001). In a large field trial, a high glucose and insulin response to a concentrate meal was associated with an increased incidence of OCD. Plasma glucose and insulin 2 h post feeding were significantly higher in weanlings with OCD than in unaffected foals (P < 0.05). Insulin/glucose ratios, however, were not significantly different (Table 2). The incidence of OCD was significantly higher in foals whose glucose and insulin values were greater than one standard deviation above the mean for the entire population (both OCD and unaffected) in the study (Table 3). Elevated insulin/glucose ratios did not appear to be correlated with an increased incidence of OCD. Glycemic responses measured in the weanlings were highly correlated with each feed's glycemic index (GI), suggesting that the GI of a farm's feed may play a role in the pathogenesis of OCD. Hyperinsulinemia may affect chondrocyte maturation, leading to altered matrix metabolism and faulty mineralization or altered cartilage growth by influencing other hormones such as thyroxine (Jeffcott and Henson, 1998). Based on the results of this study, it would be prudent to feed young horses concentrates that produce low glycemic responses such as feeds in which energy is supplied by fat and fermentable fiber sources (beet pulp and soy hulls).

Table 2. Plasma glucose, insulin, and insulin/glucose ratio two hours post feeding in weanling Thoroughbreds on six Kentucky farms (Pagan et al., 2001).

	Glucose (mg/dl)		Insulin (pmol/l)		Insulin/Glucose Ratio	
	OCD (n=25)	Unaffected (n=193)	OCD (n=25)	Unaffected (n=193)	OCD (n=25)	Unaffected (n=193)
Mean ± SE	150.1 ± 7.1	134.2 ± 1.9	130.3 ± 12.8	106.0 ± 3.4	0.85 ± 0.06	0.78 ± 0.02
Significance	P<0.01		P<0.05		P>0.10	

Mineral deficiency and/or excess of calcium, phosphorus, copper, and zinc may lead to DOD (Pagan, 2003). The ration of a growing horse should be properly fortified because commonly fed cereal grains and forages contain insufficient quantities of several important minerals. A ration of grass hay and oats would only supply about

Table 3. The relationship between glucose, insulin, and insulin/glucose ratio and the incidence of OCD in weanling Thoroughbreds on six Kentucky farms (Pagan et al., 2001).

Standard Deviation from Mean	Glucose		Insulin		Insulin/Glucose Ratio	
	% Population	% OCD	% Population	% OCD	% Population	% OCD
<1SD	11.0	0.0	10.1	0.0	15.1	6.0
±SE	72.9	10.1	78.0	11.2	68.3	12.1
<1SD	16.1	25.7	11.9	23.0	16.5	13.9

40% and 70% of a weanling's calcium and phosphorus requirement, respectively, and less than 40% of its requirement for copper and zinc. It is important to provide a balanced ration as the ratio of certain minerals (calcium to phosphorus; copper to zinc) is extremely important. The ideal ratio of calcium to phosphorus in the ration of young horses is 1.5:1 and should never fall below 1:1 or exceed 2.5:1. Too much calcium may affect phosphorus status, particularly if the level of phosphorus in the ration is marginal; conversely, high levels of phosphorus in the ration will inhibit the absorption of calcium and will lead to a deficiency, even if the amount of calcium present was normally adequate. Forage diets with high calcium levels should be supplemented with phosphorus. The ratio of zinc to copper should be 3:1 to 4:1.

Conclusion

Kentucky Equine Research (KER) has studied the growth and development of the equine athlete for nearly 20 years. The company's researchers have identified considerable differences among Thoroughbred growth patterns around the world, indicating that reference growth curves specific to location are important. Breeders aim to produce a fully-grown individual with minimal skeletal problems. To achieve this goal, reference growth curves have been formulated to help breeders monitor growth rates. Reference curves from horses raised in the same environment under similar conditions are more appropriate for breeders who wish to track the growth of their young stock than a general "Thoroughbred" curve. In addition, the use of percentiles to assess individual growth gives a much more useful comparison within a population and allows breeders to adjust nutrition and conditioning practices as necessary to affect growth.

Managing the growth and development of the athletic horse is a balancing act between achieving maximal physiological size and preventing developmental orthopedic disease. Maintaining a steady growth rate by providing appropriate amounts of correctly balanced, low-starch rations intended for growing horses and regularly weighing and measuring horses during the growth period is recommended to help maximize athletic potential before entering training.

References

Brown-Douglas, C.G., and J.D. Pagan. 2006. Body weight, wither height and growth rates in Thoroughbreds raised in America, England, Australia, New Zealand and India. In: Proc. Kentucky Equine Research Nutr. Conf. 15:15-22.

Brown-Douglas, C.G., J.D. Pagan, A. Koch, and S. Caddel. 2007. The relationship between size at yearling sale, sale price and future racing performance in Kentucky Thoroughbreds. In: Proc. Equine Sci. Soc. Symp. 20:153-154.

Brown-Douglas, C.G., J.D. Pagan, and A.J. Stromberg. 2006. Thoroughbred growth and future racing performance. In: Proc. Kentucky Equine Research Nutr. Conf. 15:125-139.

Jeffcott, L.B., and F.M. Henson. 1998. Studies on growth cartilage in the horse and their application to aetiopathologenesis of dyscondroplasia (osteochondrosis). Vet. J. 156:177-192.

Lawrence, L.A. 2003. Principles of bone development in horses. In: Proc. Kentucky Equine Research Nutr. Conf.12:69-73.

Pagan, J.D. 1998. The incidence of developmental orthopedic disease (DOD) on a Kentucky Thoroughbred farm. In: J.D. Pagan (Ed.) Advances in Equine Nutrition, Vol. I. p. 469-475. Nottingham University Press, Nottingham, U.K.

Pagan, J.D. 2003. The role of nutrition in the management of developmental orthopedic disease. In: Proc. Kentucky Equine Research Nutr. Conf. 12:40-56.

Pagan, J.D., C.G. Brown-Douglas, and S. Caddel. 2006. Body weight and condition of Kentucky Thoroughbred mares and their foals as influenced by month of foaling, season and gender. In: Proc. Kentucky Equine Research Nutr. Conf. 15:61-69.

Pagan, J.D., R.J. Geor, S.E. Caddel, P.B. Pryor, and K.E. Hoekstra. 2001. The relationship between glycemic response and the incidence of OCD in Thoroughbred weanlings: A field study. In: Proc. Amer. Assoc. Equine Practnr. 47:322-325.

Pagan, J.D., S.G. Jackson, and S. Caddel. 1996. A summary of growth rates of Thoroughbreds in Kentucky. Pferdeheilkunde 12:285-289.

Pagan, J.D., A. Koch, S. Caddel, and D. Nash. 2005. Size of Thoroughbred yearlings presented for auction at Keeneland sales affects selling price. In: Proc. Equine Sci. Soc. Symp. 19:224-225.

BODY WEIGHT, WITHER HEIGHT AND GROWTH RATES IN THOROUGHBREDS RAISED IN AMERICA, ENGLAND, AUSTRALIA, NEW ZEALAND AND INDIA

CLARISSA G. BROWN-DOUGLAS AND JOE D. PAGAN
Kentucky Equine Research, Versailles, Kentucky

Introduction

Past studies on the growth of Throughbreds have been limited to small populations located primarily in the northern hemisphere (Green, 1969; McCarthy and Mitchell, 1974; Hintz, 1978; Hintz et al., 1979; Thompson, 1995; Jelan et al., 1996; Pagan, 1996; Jones and Hollands, 2005). There are fewer data available on Southern Hemisphere populations (Grace et al., 1999 and 2001; Nash, 2001; Brown Douglas et al., 2005) and there has been no detailed comparison made between the growth patterns of Thoroughbreds in different countries.

Thoroughbred populations around the globe are of similar genetic makeup so it could be assumed that the patterns of growth would be comparable between countries, and growth curves described by scientists in one country may be applied to Thoroughbreds in another.

The purpose of this study was to obtain growth data from populations of Thoroughbreds born and raised in the USA, England, Australia, New Zealand, and India and present and compare body weight, daily weight gain, and wither height growth curves.

Materials and Method

Thoroughbreds born and raised on commercial and private farms in America, England, Australia, New Zealand, and India were weighed monthly during the years 1996 to 2006 (Table 1). Wither height was also measured in approximately 85% of the horses.

The data were split into foal-age categories: 1-15 days (7 days), 16-45 days (1 month), 46-75 days (2 months), 76-105 days (3 months), 106-135 days (4 months), 136-165 days (5 months), and so on up to 18 months of age. Splits were chosen such that the relationship between foal age and foal weight was approximately linear and to ensure that the vast majority of the foals were measured only once per age category.

Table 1. Summary of data collected from Thoroughbreds in America, England, Australia, New Zealand, and India.

Population	Number	Colts	Fillies	Sires	Farms
Kentucky	6783	3359	3424	682	76
Australia	2653	1290	1363	266	17
England	1233	607	626	235	38
India	939	468	471	110	8
New Zealand	925	374	551	136	8
Rest of USA	896	472	424	268	12
Total	**13429**	**6570**	**6859**	**1117**	**159**

Data Analysis

All growth data from each country for the ten seasons were initially analyzed separately, but as there were no significant differences for any parameter between the seasons ($p<0.05$), data were combined for further analysis.

A linear regression model with foal age as the explanatory variable and country as the response variable was used to predict weight, height, and ADG and provide a confidence interval for the mean response at a specified age within each month of age category. When gender was being considered, it was included as an explanatory variable. When a significant ($p<0.05$) main effect or interaction was found, multiple comparisons were made using the least significant difference method. Computations were done using JMP 6.0 (SAS, Inc., Cary, NC). Results are expressed as mean ± 95% confidence interval and significance is reported at the 5% level.

Results

Australian Thoroughbreds were significantly heavier and taller at 7 days and 18 months of age than Thoroughbreds in all other countries. Australian and New Zealand Thoroughbreds were significantly heavier than other populations between one and four months of age, and seven and eighteen months of age. English Thoroughbreds were significantly lighter than in all other countries except India between 7 days and 4 months of age. At 4 months of age there were no significant differences in foal body weight between countries, with the exception of foals in India, which were significantly smaller (Table 2 and 3, Figure 1 and 2).

Table 2. Body weight (kg) ± 95% confidence interval of Thoroughbreds reared in America, Australia, England, India, and New Zealand compared with the world average. Differing superscripts within a row indicate significant differences (p<0.05).

Age (mth)	Kentucky	USA (excl KY)	Australia	England	India	New Zealand	World Avg
0	67.5±0.3[b]	69.8±1.1[a]	69.6±0.5[a]	64.5±0.9[c]	62.2±0.6[d]	65.6±2.1[b]	66.9
1	99.3±0.4[b]	100.8±1.1[b]	102.4±0.7[a]	95.4±1.0[c]	90.5±0.7[d]	102.0±2.2[a]	98.6
6	250.7±0.7[a]	246.0±1.6[b]	251.4±1.3[a]	248.0±2.0[b]	224.8±1.4[c]	248.1±1.8[b]	247.1
12	353.3±1.0[b]	349.6±2.3[b]	357.8±1.6[a]	349.6±2.8[b]	326.2±2.1[c]	357.5±3.9[a]	350.7
18	453.9±1.7[b]	455.9±5.4[b]	460.7±3.9[a]	442.8±6.0[c]	408.8±2.9[d]	.	444.9

Table 3. Wither height (cm) ± 95% confidence interval of Thoroughbreds reared in America, Australia, England, India, and New Zealand compared with the world average. Differing superscripts within a row indicate significant differences (p<0.05).

Age	Kentucky	USA (excl KY)	Australia	England	India	New Zealand	World Avg
7 days	105.7±0.2[b]	105.2±0.6[bc]	110.9±0.4[a]	104.5±0.7[c]	102.2±0.5[d]	105.2±4.3[bcd]	106.1
1 mo.	112.6±0.1[a]	112.5±0.4[a]	112.2±0.4[a]	111.5±0.5[b]	108.0±0.3[c]	113.1±1.4[a]	112.0
6 mo.	135.9±0.1[a]	135.4±0.4[a]	135.0±0.4[a]	134.4±0.5[a]	131.2±0.3[b]	134.7±0.4[a]	135.0
12 mo	147.8±0.3[a]	147.8±0.5[a]	147.4±0.3[a]	145.8±0.5[b]	144.2±0.3[c]	147.4±0.6[a]	147.1
18 mo.	154.7±0.2[b]	154.4±0.8[b]	156.0±0.7[a]	153.1±0.8[b]	151.2±0.3[c]	.	153.8

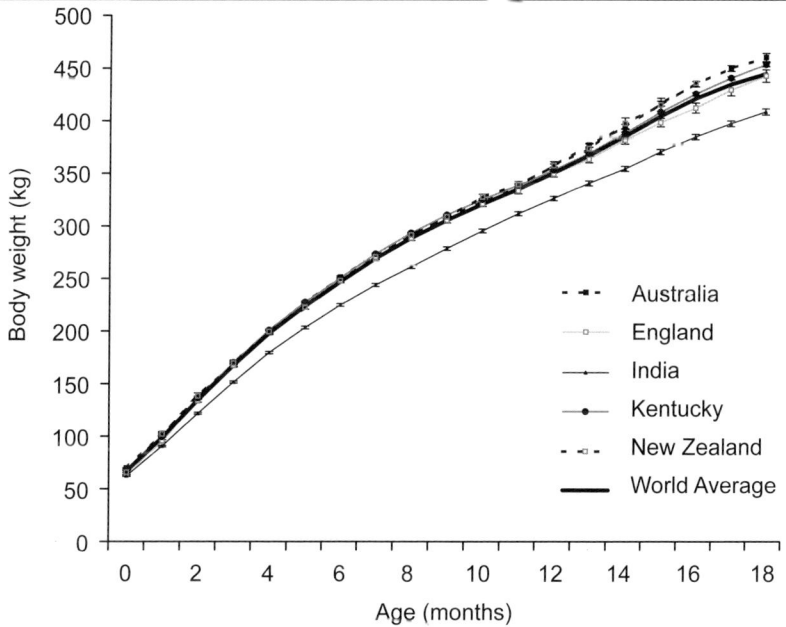

Figure 1. Body weight ± 95% confidence interval (kg) of Thoroughbreds reared in Australia, England, India, America, and New Zealand compared with the world average.

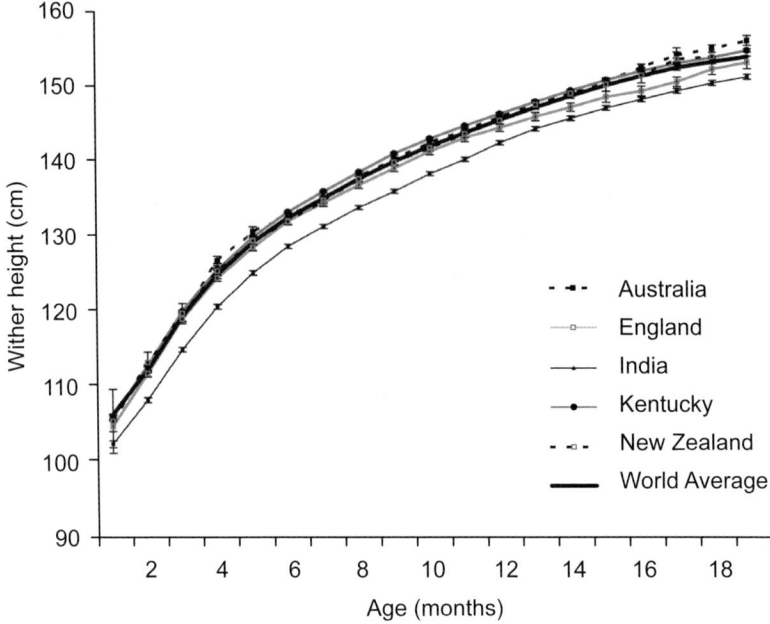

Figure 2. Wither height ± 95% confidence interval (cm) of Thoroughbreds reared in Australia, England, India, America, and New Zealand compared with the world average.

Indian Thoroughbreds were significantly smaller (lighter and shorter) than all other Thoroughbred populations throughout the study (P<0.05). Birth weights of Indian foals were significantly less than those raised in Kentucky, Australia, and England at 49.4 ± 0.5 kg (95% CI) vs. 54.4 ± 0.4 kg, 54.9 ± 0.5 kg, and 53.1 ± 0.5 kg, respectively (P<0.05).

At 6 months of age, Kentucky and Australian foals were heavier than those born in England, New Zealand, and India. However, there was no significant difference in height between foals of any countries except for those in India, which were significantly shorter. At 12 months of age Australasian (Australian and New Zealand) and American foals were heavier and taller than English and Indian foals. Between 15 and 18 months Australasian Thoroughbreds were significantly heavier than those of all other countries. There were no significant differences in height between Australian and American Thoroughbreds between 12 and 16 months, but Australian Thoroughbreds were taller at 17 and 18 months.

Thoroughbreds raised in America, England, Australia, and New Zealand exhibited a similar pattern of ADG over the first 11 months of their life (Figure 3). Over this 11-month period, ADG declined at a constant rate from maximum values immediately after birth (between 1.4 and 1.6 kg/d at 1 month of age) to reach a low of 0.5 to 0.6 kg/d at 11 months of age. Between 13 and 16 months of age Thoroughbreds in America, England, Australia, and New Zealand exhibited ADGs of between 0.7 and 1.0 kg/d.

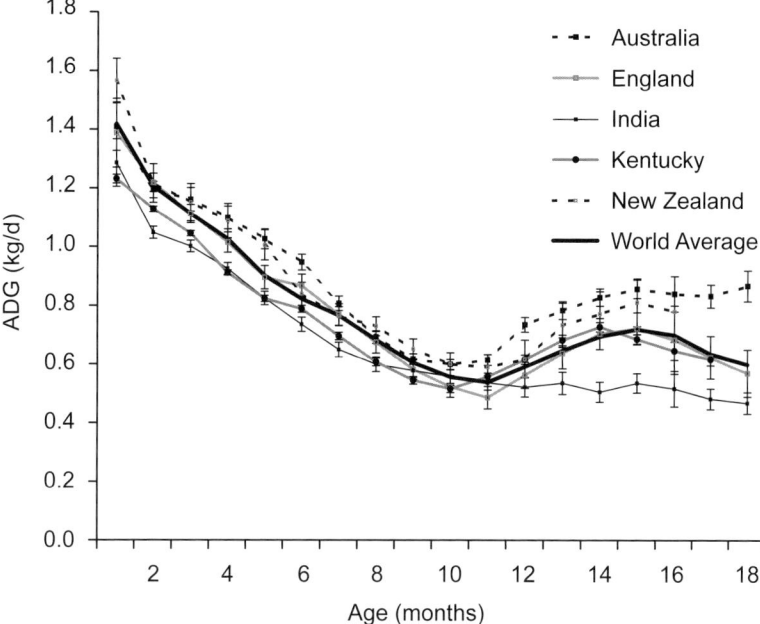

Figure 3. Average daily gain ± 95% confidence interval (kg/d) of Thoroughbreds reared in Australia, England, India, America, and New Zealand compared with the world average.

ADG in Indian horses steadily declined from 1.3 kg/d at 1 month of age to 0.5 kg/d at 18 months of age and did not exhibit the increase in ADG between 10 and 14 months of age of other Thoroughbred populations. The ADGs of Indian Thoroughbreds were significantly less than in other countries of the world between 13 and 15 months of age ($P<0.05$).

Discussion

Significant differences in body weight, wither height, and average daily gain were observed between the populations of Thoroughbreds. In general, Australian and New Zealand Thoroughbreds tended to be larger than American Thoroughbreds, which in turn were larger than those reared in England.

Body weights and wither heights for Kentucky Thoroughbreds reported in this study are within 1 to 2% of those reported in an earlier study of Kentucky Thoroughbreds (Pagan, 1996). However, in contrast to published English data collected from 200 horses (Jones and Hollands, 2005), body weights of 1233 English Thoroughbreds in this study were up to 20% heavier (Table 4). The data from our study, while still showing that English Thoroughbreds are smaller than American Thoroughbreds, indicates that large numbers of the population should be sampled to create accurate references.

Table 4. Body weight comparisons between English and Kentucky Thoroughbreds in this and prior studies. Percentages in brackets indicate the percentage difference between body weights of English Thoroughbreds in the present study and published data for English Thoroughbreds.

Country	Study	14 d	32 d	183 d	350 d	490 d
UK (n=200)	Jones and Hollands (2005)	64.2	78.9	224.4	358.5	424.5
England (n=1233)	Present study	72.6 (+12%)	97.3 (+20%)	253.5 (+11%)	345.0 (-4%)	427.4 (+1%)
KY (n=700)	Pagan (1996)	76.1-77.7	.	250.7-255.9	335.2-349.2	418.0-427.8
KY (n=6783)	Present study	74.6-76.7	99.7-101.4	249.3-254.8	339.4-354.7	423.2-438.2

At 12 months of age, American Thoroughbreds were taller but not heavier than English Thoroughbreds. However, at 18 months of age, American Thoroughbreds were significantly heavier than English Thoroughbreds, but there was no significant difference in height. A similar trend was observed between Thoroughbreds raised in Australasia compared with those raised in America. At 12 months of age, Australasian Thoroughbreds were heavier and taller than those in all other countries. Between 15 and 18 months, Australasian Thoroughbreds were significantly heavier than those in all other countries; however, there were no significant differences in height between Australasian and American Thoroughbreds. This is most likely representative of the difference in management of yearlings prepared for sale. Australasian yearlings tend to be sold in a well-rounded condition with higher condition scores compared with American yearlings which are presented as leaner, more athletic and fit. This trend is beginning to change as breeders and buyers realize the potential musculoskeletal problems associated with over-conditioned yearlings.

These observations may further be attributed to the management of growing horses for different racing industries under different growing conditions. In general, the American racing industry has significantly more short-distance dirt races than the industries of England, Australia, and New Zealand, and as a result, American Thoroughbreds are raised to be precocious sprinting horses ready to race at two years old. In contrast, the English racing industry holds turf races commonly of distances greater than 1 mile, and as a result England has traditionally produced slower-maturing Thoroughbreds bred to run on turf. Australia and New Zealand are also known to produce turf-racing Thoroughbreds; however, these southern hemisphere horses are traditionally known for their size, which may be attributed to genetics, even though shuttle stallions have had a significant impact on evening out the genetic pool between hemispheres.

Thoroughbreds in all countries except for India showed low ADGs around 10 to 11 months and increases in ADGs between 13 and 16 months. As these horses were all born in the spring and early summer, the decline in growth rate around 10 and 11 months of age coincides with the winter months of decreased pasture quality and availability. The increase in ADG after 11 months of age in these horses could be attributed to the onset of spring pasture growth.

The ADGs of Indian Thoroughbreds declined steadily between 1 and 18 months, did not increase between 10 and 14 months of age, and were significantly less than those of horses in the rest of the world at 13-15 months of age ($P<0.05$). This significant result could be attributed to differences in nutritional management of Indian Thoroughbreds as well as climatic conditions in that country. Horse farms in India rely heavily on grain and harvested forage, predominantly alfalfa, as sources of nutrition for their growing horses (Peter Huntington, personal communication). In contrast to the other countries in this study, Indian horses have restricted or no access to pasture. The climate in India ranges from a dry, cool winter (December - February) to a dry, hot summer (March - May) and heavy monsoon conditions (June - September) (National Geographic, 2003). It is therefore understandable that horses growing in these tropical monsoon conditions will not exhibit an increase in ADG between 10 and 14 months of age associated with seasonal increase in pasture growth in temperate climates. Furthermore, the effect of demanding climatic conditions on managing growing horses could contribute to the overall smaller size of the Indian Thoroughbreds compared with those raised in temperate climates under different management conditions. Indian horses are reported to spend a significant amount of time indoors due to extreme heat in the summer and monsoon season in the fall. This restricted access to pasture and exercise may hinder growth potential of these horses. Indian bloodstock is sourced predominantly from North America and most foals arrive in India in-situ with their dams following a November or January broodmare sale. Anecdotal evidence suggests these pregnant mares may experience a difficult journey from the US to India and this stress is reported to act negatively on the size and health of their foals, which is evident in their significantly lower birth weights compared with other countries. Thoroughbreds in India begin their racing career at 3-4 years of age and it is thought that by 2 to 2 1/2 years of age, these horses have caught up in size with the world population. Data from Indian yearlings were not analysed after 18 months, so this observation cannot be verified.

The considerable differences in the patterns of growth between Thoroughbreds in different geographical regions indicate that reference growth curves created specifically for each country would be beneficial.

Acknowledgements

The authors would like to thank Arnold J. Stromberg, Ph.D., Professor and Director of Graduate Studies Department of Statistics, University of Kentucky for help with the statistical analysis.

References

Brown-Douglas, C.G. Parkinson, T.J., Firth, E.C. and Fennessy, P.F. (2005) Bodyweights and growth rates of spring- and autumn-born Thoroughbred horses raised on pasture. New Zealand Veterinary Journal 53, 326-331.

Grace, N. D. Gee, E. K., Firth, E. C. and Shaw, H. L. (2002) Digestible energy intake, dry matter digestibility and mineral status of grazing Thoroughbred yearlings. New Zealand Veterinary Journal 50, 63-69.

Grace, N. D. Pearce, S. G., Firth, E. C. and Fennessy, P. F. (1999) Concentrations of macro- and micro-elements in the milk of pasture-fed Thoroughbred mares. Australian Veterinary Journal 77, 177-180.

Green, D. A. (1969) A study of growth rate in Thoroughbred foals. British Veterinary Journal 125, 539-546.

Hintz H. F., Hintz, R. L. and Van Vleck, L. D. (1979) Growth rate of Thoroughbreds: Effect of age of dam, year and month of birth, and sex of foal. Journal of Animal Science 48, 480-487.

Hintz, H. F. (1978) Growth rate of horses. Proceedings of the American Association of Equine Practitioners 24, 480-487.

Jelan, Z. A., Jeffcott, L. B., Lundeheim, N. and Osborne, M. (1996) Growth rates in Thoroughbred foals. Pferdeheilkunde 12, 291-295.

Jones, L. and Hollands, T. (2005) Estimation of growth rates in UK Thoroughbreds. Pferdeheilkunde 21, 121-123.

McCarthy, D. and Mitchell, J. (1974) A study of growth rate in Thoroughbred foals and yearlings. Irish Journal of Agricultural Research 13, 111-117.

Nash, D. G., Avery, A., Dempsey, W. and Nash, G. (2001) Growth and development of young Thoroughbred horses on temperate Australian pastures. Proceedings of the 17th Equine Nutrition Physiology Symposium 17, 196-198.

National Geographic Society (ed) (2003) National Geographic Concise Atlas of the World.

Pagan, J. D. Jackson, S. G. and Caddel, S. (1996) A summary of growth rates of Thoroughbreds in Kentucky. Pferdeheilkunde 12, 285-289.

Thompson, K. N. (1995) Skeletal growth rates in weanling and yearling Thoroughbred horses. Journal of Animal Science 73, 2513-2517.

SIZE MATTERS AT THE SALES

JOE D. PAGAN[1], ANTHONY KOCH[2], AND STEVE CADDEL[2]
[1]Kentucky Equine Research, Versailles, Kentucky
[2]Hallway Feeds, Lexington, Kentucky

Many factors affect the sale price of Thoroughbred yearlings at public auction. Pedigree, conformation, and the racing performance of siblings determine whether a yearling commands bids in the thousands or millions. But what about size? Does the yearling's body weight, height, and body condition influence how well it sells? Kentucky Equine Research (KER) and Hallway Feeds in Lexington conducted a study at the 2003 Keeneland September Yearling Sale that attempted to answer these questions.

Body weight, withers height, and body condition score measurements were taken in late August and early September from 294 yearlings that were to sell at Keeneland. The yearlings were then tracked through the sales where their session number and sale price were recorded. Yearlings that were listed as RNA (reserve not attained; horse was not sold because of low final bid) were also recorded. Yearlings in the study came from 16 different farms and were sold by 20 different consignors.

Two hundred forty-nine of the yearlings in this study were listed as sold. This represented over 8% of the total yearlings sold in this sale. The average and median prices of these yearlings were $106,810 and $40,000, respectively, compared to an average and median of $92,329 and $34,000 for the entire sale. Forty-five of the 294 yearlings (15%) were listed as RNA.

The average age of the yearlings at sale time was 538 days. The measurements used in the study were taken an average of 16 days before sale day. Not surprisingly, on average colts (n = 161) were heavier (1003 lb vs 955 lb) and taller (15.1 hands vs 15 hands) than fillies (n = 133). Colts also averaged slightly lower in body condition score than fillies (5.8 vs 5.9). Body condition score is a relative measure of the amount of body fat that the yearling is carrying. A higher condition score indicates that the yearling is carrying greater fat cover. Although the scoring system goes from 1 (emaciated) to 9 (grossly obese), all of the yearlings measured fell into a narrow range of 5.5 to 6.5.

To evaluate whether body size and condition affect sales price, the data were evaluated in two ways. First, the yearlings were divided into two groups based on whether their sale price was above or below the median price of the session in which they were sold. The rationale for this division was that the yearlings had already been assigned to a particular session based on their relative value, which was determined largely on pedigree and conformation. Therefore, if body size truly affected sales price it should be reflected by whether yearlings sold for more or less than their session median. In this primary evaluation, the last bid for RNA horses was considered as the sale price. A second evaluation compared all RNA yearlings (n = 45) with all yearlings listed as sold (n = 249).

Comparison by Session

Yearlings that brought bids above their session median were significantly heavier (995 lbs vs 970 lbs) (Figure 1) and slightly taller (Figure 2) than those below the median, but they did not have significantly higher condition scores (Figure 3).

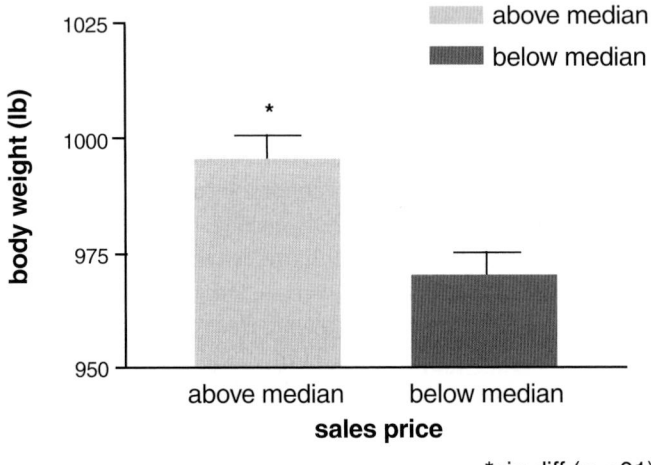

*sig diff (p <.01)

Figure 1. Body weight (lb) of all sales yearlings relative to session median price.

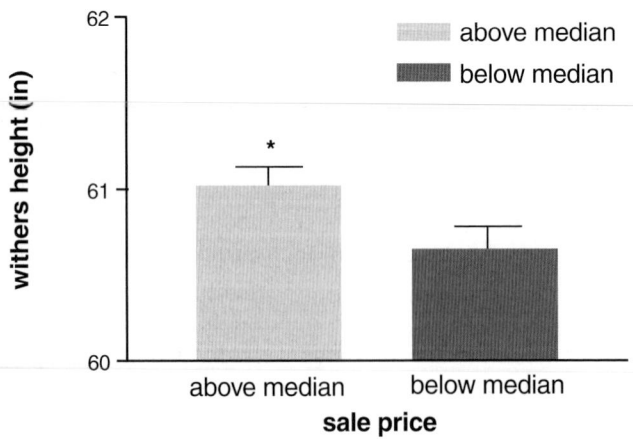

*sig diff (p <.05)

Figure 2. Withers height (in) of all sales yearlings relative to session median price.

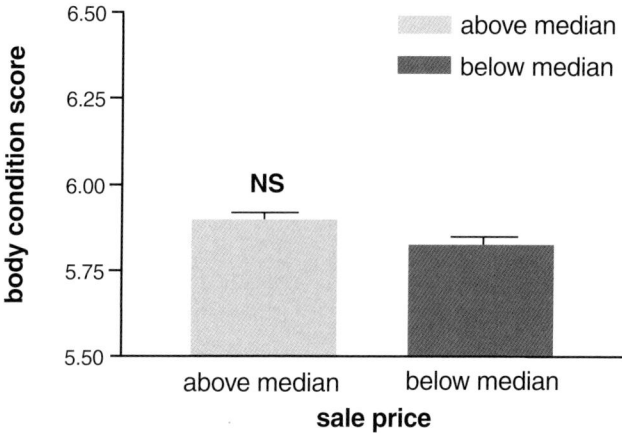

Figure 3. Body condition score of all sales yearlings relative to session median price.

Some of these difference in body weight and height were related to age (544 days vs 535 days) (Figure 4) and gender. There was a greater percentage of colts that sold above the session median than fillies (61% vs 39%).

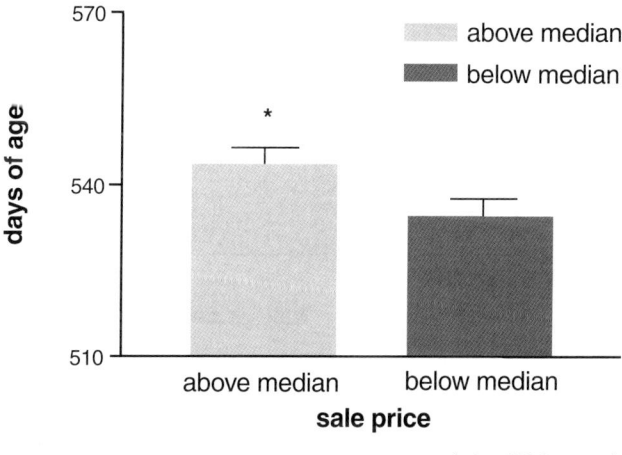

Figure 4. Age (days) of all sales yearlings relative to session median price.

Because of these age and gender effects, the data for colts and fillies were re-analyzed separately. Body weight was still significantly greater in both colts and fillies that received bids above their session median (Figure 5). Withers height, however, was no longer significantly different between groups in either colts or fillies (Figure 6).

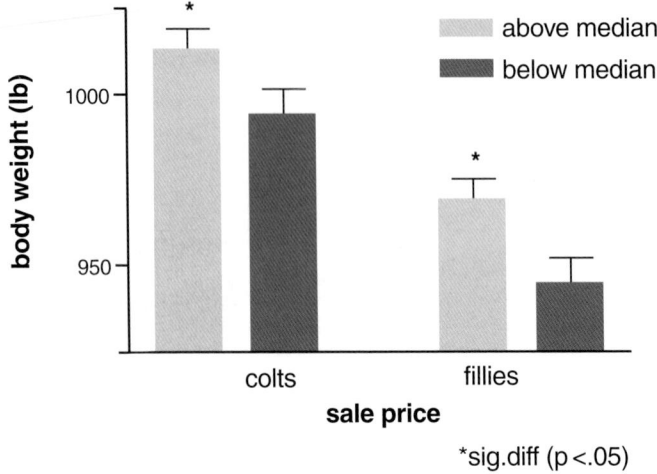

Figure 5. Body weight (lb) of colts and fillies relative to session median price.

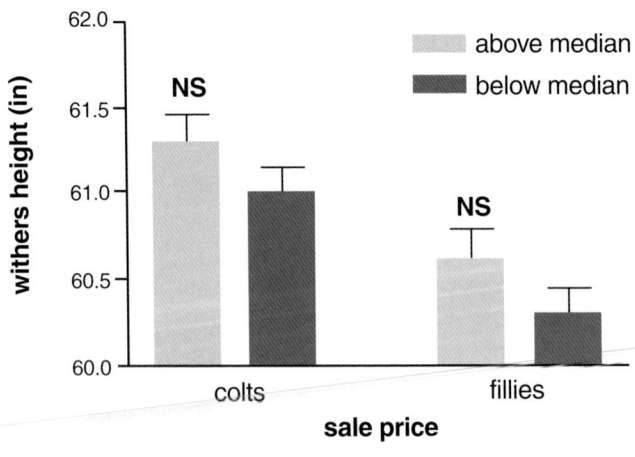

Figure 6. Withers height (in) of colts and fillies relative to session median price.

Fillies that received bids above their session median were significantly older (544 days vs 530 days) (Figure 7) than those selling below. There was no significant difference in the age of colts selling above and below their session median.

To remove the effect of age and gender from the analysis, each yearling's body weight and height were expressed as a percentage of the average for the same gender and age, which was calculated by linear regression of age vs body weight or height (Figures 8-11).

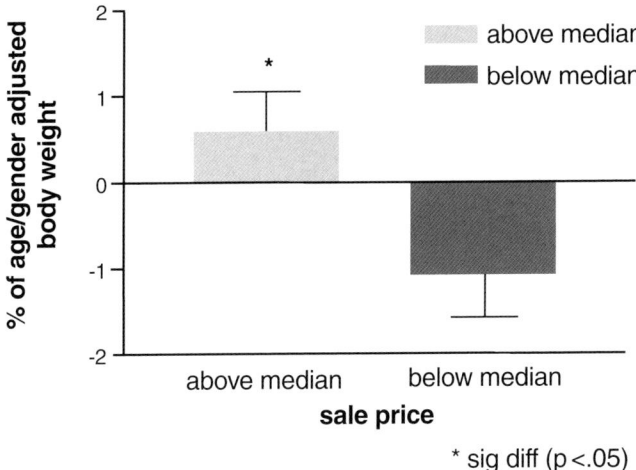

Figure 12. Body weight adjusted for age and gender relative to session median price.

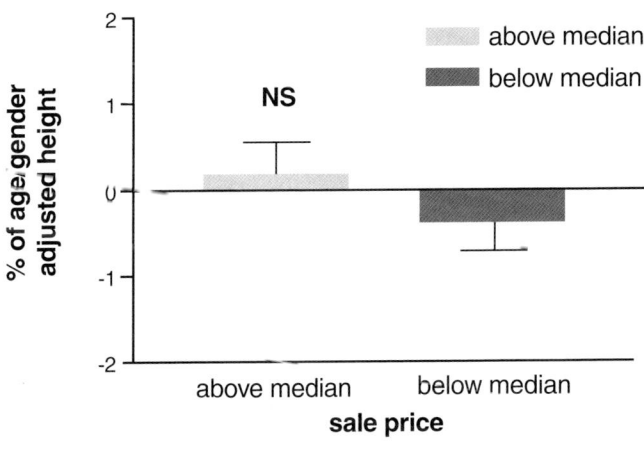

Figure 13. Withers height adjusted for age and gender relative to session median price.

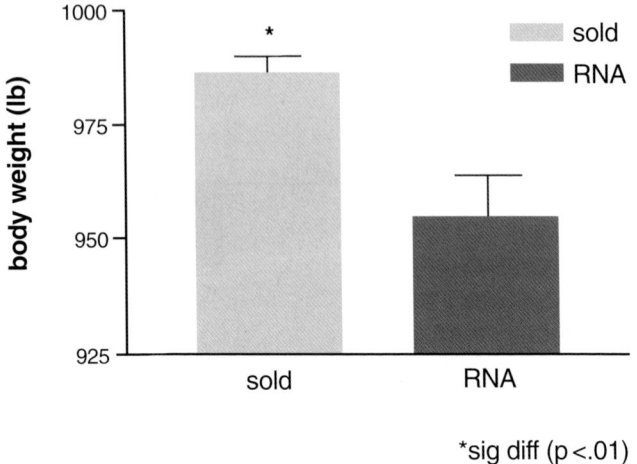

Figure 14. Body weight of yearlings listed as RNA vs yearlings listed as sold.

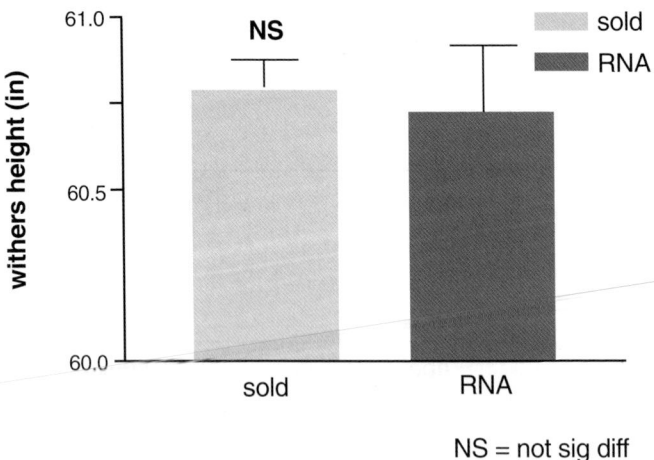

Figure 15. Withers height of yearlings listed as RNA vs yearlings listed as sold.

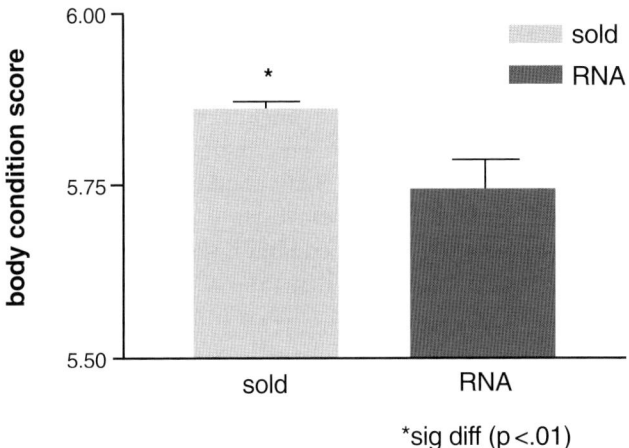

Figure 16. Body condition score of yearlings listed as RNA vs yearlings listed as sold.

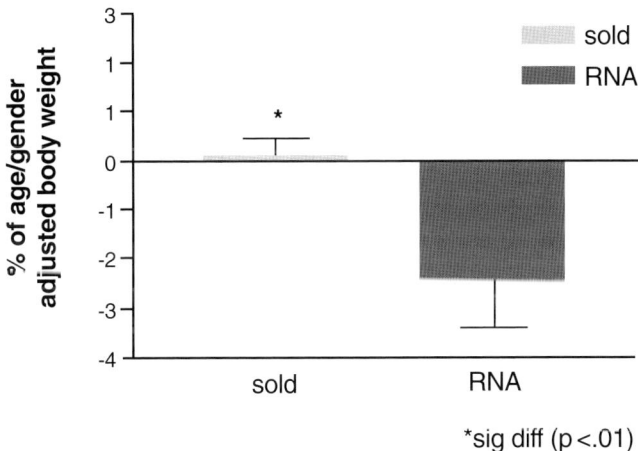

Figure 17. Body weight adjusted for age and gender in yearlings listed as sold or RNA.

Conclusions

Yearlings that commanded bids higher than the median price of the session in which they were sold tended to be heavier and slightly taller, but not fatter, than yearlings receiving bids below their session's median price. Some of this difference was related to gender, since more colts sold above the median price than fillies. Age also played a role, especially in fillies. When these measurements were adjusted to account for age and gender effects, yearlings selling above the session median were still heavier, but not taller, than those below the session median. Although it can't be determined from these data, it is likely that yearlings selling above their session median price represented individuals with more substance and a more heavily muscled, athletic physique resulting from a combination of genetics, nutrition, and exercise.

Interestingly, yearlings listed as RNA were lighter than horses listed as sold and a higher percentage of them had lower body condition scores. These data suggest that the ideal condition score for a sales yearling is 6.0 on a scale from 1 to 9. Yearlings presented for sale with lower condition scores are less likely to meet the sellers' expectations.

THOROUGHBRED GROWTH AND FUTURE RACING PERFORMANCE

CLARISSA G. BROWN-DOUGLAS[1], JOE D. PAGAN[1], AND ARNOLD J. STROMBERG[2]
[1]Kentucky Equine Research, Versailles, Kentucky
[2]University of Kentucky, Lexington, Kentucky

Introduction

The success of a Thoroughbred racehorse is determined by a multitude of factors, many of which are impossible to evaluate. Thoroughbreds are commonly selected for racing ability by pedigree and conformation analysis. There have been few studies associating growth and body size with racing performance (Pagan, 1998a; Cain, 2006; Smith et al., 2006).

The genetic make-up, or genotype, contributes to a horse's racing ability by influencing physical characteristics including conformation, lung capacity, and growth potential, and mental attributes including the "will to win." Environmental factors such as nutrition, exercise, and conditioning are difficult to quantify, and management during growth and development as well as trainer variation all influence the horse's potential for success. Many methods of anatomical or pre-competitive performance assessment are employed by Thoroughbred breeders, trainers, bloodstock agents, and owners. However, these methods are subjective and there have been no established and fail-proof methods for predicting potential success.

A large retrospective study conducted by Cecil Seaman of Thoroughbred Analysts using body measurements taken at Thoroughbred sales concluded that horses in the "underweight" to "ideal weight" (±2% optimum weight) range earned significantly more than those in the "overweight" to "obese" categories (Pagan, 1998a; Cain, 2006). However, body weights in this study were estimated and not actually measured.

A study of 260 Thoroughbreds born in 1981 and 1982 described associations between yearling body measurements and racing performance (Smith et al., 2006). It was reported that hip height, body length, and heart girth were positively correlated with win percentage (number of wins/number of starts). There were no significant correlations between any body measurement and lifetime earnings; however, the study reported a trend linking taller fillies and greater earnings. Horses that won or placed in a stakes race tended to be taller as yearlings.

Mature size and the pattern of growth are influenced by the genetic make-up of the horse and the environment, but it is inconclusive if growth plays a role in the success of a racehorse. It is known that heavier foals have a greater incidence of osteochondrosis (Pagan, 1998b). Foals that developed hock and stifle OCD tended to be heavier at birth and fast-growing between 3 and 8 months. Furthermore, it is reported that heavier but not taller yearlings command higher prices at public auction (Pagan et al., 2005).

The purpose of this study in Thoroughbreds was to make objective measurements of a horse's growth to determine if certain characteristics affect the odds of its success as a racehorse.

Materials and Method

Racing performance data were collected from 3,734 Thoroughbreds raised in the USA between 1996 and 2002 and their growth records were retrospectively examined to determine if various growth characteristics could be associated with success as a racehorse.

The population consisted of 1,850 fillies and 1,884 colts raised on 55 commercial and private farms in the states of Kentucky (n=3,199), California (n=183), and Virginia (n=352). The population was represented by 456 sires.

Growth measurements (body weight using an electronic scale and wither height) were taken approximately every 30 days; however, the number of records per horse ranged from 1 to 18. Growth variables were converted into percentiles and quartiles for analysis. Percentiles and quartiles provided a standard unit of measurement to compare an individual horse to the population. Percentiles rank the relative position of an individual in the population by indicating what percent of the reference population that individual will equal or exceed. The 50th percentile is the median. Percentiles take into account the spread of data around the mean. The reference growth population used was the USA Thoroughbred separated for fillies and colts. This reference population was created by Kentucky Equine Research using data from approximately 7000 Thoroughbreds.

Racing results were collected from the American Produce Records (Bloodstock Research Information Services Inc, Lexington, Kentucky, USA, 2006) and are complete up to October 2005. Variables recorded for each horse included registered name, total years raced and country(s) raced in, total number of starts, wins, shows and placings, total number of starts as a two-year-old, wins as a two-year-old, starts and wins on a turf track, dirt-sprint starts and wins, dirt-distance (> one mile) starts and wins, starts and wins on a muddy or sloppy track, and stakes wins and places (classified as either listed or graded stakes). Each horse's standard starts index (SSI), also known as the racing index (RI), was recorded. The SSI indicates the earning power of an individual based on average earnings per start and enables comparison of racing performance of horses regardless of year of birth or gender. An SSI of 1.00 represents the average for each crop.

To account for genetic variation, the sire index (SI), also known as the sire production index (SPI), was collected for each horse. The SI indicates the average racing class of foals sired by a stallion and is calculated by averaging the SSI of all the stallion's foals that have started three or more times in North America or Europe.

DATA ANALYSIS

Growth data were divided into four age groups: foal (1 month or 0-30 d), suckling (2-6 months or 31-180 d), weanling (7-12 months or 181-360 d), and yearling (13-18 months or 361-555 d). Within each age group, individuals had between 1 and 6 measurements. The averages of the growth percentiles were calculated so that each individual had 4 percentiles for weight and height over the study.

Percentile data were then grouped into quartiles, so that instead of dividing the data into 100 even divisions, the data were divided into 4 divisions. Animals could then be described in the first quartile (percentile of 0-25), the second quartile (percentile of 26-50), the third quartile (percentile of 51-75), and the fourth quartile (percentile of 76-100) for weight or height.

Using the racing performance data, observations were made regarding each horse's status as a racehorse. First, horses were catalogued as being "raced" or "unraced." Unraced horses were unnamed, named with no race record, or named and unraced. All the horses in the population were then classified as having started or not started as two-year-olds. Win percentage was calculated for horses that raced by dividing total number of wins by total number of starts.

The data were presented in two different ways. First, in each age group the average growth percentiles were compared between the two groups within each performance measure (raced vs. unraced, winners vs. non-winners, raced at two years old vs. not raced at two years old, stakes winners vs. not stakes winners, graded stakes winners vs. not graded stakes winners, and G1 winners vs. not G1 winners).

Second, for each age group (foal, suckling, weanling, and yearling) the percentage of raced, raced at two years old, winners, stakes winners, graded stakes winners, or G1 winners in each growth quartile (both weight and height) was calculated.

STATISTICAL ANALYSIS

Data for weight and height quartile (as the response variable) for each factor (raced, raced at two years old, winner, stakes winner, graded stakes winner, G1 winner) were analyzed using an analysis of variance with respect to age category. When a significant ($p<0.05$) main effect or interaction was found, multiple comparisons were made using the least significant difference method. Data for earnings, sire index, and number of starts for each quartile (weight and height as the factor) for each age group were also analyzed using an analysis of variance.

In each age group, the percentages of raced vs. unraced, winners vs. non-winners, raced at two years old vs. not raced at two years old, stakes winners vs. not stakes winners, graded stakes winners vs. not graded stakes winners, and G1 winners vs. not G1 winners were compared for the four quartiles using Pearson's Chi Square test statistics. P-values less than 0.05 indicate that the percentage of yes was significantly different among the four quartiles.

A logistic regression model was applied in each age group to predict the probability of being a stakes winner based on sire index, exact weight percentile, exact height percentile, and their various interactions.

Results are expressed as mean ± standard error of the mean (sem) unless otherwise indicated. Computations were done using JMP 6.0 (SAS, Inc., Cary, NC) and NCSS (Number Crunching Statistical Systems, Kaysville, UT).

Results

STUDY POPULATION AND RACING PERFORMANCE

Of the 3,734 foals, 79% (2,940) started in a race and 71% (2,088) of those won at least one race. More colts raced than fillies (82% vs. 74%) and of those, more colts than fillies won at least one race (73% vs. 69%). However, of those that raced, fewer colts started as two-year-olds than fillies (44% vs. 51%). There was no difference in the percentage of two-year-old winners (36% vs. 34% for colts and fillies respectively), but more colts than fillies won two-year-old stakes (9.2% vs. 4.6%) and G1 races at any age (1.2% vs. 0.9%) (Table 1).

Table 1. Summary of the study population.

Numbers	Colts	Fillies	Total
Born	1884	1850	3734
Starters	1544	1396	2940
Winners (horses that won at least one race)	1124	964	2088
Repeat winners	797	605	1402
Raced as two-year-old	673	714	1387
Winner as two-year-old	245	243	488
Registered names	1814	1800	3614
Named unraced	270	404	674
Unnamed	70	50	120
Total unraced	340	454	794
Two-year-old stakes winners	47	33	80
Stakes winners	143	122	265
Stakes placed	249	205	454
Graded stakes winners	67	40	107
G1 winners	18	13	31
Millionaires	13	8	21

The majority of starters (60%) had racing careers of one to two years (66% fillies and 55% colts) while 14% of fillies and 26% of colts raced for four or more years.

Only two fillies compared with 24 colts in the data set raced for more than seven years (Table 2).

Table 2. Summary of years raced in the racing careers of the study population.

Years raced in career	Colts	Fillies	Total
1	366	382	748 (25.4%)
2	477	544	1021 (34.7%)
3	299	299	598
4	197	114	311
5	119	45	164
6	62	10	72
7+	24	2	26
Average number of years raced ± SD	2.69 ± 1.50	2.24 ± 1.10	
Median number of years raced (range)	2 (1-10)	2 (1-7)	

The number of career starts ranged from 1 to 85 with a median of 11 and an average of 15 ± 13.4 (SD) (Table 3). Average earnings per starter were $79,384 (median = $27,187), and average career earnings for colts and fillies were $93,184 vs. $64,143 respectively. Colts also earned more per start than fillies ($5,913 vs. $4,730). The average SSI of all starters was 1.92 (1.96 vs. 1.87 for colts and fillies respectively).

A total of 2,565 (84.2%) starters in this study raced in the USA and of those, 56 also raced overseas. The most common racing destination after the USA was the UK (218 horses) followed by Japan (122 horses), France (57), UAE (29), Puerto Rico (31), Italy (16), Germany (3), and Panama (2). Brazil, Hong Kong, South Africa, and Turkey had one horse each from the data.

In contrast with the breed average, the population of horses in this study had a greater number of starters (79% vs. 70%), winners/foals (56% vs. 47%), repeat winners/foals (37.5% vs. 35.9%), stakes winners (7.1% vs. 3.5%), graded stakes winners (2.9% vs. 0.8%), and G1 winners (0.8% vs. 0.2%) (Table 4).

In addition, the horses in this study had fewer career starts compared with the breed average (15 vs. 21), but greater average earnings per start ($5,352 vs. $1,723). Although in both this study and in the breed average, fillies earned less per start than colts, the difference between these was greater in the current study with the average earnings per start for fillies at 80.0% of colts compared with 92.3% in the total population.

Table 3. Summary of racing statistics from the study population.

KER racehorse population	
(3734 horses born between 1996 and 2002)	
Starters/foals	78.7%
Winners/foals (starters)	55.9% (71.0%)
Repeat winners/foals (starters)	37.5% (47.6%)
Stakes winners/foals (starters)	7.1% (9.0%)
Graded SW/foals (starters)	2.9% (3.6%)
Grade 1 SW/foals (starters)	0.8% (1.1%)
Stakes-placed/foals (starters)	12.2% (15.4%)
Two-year-old starters/foals (starter)	37.1% (47.2%)
Two-year-old winners/foals (% 2yo starters)	13.1% (35.2%)
Two-year-old SW/foals (% 2yo starters)	2.1% (5.8%)
Average career starts/foals (median)	11.8 (8)
Average career starts/starter (median)	14.9 (11)
Average earnings/starter (median)	$79,384 ($27,187)
Average earnings/starter male (female)	$93,164 ($64,143)
Average earnings/start (median)	$5,352 ($2,254)
Average earnings/start male (female)	$5,913 ($4,730)
Average racing index of sires	1.48
Average SSI of all starters	1.92

Table 4. Summary of racing statistics from the USA average for the breed.

Thoroughbred Times averages for the breed	
(all registered Thoroughbreds born between 1987 and 1996)	
Starters/foals	69.9%
Winners/foals (starters)	46.9% (67.1%)
Repeat winners/foals (starters)	35.9% (51.4%)
Stakes winners/foals (starters)	3.5% (5.0%)
Graded SW/foals (starters)	0.8% (1.1%)
Grade 1 SW/foals (starters)	0.2% (0.3%)
Stakes-placed/foals (starters)	5.5% (7.8%)
Two-year-old starters/foals	34.3%
Two-year-old winners/foals (% 2yo starters)	11.5% (33.5%)
Two-year-old sw/foals (% 2yo starters)	1% (3%)
Average career starts/foal	14.9
Average career starts/starter	21.3
Average earnings/starter	$36,682
Average earnings/starter male (female)	$43,505 ($29,593)
Average earnings/start	$1,723
Average earnings/start male (female)	$1,779 ($1,642)
Average SSI of all starters	1.16

WEIGHT AND HEIGHT PERCENTILES AT DIFFERENT AGES

There was no difference in body weight percentile or height percentile between horses that were raced versus unraced as foals, sucklings, and weanlings (P>0.05). Yearlings that raced had significantly lower average weight percentiles than those that did not (46.73 ± 0.32 vs. 49.01 ± 0.65, p<0.01) (Figure 1). Horses that raced as two-year-olds were significantly shorter and lighter than those that did not start as two-year-olds in all age groups (p<0.05) (Figure 2). There was no significant difference in body weight percentile or wither height percentile between winners and non-winners in all age groups. Stakes and graded stakes winners were heavier and taller than non-stakes winners as sucklings, weanlings, and yearlings, but there was no difference in weight percentiles as foals (Figure 3). G1 winners had significantly larger weight percentiles than non-G1 winners as sucklings, weanlings, and yearlings, but not as foals. There was no difference in height percentile between G1 winners and non-G1 winners as foals, sucklings, and weanlings; however, G1 winners had significantly larger height percentiles as yearlings than non-G1 winners (Table 5).

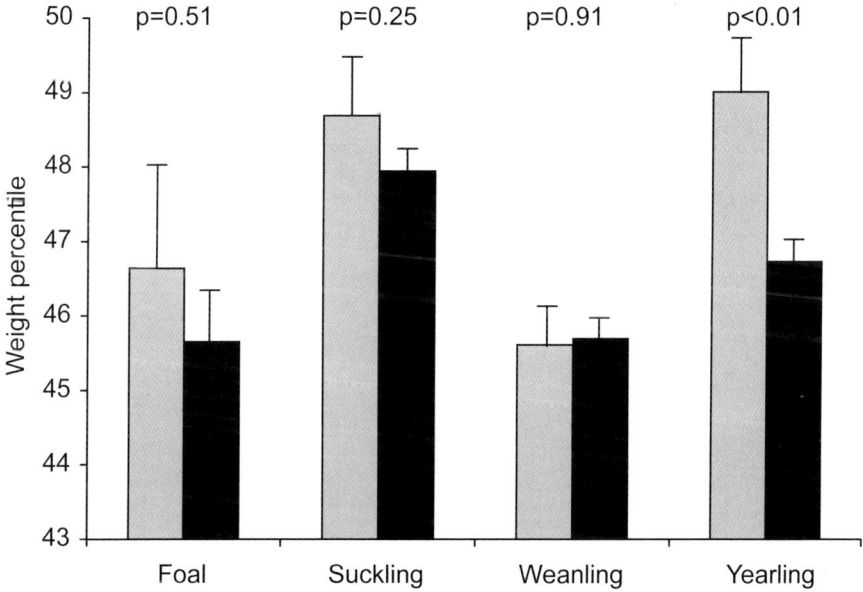

Figure 1. Weight percentile (mean ± sem) of raced (■) and unraced (□) horses as foals, sucklings, weanlings, and yearlings (p<0.01 indicates significant differences between factors).

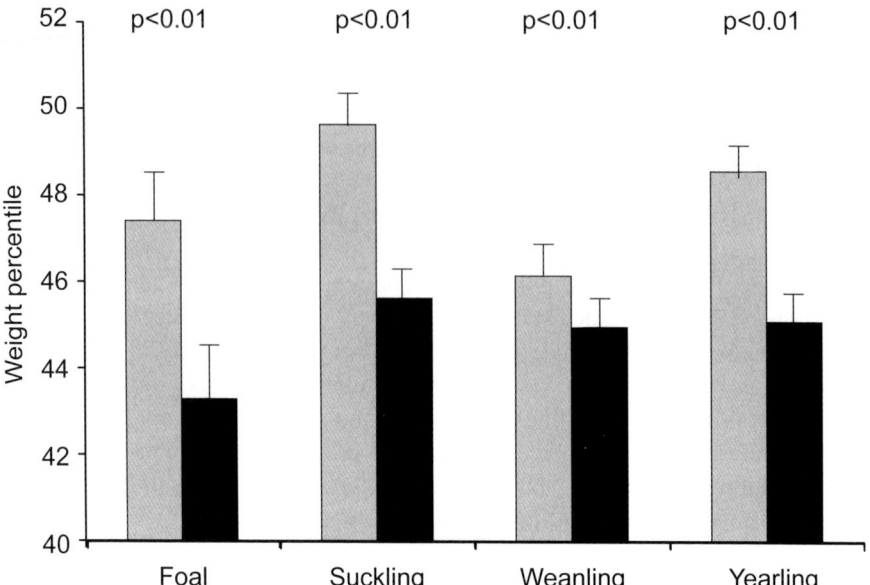

Figure 2. Weight percentile (mean ± sem) of horses that raced at two years old (■) and those that did not race at two years old (□) as foals, sucklings, weanlings, and yearlings (p<0.01 indicates significant differences between factors).

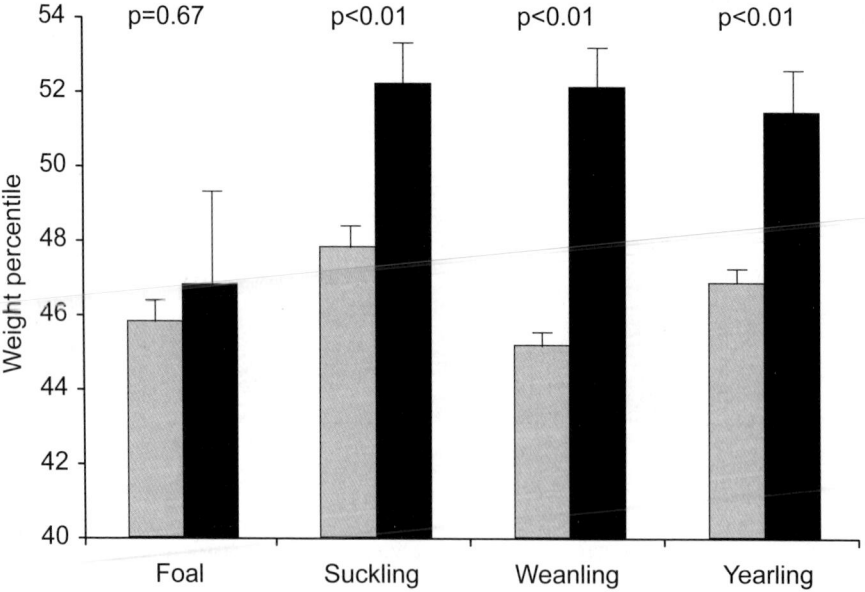

Figure 3. Weight percentile (mean ± sem) of stakes winners (■) and non-stakes winners (□) as foals, sucklings, weanlings, and yearlings (p<0.01 indicates significant differences between factors).

Table 5. Yearling weight and height percentiles (average ± sem) for each performance category.

	Weight percentile	Height percentile
All foals	47.2 ± 0.3	50.5 ± 0.3
Starters	46.7 ± 0.3	50.4 ± 0.4
Two-year-old starters	45.0 ± 0.5	48.6 ± 0.5
Winners	47.0 ± 0.4	51.0 ± 0.4
Stakes winners	51.3 ± 1.0	58.3 ± 1.2
Graded stakes winners	55.6 ± 1.6	63.6 ± 1.9
G1 stakes winners	53.8 ± 2.8	58.9 ± 3.7
Millionaires	60.9 ± 2.7	78.6 ± 3.2

SIRE INDEX

In all age groups, SI was significantly greater in the fourth weight and height quartile than in the first weight and height quartile (Figures 4 and 5). There was no significant difference in SI between raced and unraced horses as foals. However, as yearlings, raced horses had a significantly lower SI than unraced (2.23 ± 0.2 vs. 2.35 ± 0.03, $p<0.001$). Similarly, there was no difference in SI between winners and non-winners as foals, but as yearlings winners had a significantly lower SI than non-winners (2.18 ± 0.002 vs. 2.36 ± 0.002, $p<0.001$). Interestingly, horses that started as two-year-olds had significantly lower SI as foals and yearlings than those that did not ($p<0.01$).

Sire index of graded stakes winners was significantly greater in both foals and yearlings than those that did not win a graded stakes race (2.87 ± 0.11 vs. 2.33 ± 0.003 in foals and 2.60 ± 0.05 vs. 2.23 ± 0.001 in yearlings, $p<0.001$).

RACED AND RACED AS TWO-YEAR-OLDS

There was no significant difference in percentage of horses that raced across either weight or height quartiles at any age group; an even percentage of horses raced in each quartile. A greater percentage of horses ($p<0.05$) in the lower two weight and height quartiles in all age groups started as two-year-olds than in the upper two weight and height quartiles, indicating that smaller horses as foals, sucklings, weanlings, and yearlings are more likely to start as two-year-olds.

NUMBER OF STARTS

Horses in the lowest weight quartile at all age groups had significantly more starts than those in the upper weight quartile (13 vs. 9 starts in the first and fourth foal weight quartiles, and 14 vs. 10 starts in the first and fourth yearling weight quartiles, $p<0.01$).

240 *Thoroughbred Growth and Future Racing Performance*

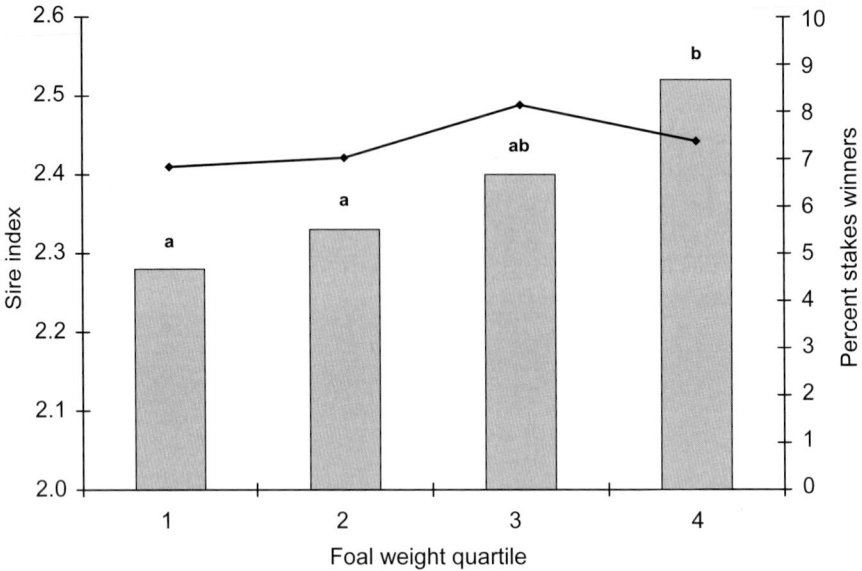

Figure 4. Sire index (□) and percent stakes winners (-♦-) in each foal weight percentile (a, b, etc.; different letters within a factor indicate significant differences).

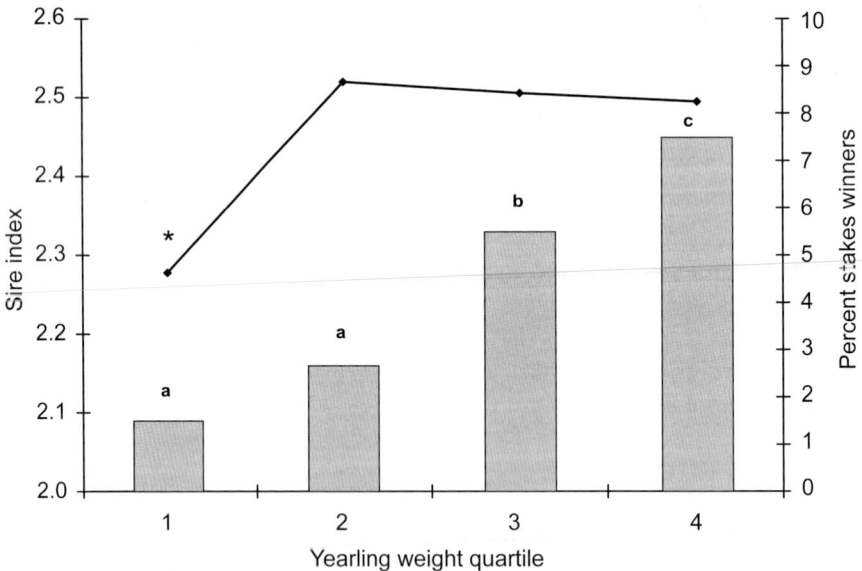

Figure 5. Sire index (□) and percent stakes winners (-♦-) in each yearling weight percentile (* $p<0.01$) (a, b, etc.; different letters within a factor indicate significant differences).

WINNERS AND WIN PERCENTAGE

Significantly fewer foals in the fourth weight quartile went on to become winners (53% versus 60%, 62% and 59% in the first, second, and third foal weight quartiles, respectively ($p<0.05$). However, as sucklings and weanlings this trend was reversed as there were significantly fewer winners in the first weight quartile ($p<0.05$) than in the second, third, and fourth quartiles. There was no significant difference in the percentage of winners in each weight quartile as yearlings, where approximately 60% in each weight quartile went on to become winners. There was no significant difference in the percentage of winners across height percentile in each of the age groups ($p>0.05$). Win percentage of horses that started in a race was significantly greater in horses that were in the third and fourth weight and height quartiles as yearlings.

STAKES WINNERS

There were significantly fewer stakes winners in the first weight quartile as sucklings, weanlings, and yearlings (but not in foals) than in the second, third, or fourth weight quartiles. Fewer horses in all age groups in the first height quartile went on to win a stakes race than in the second, third, and fourth height quartiles (Figures 4 to 7).

GRADED STAKES WINNERS

There was no difference in percentage of graded stakes winners in each foal weight quartile as foals, but in sucklings and weanlings there were fewer graded stakes winners in the first weight quartile than in the second, third, or fourth. There were fewer graded stakes winners in the first yearling weight quartile (n=13) than in the other weight quartiles (n=17, 20, and 21 for the second, third, and fourth weight quartiles, respectively) and 7 times as many graded stakes winners in the fourth height quartile as yearlings (n=20) than in the first (n=3).

EARNINGS

There was no significant difference in the average earnings among the four weight or height quartiles as foals. However, as weanlings and yearlings there were significantly fewer earnings in the first quartile than in the second, third, and fourth quartiles for both weight and height (Figures 6 and 7).

LOGISTIC REGRESSION TO PREDICT STAKES WINNERS

In foals, height percentile was the only variable included in the model that significantly predicted the probability of being a stakes winner. Foals with greater height percentiles had a higher chance of becoming stakes winners. In sucklings and yearlings, sire index,

242 *Thoroughbred Growth and Future Racing Performance*

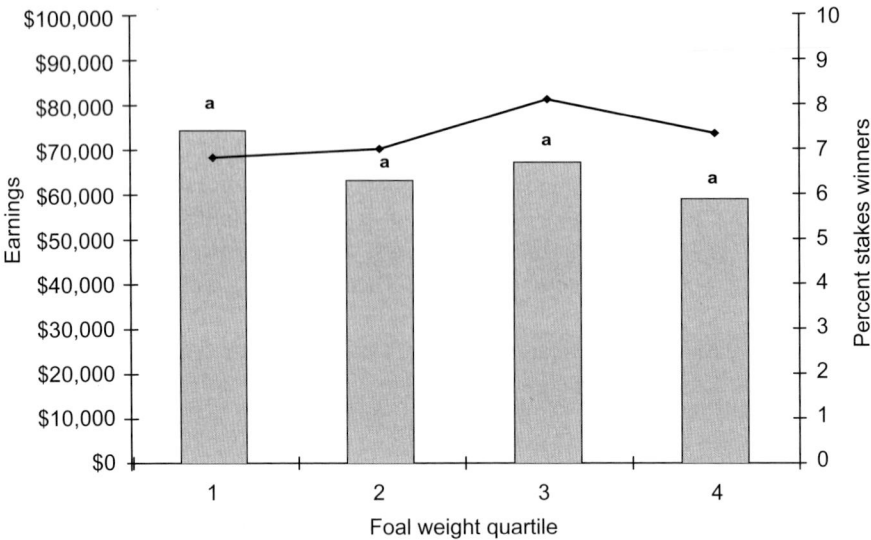

Figure 6. Average earnings (□) and percent stakes winners (-♦-) in each foal weight percentile (a, b, etc.; different letters within a factor indicate significant differences).

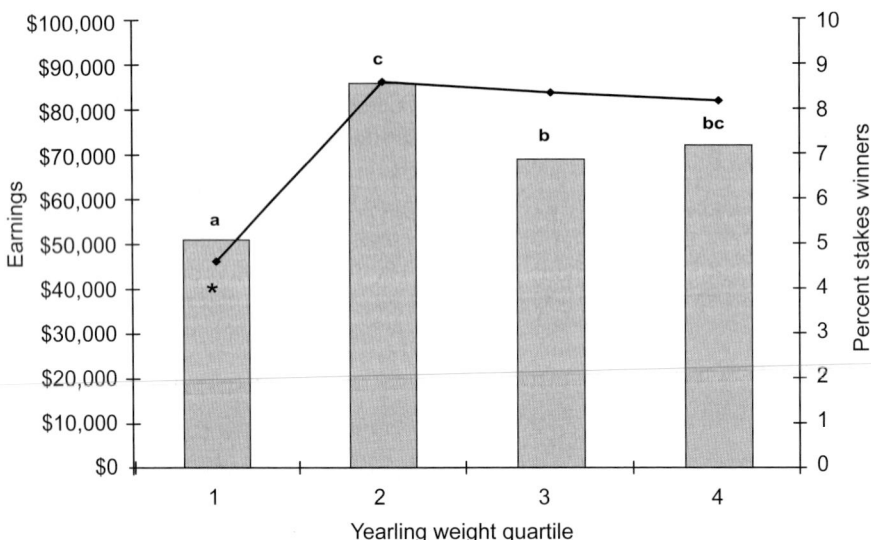

Figure 7. Average earnings (□) and percent stakes winners (-♦-) in each yearling weight percentile (* $p<0.01$) (a, b, etc.; different letters within a factor indicate significant differences).

weight percentile, height percentile, the interaction between sire index and weight percentile, and weight percentile squared were all used in the model to predict the probability of being a stakes winner. In general, the model indicated that extremes in weight percentile (low or high) gave sucklings and yearlings a lower chance of being stakes winners, whereas a greater height percentile improved chances. Sire index was only important if weight percentile was low, and therefore sucklings and yearlings with the greatest chance of becoming stakes winners were tall and not too heavy, and had high sire indexes. In weanlings the model was based on sire index and weight percentile. Weanlings with a greater chance of becoming stakes winners had a high sire index and were in the middle weight percentiles. Height percentile did not have any significant effect on the model for weanlings.

Discussion

The study population exhibited some differences from the breed average including a greater number of starters, winners/foals, stakes winners, graded stakes winners, and G1 winners. Furthermore, horses in this study had greater average earnings from fewer career starts compared with the breed average. Differences observed between the study population and the breed average probably reflect a higher quality of horses in the study.

Growth measurements taken for foals (0-30 days) gave an indication of the horses' genetic or natural size, whereas measurements taken for yearlings represent how management influences size of the horse. In foals in this study, there was no difference in average weight or height percentile between those that raced or not, won or not, won stakes races or not, and won graded stakes races or not. However, horses that won stakes and graded stakes races were significantly heavier as yearlings than those that did not.

Surprisingly, across all age groups, those that started as two-year-olds were shorter and weighed less than those that did not (Figure 2). It is generally accepted that faster-maturing, heavier horses are more likely to be raced as two-year-olds, but these results indicate the opposite and it appears that smaller horses are likely to run earlier. Furthermore, across all age groups smaller horses had more career starts, indicating possible increased skeletal soundness in smaller-sized horses.

Foals and yearlings that weighed less than half the population had significantly lower sire indexes than those in the heaviest quarter. There was no difference in the percentage of stakes winners between all weight quartiles as foals. However, as yearlings there were significantly fewer stakes winners in the lowest weight quartile than in the upper three quartiles. These results indicate that yearlings in the second weight quartile are outperforming their pedigrees (Figure 5).

Yearlings in the first weight quartile (those that weighed less than 75% of the population) had lower earnings, fewer stakes winners, and a lower sire index than the rest of the population. However, yearlings below the 50th weight and height percentiles were more likely to start as two-year-olds and had more career starts than those above the 50th percentile.

Combining sire index, weight, and height percentile into a model to predict the probability of becoming stakes winners established that taller foals had a greater probability of becoming stakes winners, whereas weanlings that were not too heavy with high sire indexes also had more chance. Yearlings with the highest probability of becoming stakes winners were tall, not too heavy, and had high sire indexes.

A study of Virginia Thoroughbreds reported no significant correlations between career earnings and any yearling body measurement, but there was a trend ($p<0.1$) for wither height to be correlated favorably with earnings in fillies (Smith et al., 2006). The current study found that average earnings increased significantly ($p<0.01$) with yearling wither height and body weight in fillies and colts. The Virginia Thoroughbred study also reported that hip height, but not wither height, was favorably correlated with win percentage and horses that won or placed in a stakes race were significantly taller as yearlings. These findings are in agreement with the results of the current work, which found that win percentage was greater in heaver and taller yearlings and stakes winners were significantly taller and heavier as yearlings.

Conclusion

Data from this study suggest tall but not heavy young growing horses are more likely to become successful athletes. We therefore recommend weighing and measuring horses during growth and development to ensure the skeleton maintains a steady rate of growth, while preventing the animal from becoming too heavy.

These data provide insight into managing horses for different strategies. Smaller horses were more likely to start as two-year-olds and have more career starts; however, elite performers (stakes winners, graded stakes winners, G1 winners, and millionaires) were taller and heavier. This does not indicate that small horses will not become elite athletes, as 40% of millionaires as yearlings weighed below the median.

Acknowledgements

The authors would like to thank Ms. Rachel Moxon, KER 2006 intern, for help with data entry.

References

Cain, G. (2006). For yearlings, it's thin to win, study says. Daily Racing Form, July 30, 2006. p. 15.

Pagan, J. (1998a) Recent developments in equine nutrition research. Advances in Equine Nutrition I, Nottingham University Press, UK. 251-258.

Pagan, J. (1998b).The incidence of developmental orthopedic disease (DOD) on a Kentucky Thoroughbred Farm. Advances of Equine Nutrition I, Nottingham University Press, UK. 469-475.

Pagan, J.D., Koch, A., Caddel, S. and Nash, D. (2005). Size of Thoroughbred yearlings presented for auction at Keeneland sales affects selling price. Proceedings of the 19th Equine Science Society Symposium: 224-228.

Smith, A.M., Staniar, W.B. and Splan, R.K. (2006). Associations between yearling body measurements and career racing performance in Thoroughbred racehorses. J. Equine Vet. Sci. 26(5):212-214.

MANAGING GROWTH TO PRODUCE A SOUND, ATHLETIC HORSE

JOE D. PAGAN AND DELIA NASH
Kentucky Equine Research, Versailles, Kentucky

Introduction

A horse's maximal mature body size is genetically predetermined, but growth rate can be influenced by a number of factors including environment, nutrition, and management. Optimal growth rate results in a desirable body size at a specific age with the least amount of developmental problems. Managing growth in horses becomes a balance between producing a desirable individual for a particular purpose without creating skeletal problems that will reduce a horse's subsequent athletic ability. Growing a foal too slowly results in the risk of it being too small at a particular age or never obtaining maximal mature body size. Growing a foal too quickly results in the risk of developmental orthopedic disease (DOD) manifestations such as physitis, angular limb deformities, and osteochondritis dissecans (OCD).

There is no single growth rate that is desirable for all types of horses. Therefore, horses should be managed differently for varying growth rates. Horses will generally reach physical maturity at around four to five years of age. Compared to Thoroughbreds, many breeds such as warmbloods are not expected to compete until later in life, so there is little incentive for rapid growth. Instead, a slow, steady growth rate that will allow the horse to reach maximal mature body size with the fewest problems is desirable.

Thoroughbred racehorses are a different story since they are expected to be competitive athletes at two years of age. Therefore, mature body size is not the most important end point that Thoroughbred breeders wish to achieve. In fact, there can be several important developmental milestones that must be reached even before a young Thoroughbred enters its first race.

Most Thoroughbreds are sold either as weanlings or yearlings at commercial auctions throughout the year. The size of the foal at auction can greatly impact its selling price, so there is strong incentive to market large weanlings and yearlings. At the Keeneland September sales, yearlings that were heavier and taller, but not fatter (measured by body condition score), sold for higher prices (Pagan et al., 2005). Just as important as size, however, is the foal's skeletal soundness at the time of the sale. A delicate balancing act exists between accelerated growth and skeletal soundness.

A horse undergoes rapid development in weight, height, and bone mineral content (BMC) within its first year of life. Within 30 minutes of birth, a foal can stand, and within hours can run at speeds no human athlete will ever achieve. However, despite this early development, a newborn foal has only 17% of its mature BMC and 10% of its mature body weight (Lawrence, 2003). Thoroughbreds will reach 84% of their mature height at 6 months of age; by 12 months they will have reached 94% of mature height; and by 22 months they will have almost finished growing in height (Lawrence, 2003). Mature body weight is reached at a slightly slower rate. During the first six months of life a foal will gain 46% of its mature weight; at 12 months it will have reached 65% of its mature weight; and by 22 months it should be at 90% of its adult body weight (Lawrence, 2003).

Like height and body weight, BMC has been reported to be closely related to age. However, the rate at which maximum BMC is achieved is much slower than height and body weight. At six months of age, horses have attained 68.5% of the mineral content of an adult horse, and by one year of age they have reached 76% of maximal BMC. However, horses do not attain maximum BMC until six years of age (Lawrence, 1994, 2003).

Numerous studies have investigated the relationship between BMC and age in young growing horses. Glade et al. (1986) reported that sound velocities measured through the mid cannon bone and the apparent ultimate breaking strengths of the metacarpal and metatarsal bones of young Thoroughbreds changed with age in a curvilinear fashion, although the relationships appeared linear until 300 days of age. This is similar to findings of El Shofra et al. (1979), Jeffcott and McCartney (1985), and Lawrence and Ott (1985).

In a study conducted by Hoffman et al. (1999) there were close correlations between BMC and age ($R^2 = 0.81$), BMC and body weight ($R^2 = 0.76$), and BMC and height ($R^2 = 0.76$) from birth up to 450 days of age. In this study BMC increased with age and season in three waves with two plateaus, one at two to three months of age and the other in the winter season between November and January at eight to ten months of age. It was concluded that these seasonal changes were due to changes in diet and exercise activity. The first plateau at two to three months of age was associated with a change in diet from the mares' milk to a pasture-based diet. The winter plateau was associated with limited winter activity due to packed snow and ice.

In a more recent study conducted by Reichman et al. (2004), where BMC was measured by means of dual photon absorptiometry in Quarter Horse foals during their first year of life, correlations with age ($R^2 = 0.83$) and height ($R^2 = 0.91$) were reported similar to previously published studies. In this study a winter seasonal influence similar to the Hoffman study was not recorded; however, this study was conducted in Brazil where milder climatic conditions exist. A weaning effect was recorded in foals weaned at 17 weeks but not in foals weaned at the ages of 19 and 24 weeks.

Kentucky Equine Research tracked body weight and skeletal growth in a group of 30 Thoroughbred foals born in 2003 and raised on a large commercial breeding farm in central Kentucky. Dorsopalmar radiographs of the third metacarpal bone (McIII) were taken on a monthly basis. An aluminum step wedge was exposed simultaneously with the McIII. This was used as a reference standard. Radiographic bone aluminum equivalencies (RBAE) were recorded at three sites: lateral and medial sites with peak densities, and a central site of least density in the medullary cavity. The bone mineral content in grams per 2-cm cross section of bone was estimated using regression equations derived by Ott et al. (1987).

Bone morphological measurements (bone width, medullary width, lateral and medial cortical width) were determined from radiographs. Body weights were also measured monthly using in-ground digital scales.

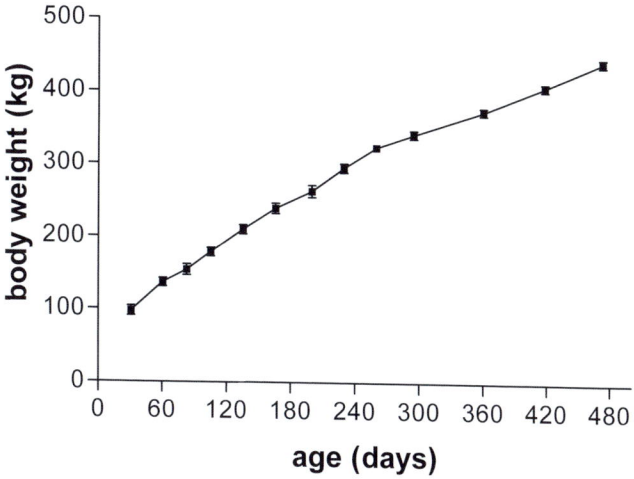

Figure 1. Body weight (kg) of Thoroughbred foals.

Table 1. Bone mineral content (BMC) and bone morphological measurements in the third metacarpal bone of Thoroughbred foals.

Month	Age	Mean BMC (g/2cm)	Width (mm)	Medial Cortical Width (mm)	Lateral Cortical Width (mm)	Medullary Bone Width (mm)
Mar-03	30.7 ± 4.6	6.7 ± 0.8	4.7 ± 0.3	4.1 ± 0.2	18.8 ± 0.6	27.5 ± 0.5
Apr-03	60.3 ± 4.6	8.3 ± 0.4	5.1 ± 0.2	4.8 ± 0.1	18.1 ± 0.3	28.0 ± 0.3
May-03	82.4 ± 6.8	10.6 ± 0.8	6.9 ± 0.3	5.8 ± 0.2	18.1 ± 0.3	30.8 ± 0.5
Jun-03	105 ± 5.9	11.0 ± 0.3	7.2 ± 0.2	5.8 ± 0.1	18.3 ± 0.3	31.3 ± 0.3
Jul-03	135.3 ± 6.1	13.6 ± 0.5	7.4 ± 0.2	7.5 ± 0.4	18.8 ± 0.4	33.8 ± 0.4
Aug-03	165.5 ± 5.9	14.0 ± 0.6	8.2 ± 0.2	6.6 ± 0.1	18.2 ± 0.3	33.0 ± 0.3
Sep-03	199.5 ± 6.3	15.8 ± 0.6	8.7 ± 0.2	7.0 ± 0.2	17.9 ± 0.3	33.6 ± 0.3
Oct-03	229.3 ± 6.5	16.2 ± 0.7	8.4 ± 0.3	6.8 ± 0.2	17.9 ± 0.5	33.2 ± 0.5
Nov-03	259.4 ± 6.3	13.7 ± 0.5	10.1 ± 0.3	7.1 ± 0.2	18.2 ± 0.3	35.3 ± 0.3
Dec-03	294.6 ± 6.2	13.9 ± 0.4	9.7 ± 0.3	7.6 ± 0.2	17.8 ± 0.3	35.1 ± 0.3
Feb-04	360.4 ± 6.6	13.6 ± 0.5	9.6 ± 0.3	7.9 ± 0.2	18.3 ± 0.4	35.7 ± 0.4
Apr-04	418.4 ± 6.3	17.2 ± 0.4	9.7 ± 0.3	7.3 ± 0.2	18.2 ± 0.4	35.2 ± 0.4
Jun-04	472.1 ± 5.9	18.3 ± 0.3	10.3 ± 0.4	7.4 ± 0.2	17.9 ± 0.3	35.6 ± 0.4

BMC increased significantly from the previous month in May 2003, July 2003, September 2003, and April 2004. November 2003 saw a dramatic reduction in values from those recorded in October (P<0.001) with values not increasing again until April 2004 (Figure 2). The reduction in BMC through the fall and winter months coincided with a reduction in body weight average daily gain (ADG), which is a typical growth pattern for Thoroughbred foals raised in central Kentucky (Pagan et al., 1996). Other factors such as pasture availability, day length, and voluntary activity may have also contributed to this reduction in BMC and warrant further investigation.

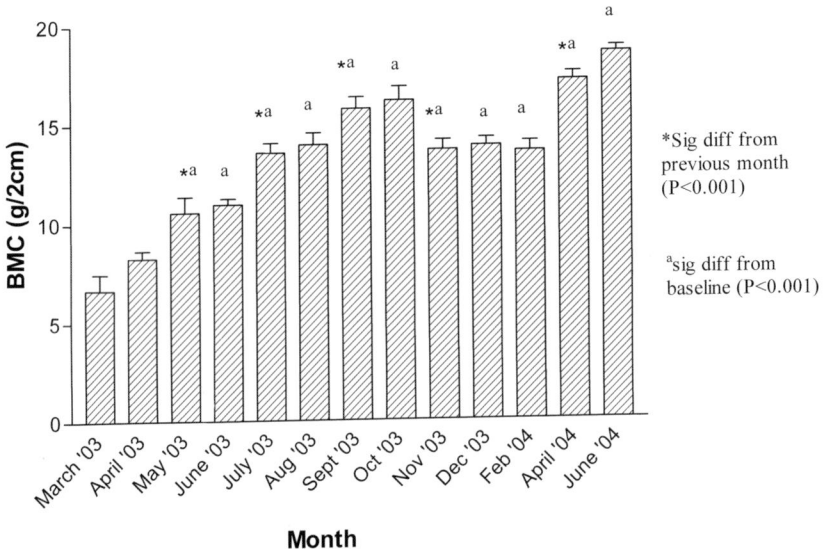

Figure 2. Bone mineral content (BMC) in the third metacarpal bone of Thoroughbred foals.

Factors Affecting DOD and Bone Strength Development

DIET

A balanced feeding regime is critical in the production of a sound equine athlete. Proper feeding begins with the pregnant broodmare. How the pregnant mare is fed will impact both the size and the skeletal soundness of the foal (Lawrence, 2006). Feeding is most important during the last trimester of pregnancy when 75% of fetal growth occurs (Huntington et al., 2003). The most critical nutrients for broodmares and foals are energy, protein, lysine, calcium, phosphorus, copper, and zinc.

ENERGY

Energy intake controls growth rate when all other nutrients are in the foal's ration in sufficient quantities. The most effective way to manage growth in foals is to adjust concentrate and/or forage intake to provide a level of calories that fuels a desired growth rate. Therefore, knowledge of energy requirements for growth is critical.

During the first two months of life, mare's milk contains enough energy and protein to meet the needs for growth. Foals with an expected mature weight of 450-500 kg require approximately 9 kg of milk for each kg of gain at seven days of age, 13 kg at one month of age, and 15 kg at two months of age (Kohnke et al., 1999).

The 1989 NRC does not give specific feeding recommendations for the suckling foal other than to say that supplemental feed prior to weaning may be desirable in foals nursing mares that are poor milkers. This differs from the previous NRC edition (1978) which recommended that a three-month-old suckling foal gaining 2.64 lb/day should receive 6.89 Mcal DE/d as supplemental feed. In a Ralston Purina study, Quarter Horse foals averaged about 2.41 lb ADG over this same time period (Pagan, 1998a). These foals consumed an average of 3.05 Mcal DE per day as supplemental feed over this two-month period. Regression analysis of these data (weighted for mare weight) yields the equation:

$$\text{Foal ADG (lb/day)} = 2.08 + 0.109 \text{ (foal DE (Mcal DE/d))}$$

Brown-Douglas and Pagan (2006) reported on growth rates in 13,429 Thoroughbred foals from around the world. These foals averaged about 2.56 lb gain/day during the second and third months of lactation. Using the above equation, foals would need to consume 4.36 Mcal of supplemental DE/day during the second and third months of lactation to fuel this rate of growth. No supplemental feeding would result in a growth rate of 2.08 lb/day. These figures agree with Doureau et al. (1982) who stated that foals require 15 kg of milk per kg live weight gain at eight weeks of lactation. Fifteen kilograms per day is the expected lactation. Thus, milk alone during this period of lactation could be expected to support a growth rate of only 2.1-2.2 lb/day, a rate which is below that desired by today's horseman.

Typical foal concentrates contain around 1.4 Mcal DE/lb. Therefore, a foal of this age would need to eat about 3.0 lb of concentrate per day to support the type of growth rate typically seen under commercial conditions. It is not known how much hay and pasture a suckling foal will consume, but these energy sources should be kept in mind when deciding how much supplemental grain to feed. Ideally, weighing the foal regularly can aid in adjusting its grain intake.

It should also be noted that higher supplemental DE intakes may result in elevated growth rates which are undesirable since accelerated growth at this early age may contribute to developmental orthopedic disease in foals. It would therefore seem unwise to allow suckling foals free access to supplemental feed in a "creep" feeding arrangement. Instead, the foal should be fed a weighed amount of supplemental feed when the mare is fed. This can easily be accomplished by simply tying up the mare at meal time. It is a good management practice to feed both the mare and the foal at least twice daily, and three or four times per day if possible.

The energy requirement for growing horses is calculated by adding the foal's maintenance requirement to the requirement for tissue energy deposition calculated using the efficiency of conversion of dietary energy for gain (Ott, 2001). The digestible energy requirement for maintenance is DE (Mcal) = 1.4 + 0.03 BW (body weight, kg) (NRC, 1989). Combining the requirements for maintenance and growth yields the following equation: DE (Mcal) = (1.4 + 0.03 BW) + (4.81 + 1.17X − 0.023X^2) (ADG), where X is age in months and ADG is average daily gain in kg.

Nutritional Factors as a Cause of Developmental Orthopedic Disease

MINERAL DEFICIENCIES

A deficiency of minerals, including calcium, phosphorus, copper, and zinc, may lead to developmental orthopedic disease. The ration of a growing horse should be properly fortified because most commonly fed cereal grains and forages contain insufficient quantities of several minerals. A ration of grass hay and oats would supply only about 40% and 70% of a weanling's calcium and phosphorus requirement, respectively, and less than 40% of its requirement for copper and zinc. The best method of diagnosing mineral deficiencies is through ration evaluation. Blood, hair, and hoof analyses are of limited usefulness.

Copper has received a great deal of attention in recent years due to its suggested role in the pathogenesis of developmental orthopedic disease. Lysyl oxidase is a copper-containing enzyme involved in the cross-linking of elastin and collagen in cartilage. Disruption to this process affects normal bone cartilage development. The 1989 NRC estimates that all classes of horses require 10 mg/kg dietary copper. This recommendation appears reasonable for horses at maintenance. However, research suggests that copper requirements of growing horses and broodmares may be considerably higher.

Two dose response studies examining the effects of increased dietary copper intake on bone and cartilage abnormalities (Knight et al., 1990; Hurtig et al., 1993) found that the incidence of DOD was decreased by increasing the copper content of the diet above NRC recommendations. van Weeren et al. (2003) examined the copper status of foals at birth and the incidence of radiographic signs of osteochondritis dissecans (OCD) in warmblood foals genetically prone to OCD. Foals with high liver copper levels at birth had decreased severity of stifle OCD from 5 to 11 months, whereas foals with low liver copper levels had more severe signs of OCD at 11 than 5 months.

Zinc is present as a component of many enzymes and the biochemical role of zinc relates largely to the functions of these enzymes. Zinc is required for the synthesis of alkaline phosphatase, an enzyme actively involved in bone development. Ciancaglini and coworkers (1990) reported a zinc deficiency can cause a decrease in the synthesis of this enzyme.

Much of the research on trace minerals, in particular copper, has focused more on bone abnormalities such as OCD than on bone strength. However, Ott and Asquith

(1995) examined the effect of trace mineral supplementation on bone mineral content. Yearlings supplemented with a complete trace mineral package had greater final BMC values than yearlings fed a basal diet containing no trace mineral supplementation. Horses fed the complete trace mineral package also had greater BMC gain than horses receiving only supplemental Cu and Zn.

MINERAL EXCESSES

Horses can tolerate fairly high levels of mineral intake, but excesses of calcium, phosphorus, zinc, iodine, fluoride, and certain heavy metals such as lead and cadmium may lead to developmental orthopedic disease. Mineral excesses may occur because of overfortification or environmental contamination.

Massive oversupplementation of calcium (>300% of required) may lead to a secondary mineral deficiency by interfering with the absorption of other minerals such as phosphorus, zinc, and iodine. Excessive calcium intake may be compounded by the use of legume hays as the primary forage source. Iodine and selenium oversupplementation occurs if supplements are fed at inappropriate levels. A ration evaluation is the best way to identify this type of mineral imbalance.

Environmental contamination is a more likely cause of developmental orthopedic disease because contamination may result in extremely high intakes of potentially toxic minerals. In addition, chemical analysis of hoof and hair samples may reveal valuable information in such a situation. Farms that are located near factories or smelters are the most likely candidates for this type of contamination. Horses grazing pastures contaminated with zinc, iron, and lead from industrial smelters in Australia were found to have enlarged joints, flexural deformities, lameness, and multiple OCD lesions (Eamens et al., 1984). On post mortem, tissue levels of zinc and lead were elevated, while copper was decreased. The authors concluded that a zinc-induced copper deficiency was responsible for the abnormalities. OCD from a zinc-induced copper deficiency has also been reported on farms using fence paint containing zinc or galvanized water pipes. If a farm is experiencing an unusually high incidence of developmental orthopedic disease or if the location and severity of skeletal lesions are abnormal, environmental contamination should be investigated. Blood, feed, and water analysis should be performed.

MINERAL IMBALANCES

The ratio of minerals may be as important as the actual amount of individual minerals in the ration. High levels of phosphorus in the ration will inhibit the absorption of calcium and will lead to a deficiency, even if the amount of calcium present was normally adequate. The ratio of calcium to phosphorus in the ration of young horses should never dip below 1:1 and ideally it should be 1.5:1. Too much calcium may affect phosphorus status, particularly if the level of phosphorus in the ration is marginal. Calcium to phosphorus ratios greater than 2.5:1 should be avoided if possible. Forage diets with high calcium levels should be supplemented with phosphorus. The ratio of zinc to copper should be 3:1 to 4:1.

DIETARY ENERGY EXCESS

Excessive energy intake can lead to rapid growth and increased body fat, which may predispose young horses to developmental orthopedic disease. A Kentucky study showed that growth rate and body size may increase the incidence of certain types of developmental orthopedic disease in Thoroughbred foals (Pagan, 1998b). Yearlings that showed osteochondrosis of the hock and stifle were large at birth, grew rapidly from three to eight months of age, and were heavier than the average population as weanlings.

The source of calories for young horses may also be important, as hyperglycemia or hyperinsulinemia have been implicated in the pathogenesis of osteochondrosis (Glade et al., 1984; Ralston, 1995). Foals that experience an exaggerated and sustained increase in circulating glucose or insulin in response to a carbohydrate (grain) meal may be predisposed to development of osteochondrosis. In vitro studies with fetal and foal chondrocytes suggest that the role of insulin in growth cartilage may be to promote chondrocyte survival or to suppress differentiation, and that hyperinsulinemia may be a contributory factor to equine osteochondrosis (Henson et al., 1997).

Research from Kentucky Equine Research (Pagan et al., 2001) suggests that hyperinsulinemia may influence the incidence of OCD in Thoroughbred weanlings. In a large field trial, 218 Thoroughbred weanlings (average age 300 ± 40 days, average body weight 300 kg ± 43 kg) were studied. A glycemic response test was conducted by feeding a meal that consisted of the weanlings' normal concentrate at a level of intake equal to 1.4 g nonstructural carbohydrate (NSC) per kilogram body weight. A single blood sample was taken 120 minutes post feeding for the determination of glucose and insulin.

In this study, a high glucose and insulin response to a concentrate meal was associated with an increased incidence of OCD. Glycemic responses measured in the weanlings were highly correlated with each feed's glycemic index (GI), suggesting that the GI of a farm's feed may play a role in the pathogenesis of OCD. Glycemic index characterizes the rate of carbohydrate absorption after a meal and is defined as the area under the glucose response curve after consumption of a measured amount of carbohydrate from a test feed divided by the area under the curve after consumption of a reference meal (Jenkins et al., 1981). In rats, prolonged feeding of high GI feed resulted in basal hyperinsulinemia and an elevated insulin response to an intravenous glucose tolerance test (Pawlak et al., 2001). Hyperinsulinemia may affect chondrocyte maturation, leading to altered matrix metabolism and faulty mineralization or altered cartilage growth by influencing other hormones such as thyroxine (Jeffcott and Henson, 1998). Based on the results of this study, it would be prudent to feed foals concentrates that produce low glycemic responses. More research is needed to determine if the incidence of OCD can be reduced through this type of dietary management.

Conclusion

Feeding and managing growing foals is a balancing act between achieving a commercially desirable level of growth and prevention of developmental orthopedic disease. The keys to success are assuring that the foal's ration is correctly balanced and then regulating feed intake to obtain a safe, desirable growth rate.

References

Brown-Douglas, C.G. and J.D. Pagan. 2006. Body weight, wither height and growth rates in Thoroughbreds raised in America, England, Australia, New Zealand and India. In: Proc. of the 2006 Equine Nutr. Confer., Lexington, KY, pp. 15-22.

Buckingham S.H.W. and L.B Jeffcott. 1990. Shin soreness; a survey of Thoroughbred trainers and racetrack veterinarians. Aust. Equine Vet., 8: 148-153.

Ciancaglini, P., J.M. Pizauro, C. Curti, A.C. Tedesco, and F.A. Leone. 1990. Effect of membrane moiety and magnesium ions on the inhibition of matrix induced alkaline phosphatase by zinc ions. Int. J. Biochem., 22:747.

Doureau, M., W., Martin-Rosset and H. Dubroeucq, 1982. Production laitiere de la jument. Liaison avec la croissance du poulain. C.R. 8eme Journee d'etude du CEREOPA, CEREOPA, Paris, pp. 88-100.

Eamens, G.J., J.F. Macadam, and E.A. Laing. (1984). Skeletal abnormalities in young horses associated with zinc toxicity and hypocuprosis. Aust. Vet. J., 61:205-207.

El Shofra, W.M., J.P. Feaster, and E.A. Ott. 1979. Horse metacarpal bone: Age, ash content, cortical area and failure stress interrelationships. J. Anim. Sci., 49:979.

Glade, M.J. and T.H. Belling. 1984. Growth plate cartilage metabolism, morphology and biochemical composition in over and underfed horses. Growth, 48:473-82.

Glade, M.J., S. Gupta, and T.J. Reimers. 1984. Hormonal responses to high and low planes of nutrition in weanling Thoroughbreds. J. Anim. Sci. 59:658-665.

Glade M.J., N.K. Luba, and H.F. Schryver. 1986. Effects of age and diet on the development of mechanical strength by the third metacarpal and metatarsal bones of young horses. J. Anim. Sci., 63:1432-1444

Henson, F.M., C, Davenport, L. Butler, et al. 1997. Effects of insulin and insulinlike growth factors I and II on the growth of equine fetal and neonatal chondrocytes. Equine Vet. J. 29:441-447.

Hoffman R.M., L.A. Lawrence, D.S. Kronfeld, W.L. Cooper, D.J. Sklan, J.J. Dascanio, and P.A. Harris. 1999. Dietary carbohydrates and fat influence radiographic bone mineral content of growing foals. J. Anim. Sci., 77(12):3330-3338.

Huntington, P.J., E. Owens, K. Crandell, and J. Pagan. 2003. Nutrition management of mares – The foundation of a strong skeleton. In: Proc. of the 2003 Equine Nutr. Confer., Sydney, Australia, pp. 144-174.

Hurtig, M.B., S.L. Green, H. Dobson, Y. Mikuni-Takagaki, and J Choi. 1993. Correlative study of defective cartilage and bone growth in foals fed a low copper diet. Equine Vet. J. Suppl., 16:66-73.

Japan Racing Association. 1999. Annual Report on Racehorse Hygiene. Number of new patients: 24-44.

Jeffcott, L.B., and F.M. Henson. 1988. Studies on growth cartilage in the horse and their application to aetiopathogenesis of dyschondroplasia (osteochondrosis). Vet. J. 156:177-192.

Jeffcott, L.B. and R.N. McCartney. 1985. Ultrasound as a tool for assessment of bone quality in the horse. Vet. Rec., 116(13):337-42.

Jenkins, D.J., T.M. Wolever, R.H. Taylor, et al. 1981. Glycemic index of foods: A physiological basis for carbohydrate exchange. Amer. J. Clin. Nutr. 34:362-366.

Knight, D.A., S.E. Weisbrode, L.M. Schmall, S.M. Reed, A.A Gabel, L.R. Bramlage, and W.I. Tyznik. 1990. The effects of copper supplementation on the prevalence of cartilage lesions in foals. Equine Vet. J., 22:426-432.

Kohnke, J.R., F. Kelleher, and P. Trevor Jones. 1999. Feeding horses in Australia: A guide for horse owners and managers. RIRDC Publication No. 99/49 RIRDC Project No. UWS – 13A. Rural Industries Research and Development Corporation.

Lawrence, L.A. 2003. Principles of bone development in horses. In: Proc. of the 2003 Equine Nutr. Confer., Sydney, Australia , pp. 69-73.

Lawrence, L.A. 2006. Nutrition of the dam influences growth and development of the foal. In: Proc. of the 2006 Equine Nutr. Conf., Lexington, KY , pp. 89-97.

Lawrence L.A. and E.A. Ott. 1985. The use of non-invasive techniques to predict bone mineral content and strength in the horse. In: Proc. 9th Equine Nutr. and Physiol. Symp., Michigan State University, MI, p.110.

Lawrence, L.A., E.A. Ott, G.J. Miller, P.W. Poulos, G. Piotrowski, and R.L. Asquith. 1994. The mechanical properties of equine third metacarpals as affected by age. J. Anim. Sci., 72(10):2617-2623.

McIlwraith, C.W. (2005) Advanced techniques in the diagnosis of bone disease. ADVANCES III pp. 373-381.

Myburgh, K.H., N. Grobler, and T.D. Noakes. 1988. Factors associated with shin soreness in athletes. Phys. Sports Med., 16(4):129.

National Research Council (NRC) (1989): Nutrient requirements of horses. 5th edition, National Academic Press, Washington D. C.

Nielsen B.D., G.D. Potter, L.W. Greene, E.L. Morris, M. Murray-Gerzik, W.B. Smith and M.T. Martin. 1998a. Characterization of changes related to mineral balance and bone metabolism in the young racing quarter horse. J. of Equine Vet. Sci., 18:190-200.

Nielsen, B.D, G.D. Potter, L.W. Greene, E.L. Morris, M. Murray-Gerzik, W.B. Smith, and M.T. Martin. 1998b. Responses of young horses in training to varying

concentrations of dietary Ca and P. J. Equine Vet. Sci., 18:397.
Nielsen, B.D., G.D. Potter, and L.W. Greene. 1997. An increased need for calcium in young racehorses beginning training. In. Proc. 15th Equine Nutr. Phys. Symp. P 153-159.
Norwood, G.L. 1978. The bucked shin complex in Thoroughbreds. In Proc. 24th Annu. Conv. Am. Assoc. Equine Pract., 319-336.
NRC. 1978. Nutrient Requirements of Horses, Fourth Revised Edition. National Academy Press, Washington, D.C.
NRC. 1989. Nutrient Requirements of Horses, Fifth Revised Edition. National Academy Press, Washington, D.C.
Nunamker, D.M., D.M. Butterweck, and M.T. Provost. 1990. Fatigue fractures in Thoroughbred racehorses: Relationship with age, peak bone strain, and training. J. Orthop. Res., 8:604.
Ott, E.A. 2001. Energy, protein and amino acid requirements for growth of young horses. In: J.D. Pagan and R.J. Geor (eds.) Advances in Equine Nutrition II. Nottingham University Press, Nottingham, U.K: 153-160.
Ott, E.A., and R.L. Asquith. 1995. Trace mineral supplementation of yearling horses. J. Anim. Sci., 73(2):466-471.
Ott, E.A., L.A. Lawrence, and C. Ice. 1987. Use of the image analyzer for radiographic photometric estimation of bone mineral content. In: Proc. 10th Equine Nutr. and Physiol. Symp., Ft. Collins, CO., p. 527.
Pagan, J.D. 1998a. Energy requirements of lactating mares and suckling foals. In: J.D. Pagan (ed.) Advances in Equine Nutrition. Nottingham University Press, Nottingham, U.K: 415-420.
Pagan, J.D. 1998b. The incidence of developmental orthopedic disease (DOD) on a Kentucky thoroughbred farm. In: J.D. Pagan (ed.) Advances in Equine Nutrition. Nottingham University Press, Nottingham, U.K: 469-475.
Pagan, J.D., R.J. Geor, S E. Caddel, P.B. Pryor, and K.E. Hoekstra. 2001. The relationship between glycemic response and the incidence of OCD in Thoroughbred weanlings: A field study In. Proc. Amer. Assn Equine Practnr., 47:322-325.
Pagan, J. D., Jackson, S. G. and Caddel, S. 1996. A summary of growth rates of thoroughbreds in Kentucky. Pferdeheilkunde 12: 285-289.
Pagan J.D., A. Koch, S. Caddel, and D. Nash. 2005. Size of Thoroughbred yearlings presented for auction at Keeneland sale affects selling price. In: Proc. Equine Sci. Soc., 19:234-235.
Pawlak, D.B., J.M. Bryson, G.S. Denyer, et al. 2001. High glycemic index starch promotes hypersecretion of insulin and higher body fat in rats without affecting insulin sensitivity. J. Nutr. 131:99-104.
Ralston, S.L. 1995. Postprandial hyperglycemica/hyperinsulinemia in young horses with osteochondritis dissecans lesions. J. Anim. Sci. 73:184 (Abstr.).
Reichmann, P., A. Moure, and H.R. Gamba. 2004. Bone mineral content of the third

metacarpal bone in Quarter horse foals from birth to one year of age. J. Eq. Vet. Sci., 24:391-396.

van Weeren, P.R., J. Knapp, and E.C. Firth. 2003. Influence of liver copper status of mare and newborn foal on the development of osteochrondrotic lesions. Equine Vet. J., 35:67-71.

PATHOLOGICAL CONDITIONS

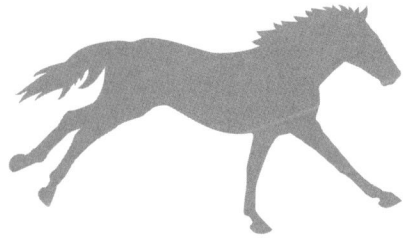

FEEDING THE ATYPICAL HORSE

LARRY LAWRENCE AND THERESA WEDDINGTON
Kentucky Equine Research, Versailles, Kentucky

Introduction

Although the majority of horses can be managed using methods that group them based on age, activity level, or stage of production (i.e., pregnant mares or weanlings), some horses fall outside of the "norm." For these atypical horses, special consideration must be given to ensure their nutritional needs are adequately met. Underweight senior horses, ailing horses, and postsurgical horses are a few of the animals that may temporarily or perpetually require specialized nutritional management in order to maintain optimal health and productivity.

Emaciation results from numerous etiologies. Refeeding the emaciated horse requires careful attention to potentially life-threatening metabolic disorders. Often just putting condition on an underweight horse (e.g., moving a horse from a condition score of 3 to 4) also presents nutritional and management challenges beyond the capabilities of the average horse owner. A thorough approach to nutritional management of the thin horse will be presented.

Excessive loss of condition can result from the effects of the aging process, malnutrition, neglect, disease, parasites, surgery, environmental stress, adrenal insufficiencies, dental problems, and temperament. In cases of extreme emaciation, a careful and complete veterinary medical examination is critical. Geor (2000) reviewed the metabolic effects of starvation and disease, two conditions that must be treated separately.

Starvation

Fasting and starvation as the result of neglect have vastly different metabolic effects as the same conditions brought about by severe illness. In the fasting or malnourished horse, metabolism slows. The body reduces energy expenditure and directs nutrients to functions necessary for survival. Initially, stored liver glycogen and glucose derived from amino acids are sources of energy. Liver glycogen stores are depleted within 24 to 36 hours of the onset of the fast. The central nervous system and red blood cells require glucose in order to support their essential functions. The body's effort to maintain blood glucose levels results in gluconeogenesis in the liver.

Glucose is synthesized in the liver from the carbon skeletons of glycerol, lactate, and some amino acids (alanine). The demand for glucose is so critical that amino acids are obtained from muscle tissue catabolism. In an effort to spare blood glucose, an increase in mobilization of fatty acids from adipose tissue occurs, as does an increased dependency on fatty acids for energy for all tissues except for the central nervous system and red blood cells. It is estimated that during a prolonged fast the body may be using fatty acids for 80-85% of its energy needs.

The driving mechanism of the metabolic response to fasting is an altered hormone profile. The most prominent change is decreased insulin production, a condition that goes hand in hand with an increased synthesis of counter-regulatory hormones such as glucogon and cortisol. These hormones promote fatty acid mobilization and the breakdown of muscle protein. In addition, the synthesis of the thyroid hormone triiodothyronine (T3) decreases, resulting in a lowered metabolic rate and energy requirement.

Disease and Emaciation

Severe stress such as disease, injury, major surgery, and sepsis affects metabolic systems much differently than starvation. While the body adapts to starvation by decreasing its metabolic rate, severe stress induces a hypermetabolic state that results in rapid breakdown of the body's reserves of carbohydrate, protein, and fat. Hyperglycemia with insulin resistance, hyperlipidemia, negative nitrogen balance, and diversion of protein (particularly glutamine) from skeletal muscle to the liver are prominent features. Protein catabolism results in severe wasting of lean body mass. Dramatic increases in the "stress hormones," including glucocorticoids, epinephrine, and glucagons along with inflammatory cytokines such as interleukin-1 and tumor necrosis factor, creates a catabolic state that results in malnutrition. These processes lead to delayed tissue repair, immune insufficiency, and declining survivability (Geor, 2000).

EFFECTS OF MALNUTRITION AND HYPERLIPIDEMIA

Hyperlipidemia is a disease syndrome in ponies, miniature horses, and more rarely in horses. The disease results in a marked increase in plasma triglycerides (7,000 mg/dl), cloudy serum or plasma, and fatty infiltration of the liver and kidneys. Starved horses not suffering from hyperlipidemia have increased plasma free fatty acids and glycerol. Plasma free fatty acids and glycerol consistently increase more dramatically than triglycerides. Hyperlipidemia is often precipitated in ponies by a primary illness that results in reduced feed intake over a period of days to weeks. Increased metabolic needs due to the illness increase fat mobilization. In addition, pregnancy, lactation, and obesity increase plasma triglycerides. Under conditions of rapid and sustained lipolysis, some of the fat is reesterified in the liver and transported to tissues as very low-density lipoproteins (VLDL). When the liver's capacity for VLDL synthesis is overwhelmed, fat is deposited in the liver. Affected animals require aggressive nutritional support and recovery is difficult.

LOW PLASMA ALBUMIN

Long periods of reduced feeding, renal disease, liver disease, and enteropathy can reduce plasma albumin. Regardless of the cause, low plasma albumin should be corrected by refeeding energy and protein. In severe cases (albumin is less than 2 g/dl), blood transfusions may be necessary (Lewis, 1995).

INTESTINAL TRACT

The gastrointestinal tract (GI) is lined with enterocytes, which have high metabolic rates. These cells also have fairly quick turnover rates, with cell replacement occurring every three days. Enterocytes prevent harmful bacteria from entering the bloodstream, while at the same time providing the mechanism for nutrient absorption. Enterocytes depend on nutrients absorbed from the GI tract for DNA transcription and synthesis of replacement cells. Periods of nutrient deprivation rapidly result in impaired digestion as the result of mucosal atrophy (Geor, 2000). Breakdown of the gut lining increases the risk of bacteria entering the bloodstream, which may set the stage for sepsis.

IMMUNE SYSTEM

Naylor and Kenyon (1981) report a severely compromised cellular and nonspecific immune function after three to five days of complete feed deprivation in horses. This decrease in immune function increases susceptibility to infection and compromises intestinal mucosal barriers, a fatal combination in horses.

HYPOTHERMIA

Anorexic horses are susceptible to hypothermia (Naylor, 1999). These horses do not have insulating fat or produce heat from the process of fiber digestion, nor do they have energy reserves. During rehabilitation, keep these horses warm, dry, and out of the wind. Provide deep bedding and blankets.

Nutritional Requirements for Emaciated and/or Sick Horses

Numerous factors affect the energy needs of compromised horses, and there is limited information available specifically for horses. Ousey et al. (1996) reported the metabolic rate of foals with neonatal maladjustment syndrome (NMS) was 50% of healthy age-matched controls. The authors state that foals with NMS were recumbent and inactive during measurement periods. Even though these foals had very low metabolism, they were in negative energy balance because of low milk intakes. Foals with hypermetabolic stress such as septicemia, diarrhea, and pneumonia will have greater energy deficits.

Data from human and animal studies have demonstrated severe trauma increases energy expenditure by a factor of 1.3 to 1.4, and expenditure in animals with sepsis or a major burn can be up to 1.4 to 1.7 times higher when compared to resting healthy humans (Geor, 2000). Pagan and Hintz (1986) reported that the resting energy expenditure (REE) of horses could be estimated from the formula: REE=21 kcal (BW kg)+975 kcal. Thus, for a 500-kg horse, REE would be approximately 11.5 Mcal/d, 30% lower than the requirement for maintenance under normal conditions (16.4 Mcal/d for a 500-kg horse). No data are available on energy requirements of sick horses. However, if regression equations for human medicine are applied, a stalled 500-kg horse with an infection or postsurgical condition would have energy requirements of 16 to 20 Mcal/d (1.5 to 1.8 x 11.5 Mcal/d).

Increased protein requirements in sick, debilitated, or injured horses due to protein catabolism should be taken into consideration. Rooney (1998) suggested that 5 g of protein be provided per 100 kcal (i.e., 800 g) of crude protein for a diet containing 16 Mcal digestible energy. This is a 25% increase over the NRC (1989) maintenance protein requirement. There are probably increased requirements for essential vitamins and minerals due to debilitation. However, without knowing specifics, meeting maintenance requirements is a reasonable goal. The main concern is to limit tissue breakdown and weight loss. Realistic goals of providing 60 to 70% of maintenance requirements should help the sick or injured horse.

Recent research in human medicine points to the therapeutic effects of certain nutrients. Arginine, glutamine, omega-3 fatty acids, and ribonucleic acid are reported to upregulate immune function in critically ill humans (Beale et al., 1999). Glutamine is a nonessential amino acid that is important in the growth and repair of the small intestinal mucosa. Glutamine also helps maintain intestinal immune function (Nappert et al., 1997). Routledge et al. (1999) reported plasma glutamine concentrations decrease following viral infection. Further research is needed on glutamine and the immune system of horses. Omega-3 fatty acids have also received a great deal of attention because of their effects on the immune system.

Determining body condition scores and evaluating horses for potential disease or injury are important in identifying those horses in need of nutritional support (Doneghue, 1992). Well-fed adult horses that are not pregnant (last trimester) or lactating can withstand up to four days of partial or complete starvation without long-term effects. However, thin horses with condition scores between 1 to 3 that have experienced a dramatic loss in weight (10% or more) need emergency nutritional support. Rapid weight loss is commonly observed in horses with sepsis, endotoxemia, pulmonary abscess, pleuropneumonia, abdominal abscesses, diarrhea, severe trauma, surgery, or intestinal disorders. Overweight horses, those with condition scores of 7 to 9, quickly develop hypertriglyceridemia (7,500 mg/dl) after even short periods of anorexia.

Foals, particularly during the first weeks of life, have limited energy stores. Conditions compromising nutritional support of foals can quickly result in hypoglycemia, weakness, and death.

Disease and Nutrition

Certain diseases result in weight loss and require specific nutritional adjustments. These include respiratory disease, laminitis, Cushing's syndrome, renal failure, hepatic disease, chronic diarrhea, and small intestinal malabsorption syndromes. Resection of the GI tract requires special feeding regimes. For performance horses that have viral or bacterial infections, minor injuries, or orthopedic surgery, the primary nutritional goal is often energy reduction. While on stall rest these horses should be fed a diet of hay at a rate of 1.5-2.0% of body weight, a vitamin/mineral supplement, and salt.

RESPIRATORY DISEASE

Chronic obstructive pulmonary disease (COPD), or heaves, in horses is caused by hypersensitivity to fungal spores present in hay or bedding, dust, molds, and occasionally grass pollen. The hypersensitivity results in bronchoconstriction, excess mucus, and inflammatory thickening of the alveoli. Often there is a prior infectious respiratory disease that increases the likelihood of the condition. COPD usually subsides when the allergen is identified and eliminated in the early stages.

Housing in barns usually makes the condition worse. Maintaining horses at pasture is usually the best management system. If horses have to be stabled, ventilation and dust-free bedding must be used. Hay is the primary source of allergens. If hay is included in the diet, it must be soaked by submersion in water for at least five minutes. Hay cubes and complete diets are good alternatives to hay. If hay cubes are used, they too must be soaked prior to feeding.

HEPATIC DISEASE

Liver dysfunction causes the plasma concentration of branched-chain amino acids (leucine, isoleucine, and valine) to decrease and aromatic amino acids (phenylalanine, tyrosine, and tryptophan) as well as ammonia to increase. These changes may be responsible for hepatoencephalopathy. Feeding diets that meet energy needs without excess protein helps minimize neurologic signs. Feeding adequate energy reduces mobilization of body glycogen, fat, and protein. Excess fat is deposited in the liver and further limits hepatic function. Readily available soluble carbohydrates are essential to the diet. In addition, the protein source should have a high branched-chain to aromatic amino acid ratio. A diet consisting of 50% steam-flaked corn or milo and 50% grass hay should be fed. Molasses can be added to provide glucose. Multiple feedings will help maintain glucose homeostasis and prevent bacterial ammonia surges. Legume hays, oats, and soybeans should be avoided because of high levels of aromatic amino acids.

RENAL FAILURE

Chronic renal failure occurs most frequently in older horses. Depression and anorexia are signs of chronic renal failure. Polyuria and polydipsia are due to an inability to concentrate urine. Renal failure in horses is also associated with hypercalcemia and elevated urea. Phosphorus excretion can also be impaired and sodium deficits might develop.

Feedstuffs high in protein (legumes, soybeans), phosphorus (wheat bran), and calcium (legumes, calcium-containing supplements) should be avoided. In some cases, hypoproteinemia can develop with chronic renal failure. In these cases, the level of protein should be increased. Horses with hypoproteinemia benefit from fat supplementation.

GASTROINTESTINAL DISORDERS

Difficult or painful swallowing can reduce intake in horses. Some of the causes of difficult swallowing include obstruction from abscesses or strangles; nerve damage from equine protozoal myeloencephalitis (EPM) and muscle weakness caused by hyperkalemic periodic paralysis (HYPP); or botulism. Scar tissue from an episode of choking can cause difficulty swallowing. If the esophagus is narrowed due to scarring from choking, a hay cube and grain slurry may need to be fed.

Gastric ulcers can cause a reduction in appetite. The incidence of ulcers in horses is high. Surveys put the incidence for racehorses near 90%. In stalled show horses, the occurrence approaches 65%. Horses maintained on pasture rarely have ulcers, but when they are confined to stalls and fed grain meals, ulcers can develop within four days. Damage to the nonglandular portion of the stomach by hydrochloric acid produced in the glandular region causes painful lesions that can reduce intake. Signs associated with gastric ulcers are irritability, chronic colic, diarrhea, weight loss, and dull hair coat.

Gastrointestinal disorders can be further divided into those associated with the small intestine including enteropathies, malabsorption syndromes, and small intestine resection, and those involving the large intestine such as colitis, diarrhea, chronic impaction, and colon resection. With small intestinal disease, the primary goal is to optimize the large bowel's digestive function. This is achieved by feeding highly digestible fiber sources such as leafy alfalfa, beet pulp, or soybean hulls while reducing grain. Feeding small meals of highly fermentable fibers (beet pulp and alfalfa), fat (rice bran), and vegetable oil has maintained body condition in horses following resection of 50% of the small intestine. Complete pelleted feeds have been fed in small amounts with positive results even after 70% of distal small intestine resection (Lewis, 1995).

Large intestinal dysfunction usually results in diarrhea. In the acute phase, many affected horses are hypophagic and need enteral nutritional support. Small intestinal function is maintained with large colon resection. Diets that are low in fiber and high in digestible energy and protein should be fed. As the horse's appetite improves, fermentable fiber should be added. Probiotics and yeast are recommended to help reestablish the gut microflora. Vitamin K and B vitamins should be supplemented because of decreased production in the hindgut. Nutritional support can be provided by parenteral (intravenous) or enteral feeding. Voluntary feeding is dependent on the condition of the horse and its appetite. Appetite stimulation is often accomplished by "cafeteria style" feeding. Lush, green grass is often the most appealing feed for horses. However, mashes, leafy alfalfa, grains, sweet feeds, and fresh fruit may also appeal to a horse when trying to encourage feed consumption.

There are a variety of enteral diets that have been developed for feeding via nasogastric tube. The Naylor diet is one of the most widely accepted (Naylor, 1977). The Naylor diet is composed of 454 g alfalfa meal, 204 g casein, 204 g dextrose, 52 g electrolyte mixture, and 5 L of water. The digestible energy (DE) is 2.77 Mcal for this mixture, and this should be fed via a nasal tube in six batches to meet the maintenance energy needs of a 500-kg adult horse (16.4 Mcal).

Once horses are eating, a simple refeeding program for starved horses has been reported by Stull (2003). The researchers at UC Davis (Stull, 2003) recommended the following program:

- Days 1-3: Feed one pound leafy alfalfa every four hours (total of 6 lb/d in 6 feedings).
- Days 4-10: Slowly increase the amount of alfalfa and decrease the number of feedings so that by day six you are feeding just over four pounds of hay every eight hours (total of 13 lb/d in three feedings).
- Days 10-several months: Feed as much alfalfa as the horse will eat and decrease feeding to twice per day. Provide access to a salt block. Do not feed grain or supplemental material until the horse returns to normal.

When rehabilitating a thin horse, sudden change from a poor-quality diet to a highly digestible diet can cause death within three to five days. Laminitis and diarrhea are common problems, but the most serious concern is when phosphorus, potassium, or magnesium are depleted and the depletion is made worse by sequestration of these minerals in newly formed cells (Whitam and Stull, 1998).

Senior Horses

Senior horses can be a challenge. After the diseases discussed above are ruled out, a checklist of management priorities for senior horses must be reviewed. More often than not, an older horse in poor condition has a dental problem. A thorough dental exam and correction of sharp teeth, wavy mouth, and/or gum or tooth infection may allow older horses to more properly grind feeds and improve nutrient digestion and absorption. If the teeth are worn and the horse is unable to chew well, pelleted or extruded feeds fed in a slurry will help improve the condition of the horse.

ENVIRONMENTAL EFFECTS

Herd dynamics and pecking order change as horses age and can result in older horses not receiving adequate nutrition in group-feeding situations. Older horses often do better when separated from the group at feeding time. Underweight horses are very susceptible to hypothermia. Table 1 illustrates the increased energy requirements of horses in inclement weather versus the normal horse.

Table 1. Effects of wind and rain on digestible energy requirements for horses at maintenance.*

Average Temperature	Wind/Rain	Additional Mcal/day	Additional Hay
32° F	10-15 mph wind	4-8 Mcal/day	4-8 lb/day
32° F	Rain	6 Mcal/day	6 lb/day
32° F	Rain and wind	10-14 Mcal/day**	10-14 lb/day

*Adapted from Anderson, 2003.
**May not be able to consume enough hay to meet requirements.

Internal parasites can cause damage to the lining of the GI tract and reduce the efficiency of digestion. Reducing parasite loads in older neglected horses should be done under veterinary supervision to avoid a rapid kill-off of parasites, which may cause impaction.

Chronic pain as a result of arthritis can interfere with grazing and affect an older horse's appetite. Depending on the seriousness of joint pain, chondroitin sulfates and glucosamine may be helpful. In more serious cases, nonsteroidal anti-inflammatory drugs and/or injectable cartilage-building drugs may be necessary.

SENIOR NUTRITION

Feed companies now offer feeds for aged horses that are supplemented with water-soluble vitamins and contain 12-16% protein, <1.0% calcium, and 0.45-0.6% phosphorus (Ralston, 1999). Also, these feeds usually contain at least 12% crude fiber. These feeds are typically extruded thereby increasing digestibility for the older horse. Alternative sources of forage such as hay cubes can be used if the horse has a dental problem that may hinder proper chewing of long-stem hay. The hay cubes should be a mixture of grass and alfalfa, rather than straight alfalfa due to the high calcium content of alfalfa.

Conclusion

Managing the atypical horse requires an individualized approach to housing, training, and nutrition. Whether horses are unusual due to illness, neglect, temperament, age, or a combination of these factors, they can be productive and healthy once they are properly diagnosed and their particular requirements are met.

References

Anderson, K. 2003. Winter care for horses. NebGuide G96-1292.

Beale, R.J., D.J. Bryg, and D.J. Bihari. 1999. Immunonutrition in the critically ill: A systematic review of clinical outcomes. Crit. Care Med. 27:2799-2805.

Doneghue, S. 1992. Nutritional support of hospitalized animals. J. Am. Vet. Med. Assoc. 200: 612-615.

Geor, R.J. 2000. Nutritional support of the sick adult horse. World Eq. Vet. Rev. 5:12, 14-22.

Lewis, L.D. 1995. Sick horse feeding and nutritional support. Equine Clinical Nutrition. p. 396. Lea and Febiger, Baltimore.

Nappert, G., G.A. Zello, and J.M. Naylor. 1997. Intestinal metabolism of glutamine and potential use of glutamine as a therapeutic in diarrheic calves. J. Am. Med. Asso. 211:547-553.

Naylor, J.M. 1999. How and what to feed a thin horse with and without disease. Proc. BEVA. 10:81-85.

Naylor, J.M., and S.J. Kenyon. 1981. Effect of total caloric deprivation on host defense in the horse. Res. Vet. Sci. 31:396-372.

NRC. 1989. Nutrient Requirements of Horses. (5th Ed.). National Research Council. National Academy Press, Washington, D.C.

Ousey, J.C., N. Holdstock, P.D. Rossdale, and A.J. McArthur. 1996. How much energy do sick neonatal foals require compared with healthy foals? Pferdeheilkunde. 12:231-237.

Pagan, J.D., and H.F. Hintz. 1986. Equine energetics. 1. Relationship between body weight and energy requirements in horses. J. Anim. Sci. 63:815-821.

Ralston, S.L. 1999. Management of geriatric horses. In: Pagan, J.D., and R.J. Geor (Eds.). Advances in Equine Nutrition, Vol. II p. 393-396. Nottingham University Press, Nottingham, UK.

Routledge, H.B.H., R.C. Harris, P.A. Harris, J.R.J. Naylor, and C.A. Roberts. 1999. Plasma glutamine status in the equine at rest, during exercise, and following viral challenge. Eq. Vet. J. Suppl. 30:612-616.

Stull, C. 2003. Nutrition for rehabilitating the starved horse. J. Eq. Vet. Sci. 23:456-459.

Whitham, C.L., and C.L. Stull. 1998. Metabolic responses of chronically starved horses to refeeding with three isoenergetic diets. J. Am. Vet. Med. Assoc. 212:691-696.

NUTRITIONAL MANAGEMENT OF METABOLIC DISORDERS

JOE D. PAGAN

Kentucky Equine Research, Versailles, Kentucky

Introduction

Several metabolic disorders are common in modern breeds of horses. Many of these disorders such as equine Cushing's disease (ECD), equine metabolic syndrome (EMS), osteochondritis dissecans (OCD), recurrent equine rhabdomyolysis (RER), and polysaccharide storage myopathy (PSSM) can be managed nutritionally by careful regulation of caloric intake with particular attention paid to the source of energy provided. Although these disorders have very different etiologies, they are all either triggered or aggravated by excessive starch and sugar intake. As in humans, excess consumption of calories from carbohydrates is one of the major problems in today's equine population. This paper will review the role various carbohydrates play in equine disease and will describe feeding programs for managing affected horses.

Carbohydrates in Horse Feed

The carbohydrates in equine feeds can be categorized by either their function in the plant or from the way they are digested and utilized by the horse. From a plant perspective, carbohydrates fall into three categories: (1) simple sugars active in plant intermediary metabolism; (2) storage compounds such as sucrose, starch, and fructans; and (3) structural carbohydrates such as pectin, cellulose, and hemicellulose. For the horse, it is more appropriate to classify carbohydrates by where and how quickly they are digested and absorbed. Carbohydrates can either be digested and/or absorbed as monosaccharides (primarily glucose and fructose) in the small intestine, or they can be fermented in the large intestine to produce volatile fatty acids or lactic acid. The rate of fermentation and types of end products produced are quite variable and can have significant effects on the health and well-being of the horse.

A physiologically relevant system to categorize carbohydrates in equine diets would be composed of three groups. (1) A hydrolyzable group (CHO-H) measured by direct analysis that yields sugars (mainly glucose) for metabolism. This includes simple sugars, sucrose, and some starches that are readily digested in the small intestine and produce fluctuations in blood glucose after feeding. (2) A rapidly fermentable group (CHO-FR) that yields primarily lactate and propionate. This group includes starches that escape digestion in the small intestine as well as galactans, fructans, gums, mucilages, and pectin. (3) A slowly fermentable group (CHO-FS) that yields mostly acetate and butyrate. This group includes the compounds captured in neutral detergent fiber (NDF) such as cellulose, hemicellulose, and lignocellulose.

Hydrolyzable carbohydrates (CHO-H) are an important component of equine diets, particularly for the performance horse, where blood glucose serves as a major substrate for muscle glycogen synthesis. Too much blood glucose, however, may contribute to or aggravate certain problems in horses such as RER, PSSM, ECD, and developmental orthopedic disease (DOD). It may also adversely affect behavior in certain individuals.

The quantity of blood glucose produced in response to a meal is a useful measure of a feed's CHO-H content. Table 1 contains the glycemic index of several equine feeds measured at Kentucky Equine Research (KER). Glycemic index characterizes the rate of carbohydrate absorption after a meal and is defined as the area under the glucose response curve after consumption of a measured amount of a test feed divided by the area under the curve after consumption of a reference meal, in this case oats.

Table 1. Glycemic index (GI) of equine feeds and forages.

Feed	Glycemic index
Sweet feed	129
Whole oats	100
Equine Senior®	100
Beet pulp + molasses	94
Crackec corn	90
Re•Leve®	81
Beet pulp (unrinsed)	72
Orchard grass hay	49
Rice bran	47
Ryegrass hay	47
Alfalfa hay	46
I.R. Pellet and orchard grass hay	34
Rinsed beet pulp	34
Bluestem hay	23

Rapidly fermentable carbohydrates (CHO-FR) such as pectin can yield propionate, which is an important gluconeogenic substrate for the horse. However, rapid fermentation can also produce latic acid, which may lead to a cascade of events culminating in laminitis. Undigested starch from cereals and fructans from pasture are the most likely compounds contributing to lactic acidosis in the hindgut.

Slowly fermentable carbohydrates (CHO-FS) from the plant cell wall are absolutely essential to maintain a healthy microbial environment in the horse. These carbohydrates alone, however, may not be able to supply enough energy to fuel a high-performance athlete. Carbohydrates in horse feeds have traditionally been estimated by measuring cell wall components as NDF and calculating the remaining carbohydrate by difference as nonfiber carbohydrate (NFC), where NFC = 100 - water - protein - fat - ash - NDF. More recently, laboratories have provided a direct analysis of additional carbohydrates in equine feeds.

Table 2 contains the chemical composition of several common equine feedstuffs as analyzed by Equi-analytical Laboratories in Ithaca, NY. In addition to NDF and the calculated values of NFC, Table 2 contains measured levels of water-soluble sugars (WSS) and starch. The sum of WSS and starch is considered the nonstructural carbohydrate (NSC). WSS in cereal grains and by-products such as beet pulp are composed of simple sugars that produce a pronounced glycemic response and fit into the CHO-H category. By contrast, much of the WSS in temperate grasses are actually fructans, which should be included in the CHO-FR fraction.

Table 2. Carbohydrate content of some common equine feeds.

	Oats	Corn	Beet pulp	Soy hulls	Legume hay	Grass hay
WSS (%)	3.9	3.5	10.6	3.6	9.0	10.7
Starch (%)	44.3	70.5	1.3	1.7	2.4	2.8
NSC (%)	50.7	73.1	12.1	5.3	11.4	13.3
NFC (%)	50.9	76.4	44.4	19.8	30.8	19.5
NDF (%)	27.9	9.8	41.9	61.7	38.5	63.8

Therefore, they would have little effect on glycemic response but may contribute to the development of hindgut acidosis and laminitis.

Starch is the predominant carbohydrate fraction in cereal grains. Although all starch is made up of glucose chains, how the starch molecule is constructed varies in different types of grain. These differences in the architecture of individual starches have a large impact on how well they are digested in the horse's small intestine.

Of the grains most commonly fed to horses, oats contain the most digestible form of starch, followed by sorghum, corn, and barley. Processing can have a huge effect on prececal digestibility, particularly in corn. In a KER study, steam flaking corn caused a 48% increase in glycemic response compared to coarse cracking. NSC is a mixture of CHO-H and CHO-FR fractions. NSC tends to be higher in CHO-H in processed cereal grains and mixes but may be high in CHO-FR in certain unprocessed cereals or high-fructan forages. NFC represents an even more mixed group of carbohydrates because in addition to the compounds found in NSC, they may also contain significant quantities of pectin and other fermentable compounds not captured in NDF. For instance, beet pulp contains only 12.1% NSC but 44.4% NFC. At present, there is no satisfactory, commercially available analytical method to segment carbohydrates into categories that are physiologically meaningful for the horse.

Metabolic Disorders

Equine Cushing's disease (ECD) or pituitary pars intermedia dysfunction (PPID) results from a tumor in the pituitary gland and is frequently recognized in older horses (Frank et al., 2006). For a review of ECD, see the article by Andrews and Frank in this volume (Andrews and Frank, 2008). The pituitary glands of horses with ECD secrete excessive amounts of adrenocorticotropic hormone (ACTH), which results in an increased secretion of cortisol from the adrenal glands. Horses with ECD are prone to laminitis and may develop cortisol-induced insulin insensitivity, which leads to elevated blood insulin (hyperinsulinemia) and elevated blood glucose (hyperglycemia).

The best dietary strategy for horses with ECD will depend on several factors. First, since these horses tend to be insulin insensitive, a ration that produces a low glycemic response is essential. Rations containing CHO-FR such as lush pasture and high grain meals should be avoided to reduce the likelihood of laminitis. Additionally, the ration must also supply the correct amount of required nutrients for the horse, and it must supply the correct caloric intake to maintain or achieve a desired body condition. For additional information about assessing and manipulating energy balance, see Dr. Laurie Lawrence's article in this volume (Lawrence, 2008).

ECD horses that are overweight should be fed a ration composed primarily of hay. Most hays have low glycemic indexes compared to cereals and sweet feeds (Table 1). Hay rations should be supplemented with a low-inclusion fortified balancer to provide nutrients that may be deficient in the forage. KER recently developed this type of product (I.R. Pellet; KERx, Versailles, KY) to balance the rations of horses requiring low-glycemic rations. In trials with Thoroughbreds, glycemic response was lower when hay was supplemented with I.R. Pellet than when only hay was given (Table 1).

If an older ECD horse has trouble maintaining weight, its ration can be supplemented with additional calories from a high-fat, low-starch product. In addition to providing a concentrated source of energy, vegetable oil has been shown to greatly reduce glycemic response to a grain meal, possibly by delaying gastric emptying (Geor et al., 2001). If beet pulp is added to the ration, it should be rinsed to reduce its glycemic index (Table 1) (Groff et al., 2001). Rice bran also has a low glycemic index (47%). Feeds that are designed for senior horses may not be desirable for ECD horses because they may contain ingredients such as molasses, which produce a high glycemic response. For example, in a recent study by Kentucky Equine Research, Purina Equine Senior had a glycemic index that was similar to oats (Table 1).

Equine metabolic syndrome (EMS) is an endocrine and metabolic disorder that results in insulin resistance (IR) and an increased risk of pasture-associated laminitis (Andrews and Frank, 2008). Horses and ponies with EMS tend to be obese with cresty necks. These animals have often had prior bouts of laminitis and are easy keepers. A feeding program for EMS horses should be focused on reducing body weight while providing adequate protein, vitamin, and mineral intake. It should be a forage-based program, but pasture intake should either be restricted with a grazing muzzle and limited turn-out, or completely avoided during times of lush growth. Since caloric restriction is important, a concentrated balancer such as I.R. Pellet should be used for supplementation.

Recurrent exertional rhabdomyolysis (RER) is a specific form of tying-up seen in Thoroughbreds, Standardbreds, and Arabians (Valberg et al., 2005). It is an inherited trait caused by abnormal intracellular calcium regulation during muscle contraction. Although the genetic predisposition for RER is evenly divided between males and females, clinical signs of the disease are more often seen in young fillies. Excitement and stress seem to be trigger factors. High grain intakes are associated with tying-up in racehorses. Research conducted at the University of Minnesota in conjunction with KER suggests that replacing much of the grain in the diet with a low-starch, high-fat feed will significantly decrease the amount of muscle damage in RER horses. In a feeding trial, five Thoroughbred horses with RER were exercised on a treadmill for five days a week while they consumed hay and a variety of energy supplements for three weeks at a time. When the daily caloric intake of a high-starch ration was kept low (21 Mcal DE/day), the horses had lower post-exercise serum creatine kinase (CK) than when this feed was increased to provide 28 MCal DE/day (MacLeay et al., 2000). In contrast, if extra calories were provided from a low-starch, high-fat feed (Re-Leve; KERx, Versailles, KY) rather than a grain supplement at 28 Mcal/day, no increase in post-exercise serum CK activity occurred. No significant differences in muscle glycogen or lactate concentrations were apparent in these studies (MacLeay et al., 1999).

Most horses with RER have medium to high energy requirements and need significant calories supplied above those found in the forage portion of the ration. An appropriate feed should be fortified to be fed at fairly high levels of intake (4-6 kg/day). It should be low in NSC (<10%), high in fat (>10%), and supply a significant portion of its energy as fermentable fiber.

Polysaccharide storage myopathy (PSSM) is another muscle disorder that is more common in Quarter Horses, warmbloods, and draft breeds (Valberg et al., 2005). It is characterized by an abnormal accumulation of glycogen in muscle resulting from a hypersensitivity of the muscle to insulin. The same type of energy sources used for RER horses is effective for PSSM horses. Research at the University of Minnesota has shown that serum CK levels, which are indicative of tying-up, were reduced when Quarter Horses suffering from PSSM were fed Re-Leve (Ribeiro et al., 2004). Since these horses have lower energy requirements than RER horses, the concentration of other nutrients needs to be greater than in feeds designed for RER. Therefore, KER has developed a more nutrient-dense feed (Re-Leve Concentrate) for managing PSSM.

Osteochondrosis can be a problem among young horses. The source of calories for young horses may also be important, as hyperglycemia or hyperinsulinemia have been implicated in the pathogenesis of osteochondrosis (Glade et al., 1984; Ralston, 1995). Foals that experience an exaggerated and sustained increase in circulating glucose or insulin in response to a carbohydrate (grain) meal may be predisposed to development of osteochondrosis. In vitro studies with fetal and foal chondrocytes suggest that the role of insulin in growth cartilage may be to promote chondrocyte survival or to suppress differentiation and that hyperinsulinemia may be a contributory factor to equine osteochondrosis (Henson et al., 1997).

Research from KER (Pagan et al., 2001) suggests that hyperinsulinemia may influence the incidence of osteochondritis dissecans (OCD) in Thoroughbred weanlings. In a large field trial, 218 Thoroughbred weanlings (average age 300 ± 40 days, average body weight 300 kg ± 43 kg) were studied. A glycemic response test was conducted by feeding a meal that consisted of the weanling's normal concentrate at a level of intake equal to 1.4 g nonstructural carbohydrate (NSC) per kilogram body weight. A single blood sample was taken 120 minutes post-feeding for the determination of glucose and insulin.

In this study, a high glucose and insulin response to a concentrate meal was associated with an increased incidence of OCD. Glycemic responses measured in the weanlings were highly correlated with each feed's glycemic index (GI), suggesting that the GI of a farm's feed may play a role in the pathogenesis of OCD. In rats, prolonged feeding of a high-GI feed results in basal hyperinsulinemia and an elevated insulin response to an intravenous glucose tolerance test (Pawlak et al., 2001). Hyperinsulinemia may affect chondrocyte maturation, leading to altered matrix metabolism and faulty mineralization or altered cartilage growth by influencing other hormones such as thyroxine (Pagan et al., 1996; Jeffcott and Henson, 1998). Based on the results of this study, it would be prudent to feed foals concentrates that produce low to moderate glycemic responses.

Summary

The five metabolic disorders discussed in this paper have very different etiologies yet are all either triggered or aggravated by excessive starch and sugar intake. Table 3 summarizes important factors to consider for each disorder. While all of these horses require rations with a low glycemic index, the most appropriate form of energy supplementation depends on the disorder and the individual's energy requirement (Table 3). Horses with ECD are insulin insensitive and need a low-GI ration, but their energy requirement may vary. Some may be relatively easy keepers and benefit from mostly forage rations while others may need extra calories in the form of fat and fermentable fiber. EMS horses and ponies tend to be obese and easy keepers and should be fed mostly forage rations with an appropriate low inclusion balancer. Both ECD and EMS sufferers are prone to laminitis that can be triggered by access to lush pasture, so pasture intake should be carefully controlled. Horses with RER and PSSM are not insulin insensitive, but both groups benefit from low-starch feeds. Fat is an important supplement for both groups, but their energy requirements are different. RER horses tend to need moderate to high energy intakes while PSSM horses typically require fewer calories. Osteochondrosis may be triggered by high-glycemic feeds, but there is no evidence that young growing horses need extremely low-GI feeds. In fact, a certain amount of starch in the ration is desirable for young horses, particularly during sales preparation. Diets for young horses should have moderate glycemic indexes and be fortified to promote optimal muscular and skeletal development.

Table 3. Variables related to feeding horses with different metabolic disorders.

Metabolic condition	Energy requirement	Insulin insensitive	Fat in feed	High laminitis risk
EDC	Low to high	Yes	Low to high	Yes
EMS	Low	Yes	Low	Yes
RER	Moderate to high	No	High	No
PSSM	Low to moderate	No	High	No
OCD	Low to moderate	No	Moderate	No

References

Andrews, F.M. and N. Frank. 2008. Pathology of metabolic-related conditions. In: Proc. Kentucky Equine Research Nutr. Conf. 95-108.

Frank, N., F.M. Andrews, C.S. Sommardahl, H. Eiler, B.W. Rohrbach, and R.L. Donnell. 2006. Evaluation of the combined dexamethasone suppression/thyrotropin-releasing hormone stimulation test for detection of pars intermedia pituitary adenomas in horses. J. Vet. Intern. Med. 20:987-993.

Geor, R.J., P.A. Harris, K.E. Hoekstra, J.D. Pagan. 2001. Effect of corn oil on solid phase gastric emptying in horses. J. Vet. Int. Med. (Abstr.).

Glade, M.J., S. Gupta, and T.J. Reimers. 1984. Hormonal responses to high and low planes of nutrition in weanling Thoroughbreds. J. Anim. Sci. 59:658-665.

Groff, L., J. Pagan, K. Hoekstra, S. Gardner, O. Rice, K. Roose, and R. Geor. 2001. Effect of preparation method on the glycemic response to ingestion of beet pulp in Thoroughbred horses. In: Proc. Equine Nutr. Physiol. Soc. Symp.

Henson, F.M., C. Davenport, L. Butler, I. Moran, W.D. Shingleton, L.B. Jeffcott, and P.N. Schofield. 1997. Effects of insulin and insulin like growth factors I and II on the growth of equine fetal and neonatal chondrocytes. Equine Vet. J. 29:441-447.

Jeffcott, L.B., and F.M. Henson. 1998. Studies on growth cartilage in the horse and their application to aetiopathogenesis of dyschondroplasia (osteochondrosis). Vet. J. 156:177-192.

Lawrence, L.M. 2008. Assessing energy balance. In: Proc. Kentucky Equine Research Nutr. Conf. 119-125.

MacLeay, J.M., S.J. Valberg, J. Pagan, J.A. Billstrom, and J. Roberts. 2000. Effect of diet and exercise intensity on serum CK activity in Thoroughbreds with recurrent exertional rhabdomyolysis. Amer. J. Vet. Res. 61:1390-1395.

Pagan, J.D., R.J. Geor, S.E. Caddel, P.B. Pryor, and K.E. Hoekstra. 2001. The relationship between glycemic response and the incidence of OCD in thoroughbred weanlings: A field study. In: Proc. Amer. Assn. Equine Practnr. 47:322-325.

Pagan, J.D., S.G. Jackson, and S. Caddel. 1996. A summary of growth rates of Thoroughbreds in Kentucky. Pferdeheilkunde 12:285-289.

Pawlak, D.B., J.M. Bryson, G.S. Denyer, and J.C. Brand-Miller. 2001. High glycemic index starch promotes hypersecretion of insulin and higher body fat in rats without affecting insulin sensitivity. J. Nutr. 131:99-104.

Ralston, S.L. 1995. Postprandial hyperglycemica/hyperinsulinemia in young horses with osteochondritis dissecans lesions. J. Anim. Sci. 73:184 (Abstr.).

Ribeiro,W.P., S.J. Valberg, J.D. Pagan, and B. Essen Gustavsson. 2004.The effect of varying dietary starch and fat content on serum creatine kinase activity and substrate availability in equine polysaccharide storage myopathy. J. Vet. Int. Med. 18:887-894.

Valberg, S.J, R.J. Geor, and J.D. Pagan. 2005. Muscle disorders: Untying the knots through nutrition. In: J.D. Pagan and R.J. Geor (Ed.) Advances in Equine Nutrition III. p. 473-483. Nottingham University Press, Nottingham, UK.

PATHOLOGY OF METABOLIC-RELATED CONDITIONS

FRANK M. ANDREWS AND NICHOLAS FRANK
The University of Tennessee, Knoxville, Tennessee

Equine Cushing's Disease (Pituitary Pars Intermedia Dysfunction [PPID])

INTRODUCTION

Equine Cushing's disease (ECD) or pituitary pars intermedia dysfunction (PPID) results from hypertrophy, hyperplasia, or a functional adenoma in the pars intermedia of the pituitary gland and is frequently recognized in older horses (Frank et al., 2006a). The pituitary produces excessive amounts of adrenocorticotropic hormone (ACTH), which results in an increased secretion of cortisol from the adrenal glands (hyperadrenocorticism). The intermediate lobe of the pituitary gland is located between the pars nervosa (posterior pituitary) and the pars distalis of the anterior pituitary gland and is the primary site of disease. ECD develops when pars intermedia cells become hyperplastic or neoplastic and biologically active. Neoplastic cells form microadenomas (<5 mm) or macroadenomas (>5 mm) that are commonly referred to as pituitary adenomas. Hormones and other products (MSH, beta-endorphins, ACTH) of these neoplastic cells are responsible for the clinical signs associated with ECD. Current diagnostic tests, the overnight dexamethasone suppression or endogenous ACTH tests, may produce false positive and false negative results, making diagnosis of ECD difficult (Schott, 2002).

CLINICAL SIGNS AND PRESENTATION

Equine Cushing's disease is commonly found in older horses and ponies, so it should always be considered when evaluating horses over 18 years of age. Younger horses also develop ECD, but currently available diagnostic tests may not be sensitive enough to detect early disease. In a recent study, we evaluated 17 horses with histopathologic evidence of ECD. The horses ranged in age from 9 to 33 years, with a median of 23 years (Frank et al., 2006a). Ponies appear to be more susceptible to ECD, but no other breed or sex predilections are recognized (Schott, 2002).

Clinical signs in horses with suspected ECD include lethargy, loss of appetite, pot-bellied appearance, laminitis, hirsutism, hyperhidrosis (excessive sweating), polydipsia (excessive water drinking), polyuria (excessive urination), increased supraorbital fat pads, and dental and foot diseases. Laminitis is the most important clinical manifestation of ECD because it results in pain and suffering, and can lead to retirement or even euthanasia when chronic problems develop. Many horses first develop laminitis when grazing on pasture and the disease is triggered by an increase in pasture grass sugar content. Sugar concentrations rise dramatically when the grass grows rapidly in the spring and summer after heavy rainfall, or when it is preparing for winter dormancy in the fall. This alters the large intestinal flora, changes intestinal permeability, and leads to the release of triggering factors into the blood. Horses with ECD may be predisposed to laminitis because they have weaker hoof tissues or altered blood flow as a result of increased blood cortisol (Johnson et al., 2002). Some affected horses are also insulin resistant, which may further lower the laminitis threshold. These predisposing factors make horses or ponies with ECD more sensitive to alterations in pasture grass sugar content, and therefore more susceptible to pasture-associated laminitis.

Horses with ECD commonly have a long, curly haircoat (hirsutism) that does not shed out during the spring or summer months. Hirsutism is sometimes considered to be pathognomonic for ECD, but protein deficiency can also lead to haircoat abnormalities in older horses. Overt hirsutism only occurs with advanced disease but careful examination will sometimes reveal the presence of long hairs along the palmar or plantar aspects of the legs or patches of longer hair on the body. Clients should also be questioned about the exact time of year that their horse sheds its winter coat and how this compares to other horses on the farm. An early sign of ECD is delayed shedding of the winter haircoat.

There are some similarities between ECD and equine metabolic syndrome (EMS, see below) because fat deposits expand in the neck region, a condition commonly referred to as a "cresty neck." Fat pads may also develop close to the tailhead and in the supraorbital area (above the eyes). Since these are common to both ECD and EMS, it is sometimes challenging to differentiate between the two conditions. As a general rule of thumb, horses with ECD have a thinner body condition because they have lost muscle mass, whereas horses with EMS tend to exhibit generalized obesity.

Corticosteroids stimulate the conversion of muscle protein into energy through gluconeogenesis. Loss of epaxial (muscle over the back) muscle mass can often be detected in older horses, but this alteration is more pronounced in animals with ECD. A pot-bellied appearance may be seen in horses with advanced ECD as the abdominal musculature thins and weakens. Because of the increased cortisol in the blood, horses and ponies with advanced ECD are more susceptible to diseases such as sinusitis, tooth root infections, or sole abscesses. This finding is attributed to the immunosuppressive actions of corticosteroids.

Hyperhidrosis (excessive sweating) is sometimes detected in animals with ECD and will persist even after the haircoat has been clipped. Polydipsia and polyuria may accompany ECD, but these signs are hard to detect until the disease is advanced.

Clients should therefore be instructed to measure water consumption with the aim of detecting polydipsia. Lethargy is detected in some animals with ECD and clients sometimes report that their horse has become more tolerant of pain. These findings are attributed to the release of beta-endorphins from the diseased pituitary gland.

Older horses are more likely to develop ECD because the dopaminergic inhibition of the pituitary gland decreases with age. Dopaminergic neurons extend from the hypothalamus to the pituitary gland and carry dopamine, which is an inhibitory neurotransmitter. Dopamine inhibits the activity of pituitary tissues and decreases ACTH secretion. It may also prevent the development of hyperplastic cells that subsequently become neoplastic. Loss of dopaminergic neurons is a normal aging process, but degeneration may be accelerated in some horses, and these animals are likely to more susceptible to ECD. Oxidative damage may be responsible for the loss of dopaminergic neurons that occurs with age (McFarlane et al., 2005a; McFarlane et al., 2005b).

Other conditions have been described in horses with ECD and include osteoporosis, delayed wound healing, central nervous dysfunction, suspensory ligament breakdown, and persistent lactation and infertility.

DIAGNOSIS

Changes in routine blood work may include increased blood glucose concentration (>100 mg/dL) and/or changes in white blood cell count (mature neutrophilia with lymphopenia). These findings are attributed to the effects of corticosteroids on glucose metabolism (insulin resistance and enhanced gluconeogenesis) and circulating leukocytes (demargination of neutrophils).

RESTING ACTH, INSULIN, AND GLUCOSE CONCENTRATIONS

We routinely screen horses for ECD by measuring plasma ACTH concentrations, and we also measure glucose and insulin concentrations to indirectly assess glucose metabolism. Elevated ACTH concentrations indicate that the horse suffers from ECD, and hyperinsulinemia accompanies insulin resistance (IR) because insulin secretion from the pancreas increases to compensate for the change in insulin sensitivity. IR is a defining feature of EMS, but also occurs in some patients with ECD. This condition is relevant to the management of ECD patients because insulin-resistant horses and ponies are more susceptible to laminitis. It is therefore important to recognize IR and improve insulin sensitivity through dietary management, exercise, and drug interventions.

For ACTH measurements, we routinely send blood samples to the Diagnostic Center for Population and Animal Health (DCPAH) laboratory at Michigan State University. According to its reference range, ECD is suspected when the plasma ACTH concentration is above 7.5 pmol/L (35 pg/mL) and is diagnosed when the concentration

280 *Pathology of Metabolic-Related Conditions*

is above 10 pmol/L (45 pg/mL). Unfortunately, it has been our experience that ACTH concentrations are not a sensitive indicator of ECD in horses and ponies. Animals with advanced disease tend to have elevated plasma ACTH concentrations, but early disease can go undetected (McFarlane et al., 2005a). Detection of hyperinsulinemia serves as a screening test for IR, but this is complicated by the fact that reference ranges vary considerably between laboratories. For instance, the DCPAH defines hyperinsulinemia as >300 pmol/L (43 mU/L; multiply by 7 to convert units), whereas the upper limit of the reference range is 30 mU/L (210 pmol/L) at the University of Tennessee Endocrinology Laboratory. Since we are screening patients for IR, we use a narrower reference range for insulin and assume that a value >20 mU/L is suggestive of IR. High-normal (>100 mg/dL or 5 mmol/L; multiply by 18 to convert units) glucose concentrations can also be detected in horses with IR. Patients with hyperinsulinemia should have a combined glucose-insulin test (CGIT) performed to further assess insulin sensitivity and document the degree of IR (Eiler et al., 2005). More subtle alterations in insulin sensitivity can also be assessed in horses or ponies with lower (<20 mU/L) serum insulin concentrations by applying glucose and insulin values to normograms that predict insulin sensitivity and pancreatic function in horses and ponies (Kronfeld, 2006).

DIURNAL CORTISOL RHYTHM TEST

Taking a single serum cortisol concentration will not help in the diagnosis of ECD, because blood concentrations fluctuate rapidly from minute to minute. However, serum cortisol concentrations generally decrease throughout the day, so the cortisol level is usually >30% lower in the evening than it is in the morning (Dybdal et al., 1994). This is referred to as the diurnal cortisol rhythm, and it is assumed that this pattern is lost when horses develop ECD because ACTH is now being released from the pars intermedia, which is not under negative feedback control. We performed a small study in which we measured and compared serum cortisol concentrations in four healthy mares every 2 weeks for 8 weeks. Of the 20 pairs of samples evaluated, the diurnal difference was <30% on 4 occasions (20% false positive rate) in healthy mares, indicating that the test has a low specificity. We do not routinely use this test in our practice, but it may be a useful screening test. However, you should only consider the negative result to be significant. Detection of a normal rhythm (>30% difference between morning and evening) indicates that ECD is unlikely to be present, but horses with positive results must undergo further testing before a diagnosis is made.

The only way to definitively diagnose ECD is to identify neoplastic tissue within the pars intermedia of the pituitary gland at postmortem examination. At present, an antemortem diagnosis of ECD can be made by (1) observing hirsutism; (2) increased plasma ACTH concentration; or (3) getting a positive result when a dexamethasone suppression test or combined dexamethasone suppression/thyrotropin-releasing hormone (TRH) stimulation test is performed (Eiler et al., 2005).

In our recent study, we found the sensitivity and specificity of hirsutism to be 71% and 95%, respectively, and only one false positive was identified (Frank et al., 2006a). The specificity of hirsutism is high, but the sensitivity is low because only animals with advanced disease are affected. In our practice, detection of overt hirsutism (long, curly haircoat) in an older horse is sufficient to begin pergolide therapy. However, protein deficiency can result in haircoat changes, so this potential problem should be addressed by feeding a protein supplement if the diet is poor.

A dexamethasone suppression test is performed by collecting a pre-injection blood sample and then injecting 0.04 mg/kg (20 mg for a 500-kg horse) dexamethasone intravenously. A second blood sample is collected 24 hours later. In a healthy horse, the plasma cortisol concentration will remain suppressed for greater than 24 hours. The plasma cortisol concentration measured 24 hours post-injection should be <10 ng/mL (1.0 µg/dL) if the horse is responding normally. The test is therefore positive for ECD if the plasma cortisol concentration is above 10 ng/mL when blood collected 24 hours post-injection is analyzed. Plasma cortisol concentrations do not remain suppressed (i.e., they "escape") in horses with ECD because neoplastic cells within the pars intermedia are not under negative feedback control. The pars distalis responds to negative feedback, so ACTH production is suppressed, but pituitary adenoma cells continue to secrete ACTH, and this is enough to raise the cortisol level above 10 ng/mL (1 µg/ml) within 24 hours.

The combined dexamethasone suppression/thyrotropin-releasing hormone test was developed at the University of Tennessee and first described 11 years ago (Eiler et al., 1997). We recently evaluated the accuracy of the test and found that combining results of both the dexamethasone suppression and TRH stimulation components of the test increased its sensitivity (Frank et al., 2006a). The sensitivity values for the two components of the test were 65% and 41%, respectively, whereas the combined test had a sensitivity of 88%. The specificity (76%) was limited by the dexamethasone suppression component of the test. These sensitivity values suggest that the dexamethasone test will fail to identify 35% of horses with ECD when used alone, but only 12% of horses with disease will be missed when the combined test is used. Inclusion of the TRH stimulation test is easily accomplished in a referral hospital setting, but this test is more difficult to perform in the field. Thyrotropin-releasing hormone is commercially available from Phoenix Pharmaceuticals, Inc. (www.phoenixpeptide.com; 25 mg vial for $35) or a reagent grade product can be purchased from Sigma Chemical, Inc. To perform this component of the test, a pre-TRH blood sample should be collected 3 hours after injecting dexamethasone and 1 mg of TRH (total dose) is injected intravenously. A post-TRH blood sample must then be collected 30 minutes later. Plasma cortisol concentrations increase by <66% over 30 minutes in healthy horses, whereas a horse with ECD has a ≥66% increase over the same time period. Although corticotropin-releasing hormone (CRH) secreted by the hypothalamus is primarily responsible for the release of ACTH, some TRH receptors are present within tissues of the pars distalis and pars intermedia. The abundance of these receptors is low in healthy pituitary tissue, so ACTH is not released in response to exogenous TRH. However, neoplastic tissues expand the size of the pars intermedia and have more TRH receptors, so they respond positively to the same challenge. Pituitary adenoma cells release more ACTH in response to TRH, which stimulates the release of cortisol. It is advantageous to administer dexamethasone 3 hours before TRH because it lowers the baseline plasma cortisol concentration and therefore makes it easier to recognize the post-injection peak.

The approach to horses suspected of having ECD involves the following steps:

(1) A horse or pony with hirsutism is assumed to suffer from ECD and pergolide therapy is initiated. Resting glucose and insulin concentrations are measured and a CGIT is ideally performed to assess insulin sensitivity, which is important for the management of laminitis.

(2) Detection of a plasma ACTH concentration above 10 pmol/L (between November and July) is diagnostic for ECD and pergolide is prescribed. Insulin sensitivity is also assessed.

(3) If there is a high suspicion of ECD, the potential risks of performing a dexamethasone suppression test are discussed with the client. Insulin sensitivity is also assessed prior to the dexamethasone suppression test because corticosteroids induce transient IR (Donaldson et al., 2005). If the client accepts the risks and there is an adequate veterinarian/client relationship, a combined dexamethasone suppression/TRH stimulation test is performed. If the client has reservations about the test, the horse's IR (if present) is managed and a 6-month trial of pergolide is prescribed.

(4) If a cresty neck is the only clinical sign detected, insulin sensitivity is assessed and the diagnosis of EMS is considered.

TREATMENT

Pergolide is the drug of choice for treating ECD. This drug increases the production of the inhibitory neurotransmitter dopamine, which has two potential effects: (1) it suppresses the activity of neoplastic pars intermedia cells, and (2) it inhibits growth of the tumor(s). This drug is administered orally at a dosage of 1 mg (total dose) per day, and the cost is approximately $2.00 per day. We usually recommend purchasing the drug through a reputable compounding pharmacy, but quality control is important and there have been anecdotal reports of compounded pergolide lacking efficacy. Side effects of pergolide seen in humans include anorexia, diarrhea, and depression, but horses generally tolerate the drug well. We have increased the dosage to 4 mg/day in some ECD patients with advanced disease. Some clients claim that they have seen a better response when pergolide is given twice daily, but this issue has not been studied. Other drugs that can be used to treat horses or ponies with ECD include cyproheptadine (a serotonin antagonist) and trilostane (a 3ß-hydroxysteroid dehydrogenase competitive inhibitor), which is currently available only from Canada. Serotonin is an excitatory neurotransmitter, so cyproheptadine suppresses pituitary activity. Trilostane inhibits the rate-limiting step in cortisol synthesis within the adrenal gland and is administered orally at a dosage of 0.5 to 1.0 mg/kg. This drug is more commonly used in Europe, but pergolide still remains the drug of choice for treating ECD in horses and ponies. The adrenocorticolytic drug o,p'-DDD (Lysodren®) used to treat Cushing's disease in dogs is not effective in horses.

MANAGEMENT

Some horses with ECD also suffer from IR, so they should be placed on diets that contain less sugar. A diet composed primarily of hay is often recommended, but if concentrates must be fed to meet energy demands in exercising horses, they should be provided without exacerbating IR. You must therefore consider the following features: (1) the NSC content of the feed, (2) its glycemic index, and (3) the amount of feed provided. The glycemic index is the degree to which blood glucose concentrations increase after the feed is consumed (area under the postprandial blood glucose curve). Feeds with both a high NSC content and high glycemic index can exacerbate IR when fed in large quantities. Grazing on pasture presents the greatest risk to the horse with IR because the NSC content of pasture grass varies widely and fluctuates with changes in rainfall and temperature. Limited grazing time or use of a grazing muzzle should be considered when managing horses with IR, and some patients must be held off pasture altogether to prevent laminitis from being triggered.

ECD VS. EMS

This is a controversial question because there is still debate about the definition of equine metabolic syndrome (EMS) in horses, and some clinicians question whether the condition is simply an early manifestation of ECD. I do not think that EMS is caused by ECD, but the two conditions are related. Horses with EMS appear to be predisposed to ECD, and it develops at an earlier age in these animals. A horse can therefore transition from EMS to ECD as it ages. This transition tends to occur when the horse is between 10 and 20 years of age and it is recognized by a shift in body condition from generalized obesity to a thinner condition because of lost muscle mass. The cresty neck remains evident and fat pads close to the tailhead may become more prominent. Other changes can include the development of abnormal shedding patterns or the growth of longer hairs on the palmar and plantar aspects of the legs. Equine metabolic syndrome begins with a genetic difference that makes the individual horse require fewer calories to maintain body weight ("easy keeper"). Current feeding and management practices cause weight gain, and adipose tissues expand quickly in these genetically susceptible horses. IR develops as a result and this combines with obesity or regional adiposity (cresty neck) to create a proinflammatory state. Chronic IR is associated with increased inflammatory adipokine release from adipose tissues and enhanced oxidative damage. This type of damage has been associated with dopaminergic neuron degeneration in horses with ECD, so EMS may accelerate the onset of disease. Until more sensitive tests become available, horses exhibiting a cresty neck should be evaluated for ECD, and those with negative results should be diagnosed with EMS. Practitioners should use their own clinical judgment when assessing patients to discern whether the horse is beginning to make the transition to ECD. In my opinion, pergolide therapy is warranted in the horse with EMS that appears to be developing ECD, even in the absence of supportive diagnostic test results.

SUMMARY

Older horses are at risk for developing ECD and pergolide is an effective treatment for the condition. Clinical signs and available diagnostic tests will confirm the presence of advanced disease, but may not be sensitive enough to detect early ECD. Horses with EMS present a diagnostic challenge because they may develop ECD at an earlier age. The owner or veterinarian must recognize the transition from EMS to ECD and initiate pergolide therapy when it occurs.

Equine Metabolic Syndrome

INTRODUCTION

Equine metabolic syndrome (EMS) is an endocrine and metabolic disorder, where insulin resistance (IR) is the primary problem encountered and this condition increases the risk of pasture-associated laminitis.

Equine metabolic syndrome is defined by the detection of chronic IR in a horse or pony. Other potential causes of IR include pituitary pars intermedia dysfunction (ECD, also called equine Cushing's disease), stress, and pregnancy, and these conditions must therefore be ruled out before the diagnosis of EMS is made. Genetic differences in energy metabolism are likely to play an important role in this disease because clients consistently report that horses are "easy keepers"with respect to their caloric needs. This syndrome is currently defined by (1) insulin resistance, (2) the presence of obesity and/or regional adiposity, and (3) prior or current laminitis. Evidence of prior laminitis comes from the history provided by the client or detection of obvious growth rings on the hooves (founder lines), which are assumed to result from previous subclinical laminitis episodes.

"Metabolic syndrome"has been used to describe this syndrome in the past, but it is preferable to use the descriptor "equine" when referring to horses and ponies (Johnson, 2002). Metabolic syndrome is a term used in human medicine to describe a set of factors that identify people who are at risk for developing coronary heart disease, stroke, or diabetes. In contrast, EMS describes a clinical syndrome that is unique to the equine species because of its connection with laminitis. In the past, some horses or ponies with EMS have also been inappropriately labeled as "hypothyroid" after low serum thyroid hormone concentrations were detected. However, it is now known that low resting thyroid hormone concentrations can occur without thyroid gland dysfunction in horses, and clinical hypothyroidism can be diagnosed only after more advanced testing (Breuhaus et al., 2006). Equine metabolic syndrome occurs in horses and ponies. No published information is available regarding the prevalence of EMS in different breeds of horses, but based upon our experience, the disorder is most common in pony breeds, Morgans, Paso Finos, and Norwegian Fjords. We have also diagnosed EMS in Arabians, Quarter Horses, American Saddlebreds, Tennessee Walking Horses, Thoroughbreds, and warmbloods, which suggests that many breed groups are represented (Frank et al., 2006b).

Affected animals are often middle-aged (10 to 20 years of age) when EMS is first recognized, but the condition can also affect younger (5 to 10 years of age) horses. EMS is often first recognized when laminitis develops. The horse is usually being kept on pasture, and the episode occurs after the pasture has gone through a period of rapid growth (spring) or entered winter dormancy (fall). Upon closer examination, founder lines are seen on the hooves, which indicate prior subclinical laminitis episodes. Horses with EMS are predisposed to hyperlipemia, and mares may have abnormal reproductive cycles (Vick et al., 2006).

Veterinarians or farriers will sometimes recognize the physical characteristics of horses and ponies with EMS. Affected animals either suffer from generalized obesity and have an overall overweight appearance, or look more normal in appearance but have enlarged fat deposits in the neck and tailhead regions. The presence of enlarged fat deposits in these locations is referred to as regional adiposity and the thickened neck region is often called a "cresty neck."

The final part of the clinical picture comes from the history and cannot be easily measured. Horses and ponies with EMS are described as "easy keepers" because they seem to require fewer calories to maintain their body weight. This is likely to be a reflection of genetic susceptibility. Insulin is a hormone secreted by the pancreas that stimulates the uptake of glucose by tissues when sugar is abundant (i.e., after feeding). Skeletal muscle and adipose tissues are the major sites of insulin-mediated glucose uptake, but the liver also responds to insulin by increasing uptake of glucose from the blood. Insulin binds to receptors on the surface of plasma membranes and triggers a series of internal events that result in the movement of glucose transporter proteins (GLUT4) to the cell surface, facilitating rapid glucose uptake. Insulin plays an important role in the storage of energy by moving glucose into cells where it can be stored as glycogen or converted into fat.

INSULIN RESISTANCE

This condition is defined as the failure of tissues to respond appropriately to insulin. There are numerous mechanisms responsible for IR including a reduction in the density of insulin receptors on the cell surface, malfunction of insulin receptors, defective internal signaling pathways, and interference with the translocation or function of GLUT4 proteins.

We do not know the exact path physiology of EMS, but it begins with a combination of genetic and dietary factors. Evidence for a genetic component of EMS comes from a published study examining the heritability of IR in ponies (Treiber et al., 2006) and from our own observations that the dam or sire of the patient with EMS also suffers from the disorder. The easy keeper concept is relevant to this issue of genetic susceptibility. Certain breeds or genetic lines may have undergone evolutionary adaptations to survive in harsher environments, and these horses or ponies can more efficiently convert poorer quality forages into energy. Under modern circumstances, these adaptations are unnecessary and are likely to predispose the animal to obesity. Equine metabolic syndrome may therefore begin with the genetically susceptible horse or pony grazing on lush pasture or being fed large amounts of concentrates.

As excess energy is stored as fat, adipose tissues expand through an increase in the number and size of adipocytes. Cellular functions are negatively impacted and adipose tissues release factors called adipokines that act locally and enter the circulation. Some of these adipokines exert proinflammatory effects that may contribute to the development of laminitis. Skeletal muscle tissues also accumulate lipid, which means that both of the major sites of insulin-stimulated glucose uptake become affected, and IR develops as a result. All of the pieces of the puzzle must be assembled before we can fully understand the association between IR and pasture-associated laminitis in horses and ponies. However, there are three broad mechanisms by which IR could predispose horses to laminitis: (1) insulin resistance might impair glucose delivery to hoof keratinocytes, (2) insulin resistance could alter blood flow to the foot, or (3) obesity and IR could lead to a proinflammatory state. The first theory is supported by results of a study performed by Pass et al. (1998) in which it was demonstrated that hoof tissue explants separated at the dermal-epidermal junction when deprived of glucose. Furthermore, Mobasheri et al. (2004) determined that GLUT4 proteins are found in equine keratinocytes, which suggests that insulin-stimulated glucose uptake occurs in the hoof. Studies examining the relationship between IR and blood flow have not been performed to date in horses, but insulin is known to act as a slow vasodilator in humans, and IR has been associated with a decrease in peripheral vasodilation (Yki-Jarvinen and Westerbacka, 2000). If IR is a determinant of susceptibility to pasture-associated laminitis, then what triggers the laminitis episode itself? It appears that nonstructural carbohydrates (WSC) within pasture grasses play an important role in this process. Nonstructural carbohydrates include simple sugars, starch, and fructans (polymers of fructose), and levels of these components vary considerably within grass according to geographical location, soil type, weather conditions, and time of day (Hoffman et al., 2001). These carbohydrates are likely to affect the susceptible horse in two ways. First, excessive sugar consumption could exacerbate IR as it does in diabetic humans, and second, consumption of large quantities of WSC might alter the

thyroxine concentration in horses by equilibrium dialysis. J. Vet. Intern. Med. 20:371-376.
Donaldson, M.T., S.M. McDonnell, B.J. Schanbacher, S.V. Lamb, D. McFarlane, and J. Breech. 2005. Variation in plasma adrenocorticotropic hormone concentration and dexamethasone suppression test results with season, age, and sex in healthy ponies and horses. J. Vet. Intern. Med.19:217-222.
Dybdal, N.O., K.M. Hargreaves, J.E. Madigan, D.H. Gibble, P.C. Kennedy, and G.H. Stabenfeldt. 1994. Diagnostic testing for pituitary pars intermedia dysfunction in horses. J. Amer. Vet. Med. Assoc. 204:627-632.
Eiler, H., N. Frank, F.M. Andrews, J.W. Oliver, and K.A. Fecteau. 2005. Physiologic assessment of blood glucose homeostasis via combined intravenous glucose and insulin testing in horses. Amer. J. Vet. Res. 66:1598-1604.
Eiler, H., J.W. Oliver, F.M. Andrews, K.A. Fecteau, E.M. Green, and M. McCracken. 1997. Results of a combined dexamethasone suppression/thyrotropin-releasing hormone stimulation test in healthy horses and horse suspected to have a pars intermedia pituitary adenoma. J. Amer. Vet. Med. Assoc. 211:79-81.
Frank, N., F.M. Andrews, C.S. Sommardahl, H. Eiler, B.W. Rohrbach, and R.L. Donnell. 2006a. Evaluation of the combined dexamethasone suppression/thyrotropin-releasing hormone stimulation test for detection of pars intermedia pituitary adenomas in horses. J. Vet. Intern. Med. 20:987-993.
Frank, N., S.B. Elliott, L.E. Brandt, and D.H. Keisler. 2006b. Physical characteristics, blood hormone concentrations, and plasma lipid concentrations in obese horses with insulin resistance. J. Amer. Vet. Med. Assoc. 228:1383-1390.
Hoffman, R.M., J.A. Wilson, D.S. Kronfeld, W.L. Cooper, L.A. Lawrence, D. Sklan, and P.A. Harris. 2001. Hydrolyzable carbohydrates in pasture, hay, and horse feeds: Direct assay and seasonal variation. J. Anim. Sci. 79:500-506.
Johnson, P.J. 2002. The equine metabolic syndrome peripheral Cushing's syndrome. Vet. Clin. N. Amer. Equine Pract. 18:271-293.
Johnson, P.J., S.H. Slight, V.K. Ganjam, and J.M. Kreeger. 2002. Glucocorticoids and laminitis in the horse. Vet. Clin. N. Amer. Equine Pract. 18:219-236.
Kronfeld, D. 2006. Insulin resistance predicted by specific proxies. J. Equine Vet. Sci.26:281-284.
McFarlane, D., and A.E. Cribb. 2005a. Systemic and pituitary pars intermedia antioxidant capacity associated with pars intermedia oxidative stress and dysfunction in horses. Amer. J. Vet. Res. 66:2065-2072.
McFarlane, D., N. Dybdal, M.T. Donaldson, L. Miller, and A.E. Cribb. 2005b. Nitration and increased alphasynuclein expression associated with dopaminergic neurodegeneration in equine pituitary pars intermedia dysfunction. J. Neuroendocrinol. 17:73-80.
Mobasheri, A., K. Critchlow, P.D. Clegg, S.D. Carter, and C.M. Canessa. 2004. Chronic equine laminitis is characterized by loss of GLUT1, GLUT4 and ENaC positive laminar keratinocytes. Equine Vet. J. 36:248-254.

Pass, M.A., S. Pollitt, and C.C. Pollitt. 1998. Decreased glucose metabolism causes separation of hoof lamellae in vitro: A trigger for laminitis? Equine Vet. J. Suppl. 133-138.

Schott, H.C. 2002. Pituitary pars intermedia dysfunction: Equine Cushing's disease. Vet. Clin. N. Amer. Equine Pract. 18:237-270.

Treiber, K.H., D.S. Kronfeld, T.M. Hess, B.M. Byrd, R.K. Splan, and W.B. Stanier. 2006. Evaluation of genetic and metabolic predispositions and nutritional risk factors for pasture-associated laminitis in ponies. J. Amer. Vet. Med. Assoc. 228:1538-1545.

Vick, M.M., D.R. Sessions, B.A. Murphy, E.L. Kennedy, S.E. Reedy, and B.P. Fitzgerald. 2006. Obesity is associated with altered metabolic and reproductive activity in the mare: Effects of metformin on insulin sensitivity and reproductive cyclicity. Reprod. Fertil. Dev. 18:609-617.

Yki-Jarvinen, H., and J. Westerbacka. 2000. Vascular actions of insulin in obesity. Int. J. Obes. Relat. Metab. Disord. 24:S25-28.

RECENT RESEARCH INTO LAMINITIS

PETER HUNTINGTON,[1] CHRIS POLLITT,[2] AND CATHERINE MCGOWAN[3]
[1]Kentucky Equine Research, Victoria, Australia
[2]Australian Equine Laminitis Research Unit, Queensland, Australia
[3]Department of Equine and Small Animal Medicine, University of Helsinki, Finland

Introduction

Laminitis is a major disease of horses because of the associated pain and debilitating nature that make it a life-threatening condition. A complete understanding of laminitis and its complex pathophysiologic processes remains elusive despite substantial efforts and recent advances by many scientists over the last few decades. For this reason, preventative and therapeutic management strategies remain largely empirical and anecdotal with little information from evidence-based medicine. Laminitis may occur as a consequence of three broad categories of disorders: systemic disease, hormonal disturbances, or trauma. Laminitis research has been confounded by apparently disparate results and theories on pathogenesis. However, recent research has shown that many of these differences may in fact represent different stages of the disease, or different original underlying causes. Recent inflammatory, vascular, and enzymatic research in acute inflammatory or gastrointestinal illness has shown links between these mechanisms, and advances in techniques and early time-course studies have helped elucidate such links. A major trend in recent research on laminitis in the past few years has been the increasing interest in metabolic/endocrine events resulting in laminitis, and interestingly, despite the lack of systemic or gastrointestinal clinical illness in these animals, the laminitis may also involve many of the same mechanisms as those occurring in acute laminitis. This article will review recent research into the pathophysiology of laminitis as well as preventive strategies.

Incidence

The USDA NAHMS report covering 1200 operations and 28,000 horses in 2000 estimated that 13% of operations had encountered at least one case of laminitis in the last 12 months, and the overall incidence was 2.1% (USDA, 2000). The condition is responsible for 15% of all equine lameness and occurs most commonly in horses at pasture. Grazing lush pasture was the most commonly listed cause (45%) followed by complications linked with diet, injury, obesity, and pregnancy. In geriatric horses, the incidence was recorded at 6.4% (Brosnahan and Paradis, 2003) and in the UK a survey of over 100,000 horses found an incidence of 7.1% (Hinckley and Henderson, 1996).

Predisposing Causes

Laminitis is a systemic disease that occurs secondary to the following conditions:

1. Inflammatory/acute gastrointestinal illness
   - grain-based carbohydrate overload
   - pasture-induced carbohydrate overload
   - colic
   - endotoxemia and/or septicemia
   - pleuropneumonia
   - enterocolitis
   - metritis
   - contact with black walnut shavings

2. Metabolic/endocrine (hormonal) disturbances
   - insulin resistance
   - equine Cushing's syndrome
   - obesity
   - glucocorticoid administration

3. Traumatic events
   - excessive weight-bearing on one limb
   - excessive concussion

The pathologic changes that occur in the laminitic hoof are not fully understood, but the following processes are believed to occur at various times during the disease:

- decreased blood flow to the foot and perfusion of the lamellae with possible hypoxia of the lamellae
- injury due to reperfusion after an ischemic episode
- hyperemia
- inflammation
- altered metabolism
- apoptosis
- enzymatic degradation
- edema
- necrosis
- laminar shearing/tearing
- structural failure
- disruption and collapse

Pathology

Key pathologic changes include loss of cellular shape of the secondary epidermal lamellae and loss of attachment of the basement membrane of the lamellae, which is then lysed by matrix metalloproteinase enzymes (MMPs) (Pollitt, 1996). The basement membrane is the key structure bridging the epidermis of the hoof to the connective tissue of the third phalanx, so it follows that the loss and disorganization of basement membrane leads to the failure of hoof anatomy seen in laminitis. These changes are seen on hoof wall biopsies as early as 12 hours after induction of laminitis using the oligofructan induction model, and well before clinical signs (Croser and Pollitt, 2006). The earliest changes of loss of secondary digital lamellae structure and elongation of secondary epidermal lamellae coincided with the onset of a bounding digital pulse. Another component is loss of the lamellar capillaries, which may explain the resistance to blood flow increases and the bounding digital pulse seen during early laminitis. However, very few thrombi were evident and there were no signs of intercellular edema.

Pathophysiologic Theories

The pathogenesis of laminitis is uncertain (Bailey, 2004; Moore et al., 2004). There are at least five hypotheses of how laminitis initially damages the hoof's lamellae, ultimately resulting in changes to the foot's structure and microanatomy, weakening of the laminar bond, rotation/sinking of the pedal bone, and clinical signs of laminitis. However, recent research is now elucidating links between the different theories, and these may actually represent different events in the complex time course of laminitis rather than opposing theories. They include the enzymatic, inflammatory, vascular, metabolic/ endocrine, and mechanical/traumatic theories.

ENZYMATIC THEORY

It has been established that activation of lamellar MMPs is important in the separation of the lamellar cells from their basement membrane and a break in the bond which holds the dermal and epidermal lamellae together (Pollitt and Daradka, 1998; Pollitt et al., 1998; Johnson et al., 1998). This hypothesis, originally developed by the Australian Equine Laminitis Research Unit, postulates that increased digital blood flow delivers circulating cytokines or some other laminitis trigger factors to the digit, where they evoke the production and activation of MMPs.

INFLAMMATORY THEORY

Research at several American institutions using the black walnut extract model and the starch models has shown a marked upregulation of inflammatory cytokines. Increased neutrophil and platelet levels found in laminitic horses can have inflammatory roles and are thought to play a role in the development and progression of laminitis. Inflammatory mediators including cytokines, interleukins 1-beta, 6 and 8, cyclooxygenase-2 (COX-2), and endothelial and intracellular adhesion molecules are involved at an early stage (Blikslager et al., 2006; Loftus et al., 2007a). MMP upregulation has been found at a later stage in these models (Loftus et al., 2007a), indicating that the enzymatic and inflammatory theories may be simply two steps in the pathophysiological process of laminitis.

VASCULAR THEORY

The clinical signs of acute laminitis, including a bounding digital pulse and increased hoof temperature, suggest a vascular component. It is postulated that there are blood flow abnormalities including increased capillary pressure, flow in arteriovenous anastomoses, and venoconstriction so lamellae are deprived of blood flow. It has also been suggested that fluid leaks from the capillaries into the restricted soft tissue space, which leads to edema and ischemia by compressing the small blood vessels. With carbohydrate-induced laminitis models, research has been conflicting with both increased and decreased hoof temperature before the onset of lameness, suggesting increased or decreased digital blood flow. However, increased hoof temperature with the onset of lameness suggests subsequent increased blood flow. Despite these discrepancies, there is little doubt that part of the inflammatory process within the lamellae during laminitis involves endothelial activation (Loftus et al., 2007a) and dysfunction (Eades et al., 2007).

Vasoactive amines have been proposed by the Royal Veterinary College group to play a role in pasture-associated laminitis, with their vasoconstrictive effects shown in vitro (Elliot et al., 2003) and increases in their concentrations in the feces of horses fed fructan-rich diets (Crawford et al., 2007).

METABOLIC/ENDOCRINE THEORY

Insulin is a major regulatory hormone in glucose and fat metabolism, vascular function, inflammation, tissue remodeling, and growth. Insulin resistance alters insulin signaling by decreasing insulin action in certain resistant pathways while increasing insulin signaling in other unaffected pathways via compensatory hyperinsulinemia. In humans, altered insulin signaling is implicated in reduced glucose availability to insulin-sensitive cells, vasoconstriction and endothelial damage, and inflammatory response. Insulin resistance was first implicated in the pathogenesis of laminitis in the 1980s using tolerance tests, but recent research in ponies has established a direct link with insulin (Asplin et al., 2007b).

MECHANICAL/TRAUMATIC THEORY

Laminitis has also been known to result from mechanical overload situations, such as excessive concussion on very hard surfaces or one leg bearing excessive weight when the contralateral limb has a severe, non-weight-bearing injury such as a fracture. In the former case, the mechanism is thought to be damage to the lamellae from direct mechanical trauma, while in the latter, the excessive weightbearing is thought to either directly damage the lamellae or alter blood supply.

Recent Research

INFLAMMATORY AND VASCULAR EVENTS

Recent research in several institutions has started to unravel the mystery surrounding the complex inflammatory pathways involved in laminitis and, importantly, their time course in different models of acute disease.

While the type of inflammatory cytokine response during inflammation within the lamellae differs from other organs due to an absence of resident tissue macrophages, especially in respect to the lack of a TNF alpha response from lamellae (Rodgerson et al., 2001; Loftus et al., 2007a), there are a number of inflammatory events occurring in models of equine laminitis including inflammatory signaling, endothelial activation, leucocyte extravasation, activation of degradative enzymes (MMPs), and the presence of oxidative stress that indicate a similarity to remote organ dysfunction occurring in human sepsis (Belknap et al., 2007; Loftus et al., 2007a). This is supported by a recent study on risk factors for laminitis where endotoxemia, diagnosed on the basis of clinical signs and supportive laboratory findings, was the only factor in the multivariate model associated with a significantly increased risk of laminitis (Parsons et al, 2007).

The inflammatory events in the lamellae occur at an early time point in laminitis induction models including black walnut extract and oligofructose models (Belknap et al., 2007; Loftus et al., 2007a). Recent research has shown that the lamellae have a decreased antioxidant activity (Loftus et al., 2007b), with absent superoxide dismutase indicating its susceptibility to oxidative stress produced during tissue inflammatory events and myeloperoxidase activity from emigrant neutrophils (Riggs et al., 2007).

Many studies have confirmed the in vitro effects of vasoconstrictors (including 5 hydroxytryptamine, $PGF_2\alpha$ and endothelin-1) of digital vessels, especially digital veins (Peroni et al., 2006). Coincident with pro-inflammatory and pro-oxidative effects during the induction of laminitis is upregulation of endothelial and intracellular adhesion molecules (Loftus et al., 2007a). However, in a recent study using the carbohydrate-overload model, changes in endothelin occurred much later than the inflammatory response and endothelial dysfunction (11 hours compared with 1.5 hours) (Eades et al., 2007), and further in vivo work on the time course of vascular events is warranted.

ENZYMATIC THEORY

Enzymes capable of destroying key components of the hoof lamellar attachment apparatus (Pollitt and Daradka, 1998) have been isolated from normal lamellar tissues and in increased quantities from lamellar tissues affected by laminitis (Pollitt et al., 1998). The enzymes are metalloproteinase-2 and metalloproteinase-9 (MMP-2 and MMP-9). Lamellar tissues affected by laminitis increase transcription of MMP (Kyaw-Tanner and Pollitt, 2004), and increased amounts of active MMP are found in laminitis-affected tissues (Pollitt et al., 1998). More recent evidence suggests MMP-9 is associated with neutrophil migration into the lamellae rather than local production (Loftus et al., 2006) and that the activation of these MMP enzymes may be a later event in laminitis, the end result of the inflammatory cascade, rather than an initiating factor (Loftus et al., 2007a,b).

Microbiology

Carbohydrate-induced laminitis is characterized by marked changes in the composition of the hindgut microflora, with gram positive bacteria dominating an environment that is usually predominantly gram negative. An oligofructose induction model was used to study the changes in the bacterial population of the cecum and feces (Millonovich et al., 2007).

Prior to the onset of histological signs (begins at 12 hours) and clinical signs (begins at 24 hours) of laminitis, there was a proliferation of *Streptococcus bovis/equinus* complex. This began two hours after induction and remained high until the 24-hour point in cecal fluid when numbers began to decline. *Lactobacillus* spp. numbers did not increase until 16 hours after induction and numbers were higher in feces than cecal fluid, indicating a secondary proliferation in the ventral colon rather than the cecum. *Enterobacteria* numbers were low and significant increases were not seen until 16 hours after induction, so the proliferation or disappearance of *Enterobacteria* is unlikely to have a key role in laminitis pathophysiology. One unidentified large gram negative rod proliferated consistently in cecal fluid and feces prior to the onset of laminitis. Other bacteria did not establish significant populations in the hindgut before the onset of laminitis and are thought not to have a role in pathogenesis. While these studies confirmed the key role played by *Streptococcus bovis* in the cecum of horses during laminitis induction, it is not known if laminitis trigger factors are produced by proliferation or death of the bacteria or by a host inflammatory response to these changes.

Metabolic/Endocrine Events

A major trend in recent research on laminitis in the past few years has been the increasing interest in metabolic/endocrine events resulting in laminitis. Conditions associated with insulin resistance in horses include equine Cushing's syndrome (ECS), also called pituitary pars intermedia dysfunction (PPID); equine metabolic syndrome (EMS) (or pasture-associated laminitis); and iatrogenic corticosteroid administration.

OBESITY AND EMS

Insulin resistance in horses manifests differently from that in man, although obesity is also a major risk factor in horses with insulin resistance. Obesity has long been associated as a major risk factor for laminitis and this is quantified in the section on risks below. It is difficult for many horses and ponies to lose weight and the syndrome associated with insulin resistance, obesity, and laminitis has recently been termed EMS. EMS was first reported in "Laminitis, hypothyroidism and obesity: A peripheral cushingoid syndrome in horses" (Johnson, 1999). This referred to a syndrome of obese, cresty horses with laminitis. These horses are not hypothyroid as determined by testing for thyroid function (Johnson et al., 2004), but long-term thyroid hormone supplementation can induce weight loss and improve insulin sensitivity (Frank, 2006). The pathogenesis was related back to omental Cushing's in man, which is a syndrome of obesity and abnormal cortisol activity due to activation by the adipose tissue, especially omental adipose tissue as the name suggests. It is thought that fat acts like a gland to produce bioactive substances (adipokines) that reduce insulin sensitivity, cause vascular injury, lead to vasoconstriction, and establish a pro-inflammatory state. There are more than 100 adipokines including leptin, resistin, interleukins, and TNF-α (Johnson et al., 2006). Visceral fat is more biologically active than subcutaneous fat in humans, but of course is harder to assess in the horse or pony. However, it is speculated that fat accumulations in the crest may play the same role as visceral fat in man.

There is a complex relationship between cortisol and adipose tissue production. Situations such as stress or Cushing's disease lead to high cortisol levels that stimulate expansion of adipose tissue and active adipocytes. Active adipose tissue, especially visceral fat, contains the enzyme 11ßHSD-1 that can activate cortisol. This leads to further adipogenesis and contributes to insulin resistance by accumulation of fat within skeletal muscle (Davis, 2005; Johnson et al., 2006).

However, irrespective of the name of the condition, the EMS seen clinically is defined by insulin resistance, recurrent painful laminitis despite good management and veterinary care, and often obesity (historically or currently). Despite sometimes appearing similar to horses with ECS, horses with insulin resistance test negative for ECS on specific endocrine tests (i.e., low-dose dexamethasone suppression or basal [ACTH]), are not hirsute and are younger than horses with ECS (McGowan and Riley, 2004). Of potentially greater interest is that these severe clinical cases probably represent the tip of the iceberg, and there are a number of horses with subclinical disease waiting for the right pasture conditions to develop overt pasture-associated laminitis. These horses have been described by Treiber et al. (2005, 2006) as having "prelaminitic metabolic syndrome," and among other signs, ponies with this syndrome had twice the normal blood concentration of insulin when grazing on winter pasture. In spring, when lush pasture was available, these ponies developed laminitis and had even greater insulin concentrations on basal testing (more than five times the normal values) (Treiber et al., 2006). In more recent studies, it appears that the prevalence of some degree of insulin resistance in horses is 10% (Geor et al., 2007), and even higher (28%) in predisposed breeds such as ponies (McGowan et al., 2008).

ROLE OF INSULIN IN THE PATHOPHYSIOLOGY OF METABOLIC/ENDOCRINE LAMINITIS

Insulin has been shown to be the final triggering event in causing endocrinopathic laminitis in ponies (Asplin et al., 2007b). In a study using nine ponies, laminitis could be induced in 100% of ponies exposed to high concentrations of insulin (mean 1036 ± 55 µIU/mL) while maintaining normal blood glucose concentrations (5.2 ± 0.1 mmol/L) using a modified euglycemic-hyperinsulinemic clamp technique (Asplin et al., 2007b). All ponies were healthy, young (mean 6.5 years), and nonobese, with no history of laminitis and no evidence of endocrine or other abnormalities on blood tests. Laminitis occurred slowly and in all four limbs, with ponies developing mild signs without actual lameness (Obel grade 1) by 32.6 ± 5.4 hours and the onset of lameness associated with laminitis (Obel grade 2) by 55 ± 6 hours. As soon as lameness indicative of laminitis was detected, the infusions were stopped and the ponies were treated with analgesics, resulting in reduction of laminitis by one Obel grade in all cases. Laminitis was confirmed histopathologically in treated ponies. There was no evidence of gastrointestinal involvement and ponies showed no signs of systemic illness throughout the trial (Asplin et al., 2007b).

The common link in endocrinopathic laminitis is insulin resistance, which is manifested as hyperinsulinemia in horses, most commonly with euglycemia (McGowan and Riley, 2004). This new model of laminitis has shown the crucial role insulin plays in laminitis, and shows insulin to be essential in triggering endocrinopathic laminitis. Of importance is that the induction of laminitis occurred independently of glucose or (direct) dietary factors, and also without any evidence of gastrointestinal disturbance. The ponies used were young and had no prior or current obesity. Horses in the study had routine blood tests performed both before and at the onset of laminitis and no changes were found, nor were there any clinical signs indicative of systemic illness or inflammation (Asplin et al., 2007b).

Insulin levels reached in this study are higher than those typically seen in grazing horses (Treiber et al., 2005, 2006). Yet in horses with chronic insulin resistance and endocrinopathic laminitis, insulin concentrations of over 800 µIU/ml were reported in response to glucose administration by Field and Jeffcott (1989) and baseline values over 1000 µIU/ml have been seen frequently in naturally occurring cases of severe insulin resistance syndrome (McGowan and Riley, 2004). However, whether the effect is the same for longer-term exposure to lower levels of insulin or not remains to be determined with further study.

The mechanism by which insulin has triggered laminitis in the model has not yet been determined. However, there are three main theories of the mechanism of laminitis due to the effects of insulin resistance. These are glucose uptake impairment, vascular effects, and pro-inflammatory effects, although the latter two may well be linked as the vascular endothelium is typically a target tissue for the proinflammatory/pro-oxidative effects of insulin resistance.

GLUCOSE UPTAKE IMPAIRMENT

Glucose uptake impairment is the classical sign of insulin resistance, due to the principal effects of insulin in stimulating glucose dispersal into the tissues via GLUT4 transport proteins, particularly in muscle and adipose tissue. The underlying problem of insulin resistance is then potential glucose deprivation of tissues, starving them and causing cell death or damage. In support of this, research has shown that healthy hoof tissue has an absolute requirement for glucose such that when hoof explants are incubated in the absence of glucose, or in the presence of a glucose uptake inhibitor, the layers of tissue separate rapidly, as they do when laminitis occurs (Pass et al., 1998). Additionally, the hoof utilizes glucose at an exceptionally fast rate compared with most other tissues (Wattle and Pollitt, 2004) so, in theory, even a small decrease in the rate of glucose uptake could be extremely damaging. Further to classic glucose uptake impairment due to insulin resistance, there could be a combination of hormonal influences including the activity of catecholamines, which can also reduce glucose uptake synergistically to corticosteroids (Hunt and Ivy, 2002). Since corticosteroids also have the potential to increase adrenergic receptors, this synergism could further impair glucose uptake (Huang et al., 1998).

However, recent research has shown that the hoof lamellae are insulin-independent (Asplin et al., 2007a) based on a number of experiments that indicated that glucose uptake in the hoof is neither dependant on insulin, nor is it influenced by the presence of insulin. Further, when the glucose transport proteins were examined, there was a predominance of GLUT1 in lamellae, which are insulin independent, consistent with the hoof having such a high metabolic demand for glucose (Wattle and Pollitt, 2004; Asplin et al., 2007a). Wattle and Pollitt (personal communication) have also shown that the insulin receptor is not even present on lamellar cells, although it is present in the blood vessel walls. Together, these results provide compelling evidence that laminitis cannot be caused by glucose deprivation resulting from insulin resistance.

INFLAMMATION AND ENDOTHELIAL CELL DYSFUNCTION

The pro-inflammatory changes and effects on the microvasculature are a major problem in human diabetics and sufferers of insulin resistance syndrome. Vascular dysfunction is manifested as both vasoconstriction and pro-coagulant activity, and chronically involves vascular remodeling. Insulin resistance and obesity in man result in a pro-inflammatory state, with increased production of pro-inflammatory cytokines and cytokine-like substances (leptin, resistin), impaired endothelial nitric oxide (NO) production, and endothelial dysfunction (Singer and Granger, 2007). Exacerbating the vascular dysfunction in diabetic patients is the accumulation and glycation of glucose in endothelial cells (glucotoxicity). Glucotoxicity promotes the formation of advanced glycation end products (AGEs), further reducing NO production, and leads to an induction of reactive oxygen species and encourages endothelial expression of inflammatory mediators (Hartge et al., 2007). Insulin also has effects on blood flow in both small and large vessels and insulin resistance (Rattigan et al., 2007). Insulin resistance results in both reduced capillary recruitment and reduced vasodilation in animal models and in humans (Rattigan et al., 2007).

While pro-inflammatory effects and vascular effects of insulin resistance may be difficult to separate, it is clear that either or both occurring in horses with insulin resistance could precipitate laminitis by affecting blood flow or by the induction of a pro-inflammatory state and oxidative stress.

Oxidative Stress

The link between oxidative stress and laminitis has recently been studied by a number of groups at the whole-horse level. Neville at al. (2004) found that 20 ponies with chronic laminitis had significantly higher ($P<0.01$) levels of a marker of lipid peroxidation. These ponies had three times the average level of plasma thiobarbituric acid reactive substances (TBARS) which are an indicator of free radical damage.

Horses with clinical or subclinical Cushing's disease with a previous history of laminitis were found to have significantly lower levels of plasma thiol levels indicative of oxidative stress. However there was no difference in other markers of antioxidant function (glutathione peroxidase) or lipid peroxidation (malondialdehyde) (Keen et al., 2004).

Treiber et al. (2007) studied oxidative stress in a pony herd of 42 laminitis-prone ponies and 34 ponies with no history of laminitis. Ponies with a previous history of laminitis did not show reduced antioxidant function or increased oxidative stress when compared to control ponies. However it was considered that ponies may have lower antioxidant capacity than horse breeds. This study found a significant ($P<0.001$) elevation in levels of tumor necrosis factor-alpha (TNF-α) in the laminitis-prone group. This is a pro-inflammatory adipocytokine, which may limit fat accumulation by inducing insulin resistance and thus have a role in the development of laminitis.

Free radical accumulation is thought to result from a number of factors including ischemia during the initial stages of the disorder, reperfusion injury, neutrophil activity in chronic laminitis, and insulin resistance (Neville et al., 2004). Reactive oxidative species (ROS) produced in situations of oxidative stress activate MMP-2 and MMP-9 and high glucose levels can increase production of ROS and MMP-9 by vascular endothelial cells. This glucotoxic action can be reversed by antioxidants (Johnson et al., 2004). More study is needed to determine the extent to which oxidative stress plays a role in laminitis and how antioxidant function may assist in prevention. Supplementation with 8,000-10,000 IU of vitamin E per day has been recommended in the clinical management of EMS (Davis, 2005).

Forages

Grazing lush pasture is the most common perceived cause of laminitis although recent research would indicate insulin resistance is a key risk factor in the development of the disorder. It was thought that high levels of fructans accumulated in grasses under certain conditions (Longland et al., 1999) and that these were not digested in the small intestine, but were instead fermented in the large intestine to produce acid, which decreases pH and can launch a cascade of events leading to laminitis.

Routine analyses of forages do not include fructan levels. However, recent changes in reporting of forage analyses may provide more information on the starch, simple sugar, and fructan content of feeds. Some recent changes in available assays and terminology offer greater evaluation of the carbohydrate content of forages, but this means that comparison of research results from different testing eras is difficult. Dairy One Laboratory in New York now measures carbohydrates by NIR as ethanol soluble carbohydrates (ESC), which are simple sugars; water-soluble carbohydrates (WSC), which combines simple sugars and fructans; and nonstructural carbohydrates (NSC) as starch plus WSC. Thus it is possible to crudely estimate the fructan content of a forage as WSC - ESC. Nonfiber carbohydrate (NFC) numbers are calculated by subtraction; however, to complicate matters, this was previously referred to as NSC.

Analysis of grass/legume pastures in Germany found that fructan levels varied from 5.7% in spring to 1.8% in late summer (Vervuert et al., 2005). There was a significant negative relationship between fructan and protein content of the pastures. Fructan concentrations were lower in hay and silage than pasture, and these levels were much lower than those recorded by Longland et al. (1999). In addition, the calculated daily maximum intake of 2.5 g fructan/kg BW based on a pasture intake of 3% BW is much lower than the levels of fructans shown to induce laminitis (Pollitt and Van Eps, 2002).

Treiber et al. (2006) also cast doubt on the "fructan in pasture leads to laminitis" model. In a study with a single herd of 150 ponies on a farm in Virginia, they found there was no change in water-soluble carbohydrate (WSC) levels in samples taken in March and May. There was a dramatic increase in pasture availability and clover content from March to May and clinical cases of laminitis were detected in May. It was assumed that no change in WSC content equated with no change in fructan content, but there was a significant increase in starch content of the pastures sampled, from 4.2% in March to 7.8% in May. On this basis, the authors hypothesized that starch may be more important than sugars and fructans in the pathophysiology of laminitis. However, the starch levels recorded were very low compared to those found in grains.

McIntosh et al. (2007a,b) investigated circadian and seasonal patterns in sugar, starch, and fructan and the relationship to glucose and insulin values in grazing Thoroughbred mares. Strong circadian rhythms were seen in pasture NSC content, with lowest levels seen between 4:00 a.m. and 5:00 a.m. and peak levels 12 hours later. Pasture NSC levels were strongly correlated ($P<0.001$) with temperature, humidity, and solar radiation. Samples taken in April contained 20% NSC, but this dropped to 13% in May and less than 10% in August, October, and January. Simple sugar content was much higher than fructan content and starch contents were low in all samples taken. Peak fructan level was 5.5% in April and this dropped to 3.9% in May and was below 3% in other months. Ten mares were assigned to grazing and compared with four stabled controls fed timothy/alfalfa hay. Plasma insulin was highest in grazing horses in April followed by May and was significantly higher than controls in those months. Plasma glucose in grazing horses was higher in April than controls and other sample times. A circadian pattern was seen in plasma insulin levels in April with peak levels seen in the evening. Plasma insulin was significantly correlated with NSC and sugar content in April, May and January. It was thought that in susceptible horses, this change in glucose and insulin dynamics could increase the risk of laminitis.

Soaking hay has been shown to reduce the starch and sugar content and this resulted in a reduced glucose and insulin response to feeding (Cottrell et al., 2005). Soaking two orchard grass hay samples for 30 minutes in cold water reduced the sugar content from 12% to 5.6% and 22% to 13.4%. The starch content was unaffected. To test the effect of soaking on the glycemic index of the hay, it was fed to 12 weanling fillies in a crossover study. This led to a significant ($P<0.01$) reduction in area under curve for plasma glucose and insulin. This practice is an important management aid to reduce the glucose/insulin response to feeding hay in insulin-resistant horses that are prone to laminitis.

Recognition of Horses at Risk of Laminitis

Research at Virginia Tech has examined risk factors for laminitis in ponies to allow the identification of ponies with pre-laminitic metabolic syndrome (PLMS) at high risk of developing the disorder (Treiber at al., 2006; Carter et al., 2007). The initial study identified ponies with three of a possible four criteria at risk of developing laminitis. The criteria were obesity (body condition score (BSC) >6), insulin resistance, hypertriglyceridemia, and increased insulin secretory response.

In the follow-up study, 76 pony mares on one farm were assessed. Thirty-four ponies had no history of laminitis (NL) and 42 had previously had laminitis (PL). In the spring, six of the PL ponies developed laminitis and the criteria picked four of the six as at-risk horses with PLMS. The odds ratio for prediction of laminitis risk was 3.75, so horses chosen as PLMS cases were nearly four times more likely to develop laminitis than those not identified. There was no difference between NL and PL ponies in plasma glucose, cortisol, and leptin, although plasma leptin was positively correlated ($P<0.001$) with BCS on a 1-9 scale and cresty neck score (CNS) on a 1-5 scale.

Assessment of obesity provided a simpler and more accurate means of diagnosing PLMS. Criteria of BCS >6 and CNS >3 predicted the same number of cases but with a higher specificity and predictive power (75% vs. 65%) and odds ratio (6.12 vs. 3.75). To reduce subjectivity in BCS and CNS assessments, morphometric measurements could be substituted. A girth-to-height ratio of >1.28 can replace BCS and crest height >10 cm could replace CNS. The authors concluded that further study in other populations and seasons is warranted.

Genetics

In dairy cattle, the heritability of laminitis is estimated to be between 0.1 and 0.15, although no clear mode of inheritance has been determined (Huang and Shanks, 1995a,b). A recent study in Virginia examined the heritability of grass founder in an inbred herd of Welsh and Dartmoor ponies (Splan et al., 2005). The pedigrees of 257 ponies born from 1933 to 2002 were traced back up to 10 generations. Ninety-five ponies (36.7%) were reported to have suffered laminitis and nearly half the affected ponies had a parent that was recorded as laminitic. Increased severity was noted when a pony's sire and dam had both suffered laminitis. This analysis suggests a major gene with a dominant action. In theory, a dominant gene would mean that 100% of cases needed to have an affected parent, but the researchers postulated that the number was reduced by incomplete recording of cases born earlier in the study population and ponies having a genetic predisposition but environmental thresholds for clinical disease not being crossed.

The development of a test to identify those ponies with a genetic predisposition to laminitis would assist the management of these ponies so that the incidence of the disorder can be reduced.

Cryotherapy for Prevention

Continuous cryotherapy by keeping the foot in an iceboot containing water at 1°C for 48-72 hours is well tolerated and has been proven an effective and safe method in horses at risk of laminitis, when applied *before* lameness develops. One study that cooled one foot on normal and oligofructan laminitisinduced horses for 48 hours found slightly elevated activity of MMP-2 in treated vs. normal feet, but the activity in cooled feet was significantly lower ($P<0.05$) than in untreated feet. The cooled feet showed no lameness and better tissue architecture scores than untreated feet (Van Eps and Pollitt, 2004).

A later study by the same authors used 72 hours of cryotherapy after experimental oligofructan-induced laminitis to significantly reduce ($P<0.05$) the lameness score and total epidermal length in treated horses compared to controls at seven days after induction (Van Eps and Pollitt, 2006a,b). The use of water at 1°C maintained internal hoof temperatures at 1.8°C to 3.6°C for the majority of the period in six normal horses also undergoing cryotherapy. Lamellar histology was normal in these horses.

This is not a new concept for preventing/moderating laminitis and many horses with clinical laminitis have been observed to stand in cold water. Potential benefits include vasoconstriction, resulting in decreased blood flow and decreased delivery of LTFs; decreased cell and tissue metabolism in lamellae; decreased activation of MMPs; and anti-inflammatory activity. Cryotherapy is an effective preventative strategy for horses at risk of developing acute laminitis.

However, the optimum temperature has not been established. The treatment period may be extended in association with some clinical conditions such as metritis and pleuritis. It is important to cool horses to at least midcannon to cool arterial blood. Horses tolerate cryotherapy well with no signs of discomfort.

Intracecal Buffering

The pH of the cecum drops dramatically related to the production of D-lactate in the period before the onset of clinical signs of carbohydrate-overload laminitis. Souza et al. (2006) examined the effect of an intracecal buffer (CB) or saline (CS) administered eight hours after induction of a carbohydrate-induced laminitis model. Both treatments were also administered to control horses (WB and WS). The buffer was 3.5 g aluminum hydroxide and 65 g magnesium hydroxide administered through a surgically inserted cecal cannula.

Horses receiving the buffer had delayed onset of clinical signs, increased cecal pH, decreased growth of *Streptococcus* and *Lactobacillus*, and reduced expression of MMP-2 and MMP-9 in the hoof after 48 hours, but horses were not protected against laminitis in this model. Expression of MMP-2 and MMP-9 was higher in laminitic tissues than control tissues. MMP-2 expression was 2.25-fold higher in the CS group and 1.18-fold higher in the CB group than the WS group. MMP-9 followed a similar pattern, with CS tissues 17.8-fold higher and CB only 5.1-fold higher than WS tissues. Further studies are warranted to assess the potential of intracecal buffering in management of horses with carbohydrate-overload laminitis.

Intracecal administration of sodium bicarbonate has been shown to be effective in raising the pH of the cecum when administered by intracecal cannula after a starch-rich grain meal that caused a significant drop in cecal pH (Willard et al., 1977). However, oral administration of sodium bicarbonate will not protect against the pH drop, as it will be digested and absorbed before it gets to the cecum.

Kentucky Equine Research has recently examined the effect of an orally administered hindgut buffer on fecal pH and lactate levels in horses on normal grain and hay diets. Thoroughbred horses in training were fed 4 or 6 kg of an unfortified sweet feed and 4 kg of hay in a switchback study. Administration of the protected sodium bicarbonate buffer EquiShure (KERx, Versailles, KY) in each of two grain feeds prevented the significant (P<0.05) drop in fecal pH seen in control horses after feeding, and fecal D- and L-lactate levels were significantly lower (P<0.05) in treated horses at six hours after feeding (Pagan et al., 2007). While cecal measurements were not performed in this study, cecal pH has been correlated with fecal pH. It can reasonably be assumed that the protected sodium bicarbonate attenuated the drop in cecal pH seen after a grain meal, and it may have value given by stomach tube in grain overload cases.

References

Asplin, K.E., C.M. McGowan, C.C. Pollitt, J. Curlewis, and M.N. Sillence. 2007a. Role of insulin in glucose uptake in the equine hoof. In: Proc. Forum Amer. Coll. Vet. Int. Med.

Asplin, K.E., M.N. Sillence, C.C. Pollitt, and C.M. McGowan. 2007b. Induction of laminitis by prolonged hyperinsulinaemia in clinically normal ponies. Vet J. 174:530-535.

Bailey, S.R. 2004. The pathogenesis of acute laminitis: Fitting more pieces into the puzzle. Equine Vet. J. 36:199-203.

Belknap, J.K., S. Giguère, S., A. Pettigrew, A.M. Cochran, A.W. Van Eps, and C.C. Pollitt. 2007. Lamellar proinflammatory cytokine expression patterns in laminitis at the developmental stage and at the onset of lameness: Innate vs. adaptive immune response. Equine Vet. J. 39:42-47.

Blikslager, A.T., C. Yin, A.M. Cochran, J.G. Wooten, A. Pettigrew, and J.K. Belknap. 2006. Cyclooxygenase expression in the early stages of equine laminitis: A cytologic study. J. Vet. Intern. Med. 20:1191-1196.

Brosnahan, M.M., and M.R. Paradis. 2003. Demographic and clinical characteristics of geriatric horses. J. Amer. Vet. Med. Assoc. 223:93-98

Carter, R.A., K. H. Treiber, P.A. Harris, and R.J. Geor. 2007. Evaluation of criteria for pre-laminitic metabolic syndrome. In: Proc. Equine Sci. Soc. 139-141.

Cottrell, E., K. Watts, and S. Ralston. 2005. Soluble sugar content and glucose/insulin responses can be reduced by soaking chopped hay in water. In: Proc. Equine Sci. Soc. 293-298.

Crawford, C., M.F. Sepulveda, J. Elliott, P.A. Harris, and S.R. Bailey. 2007. Dietary fructan carbohydrate increases amine production in the equine large intestine: Implications for pasture-associated laminitis. J. Anim. Sci. 85:2949-2958.

Croser, E.L., and C.C. Pollitt. 2006. Acute laminitis: Descriptive evaluation of serial hoof biopsies. In: Proc. Amer. Assoc. Equine Practnr. 542-546.

Davis, E.G. 2005. Equine metabolic syndrome. In: Proc. North Amer. Vet. Conf. 140-142.

Eades S.C., A.M. Stokes, P.J. Johnson, C.J. LeBlanc, V.K. Ganjam, P.R. Buff, and R.M. Moore. 2007. Serial alterations in digital hemodynamics and endothelin-1 immunoreactivity, platelet-neutrophil aggregation, and concentrations of nitric oxide, insulin, and glucose in blood obtained from horses following carbohydrate overload. Amer. J. Vet. Res. 68:87-94.

Elliott, J., Y. Berhane, and S.R. Bailey. 2003. Effects of monoamines formed in the cecum of horses on equine digital blood vessels and platelets. Amer. J. Vet. Res. 64:1124-1131.

Field, J.R., and L.B. Jeffcott. 1989. Equine laminitis: Another hypotheses for pathogenesis. Med. Hypotheses. 30:203-210.

Frank, N. 2006. Insulin resistance in horses. In: Proc. Amer. Assoc. Equine Practnr. 52:51-54.

Geor, R.J., C.D. Thatcher, R.S. Pleasant, F. Elvinger, and L. Gay. 2007. Prevalence of hyperinsulinemia in mature horses: Relationship to adiposity: In: Proc. Ann. Forum Amer. Coll. Vet. Int. Med.

Hartge, M.M., T. Unger, and U. Kintscher. 2007. The endothelium and vascular inflammation in diabetes. Diab. Vasc. Dis. Res. 4:84-88.

Hinckley, K.A., and I.W. Henderson. 1996. The epidemiology of equine laminitis in the UK. In: Proc. BEVA Congress. 62.

Huang, Y.C., and R.D. Shanks. 1995a. Within herd estimates of heritabilities for six hoof characteristics and impact of dispersion of discrete severity scores on estimates. Livest. Prod. Sci. 44:107-114.

Huang, Y.C., and R.D. Shanks. 1995b. Visualization of inheritance patterns from graphic representation of additive and dominance relationships between animals. J. Dairy Sci. 78:2877-2883.

Hunt, D.G., and J.L. Ivy. 2002. Epinephrine inhibits insulin-stimulated muscle glucose transport. J. App. Physiol 93:1638-1643.

Johnson, P.J., S.K. Ganjam, N.T. Messer IV, et al. 2006. Obesity paradigm: An introduction to the emerging discipline of adipobiology. In: Proc. Amer. Assoc. Equine Pract. 52:41-50.

Johnson, P.J., and V.K. Ganjam, 1999. Laminitis, hypothyroidism, and obesity: A peripheral cushingoid syndrome in horses. In: Proc. Ann. Forum of Amer. Coll. Vet. Int. Med. 192-194.

Johnson, P.J., N.T. Messer, S.H. Slight, C. Wiedmeyer, P. Buff, et al. 2004. Endocrinopathic laminitis in the horse. Clin. Tech. Equine Pract. 3:45-56.

Johnson, P.J., S.C. Tyagi, L.C. Katwa, V.K. Ganjam, L.A. Moore, J.M. Kreeger, and N.T. Messer. 1998. Activation of extracellular matrix metalloproteases in equine laminitis. Vet. Rec. 142:392-396.

Keen, J.A., M. McLaren, K.J. Chandler, and B.C. McGorum. 2004. Biochemical indices of vascular function, glucose metabolism and oxidative stress in horses with equine Cushing's disease. Equine Vet. J. 36:226-229.

Kyaw-Tanner, M., and C.C. Pollitt. 2004. Equine laminitis: Increased transcription of matrix metalloproteinase- 2 (MMP-2) occurs during the developmental phase. Equine Vet. J. 36:221-225.

Loftus, J.P., S.J. Black, A. Pettigrew, E.J. Abrahamsen, and J.K. Belknap. 2007a. Early laminar events involving endothelial activation in horses with black walnut-induced laminitis. Amer. J. Vet. Res. 68:1205-1211.

Loftus, J.P., J.K. Belknap, K.M. Stankiewicz, and S.J. Black. 2007b. Laminar xanthine oxidase, superoxide dismutase and catalase activities in the prodromal stage of black-walnut induced equine laminitis. Equine Vet. J. 39:48-53.

Longland, A.C., A.J. Cairns, and M.O. Humphreys. 1999. Seasonal changes in fructan concentration in *Lolium perenne*: Implication for the grazing management of equine predisposed to laminitis. In: Proc. Equine Nutr. Physiol. Soc. 258-259.

McGowan, C.M., R.J. Geor, and T.W McGowan. 2008. Prevalence and risk factors for hyperinsulinemia in ponies. In: Proc. Ann. Forum Amer. Coll. Vet. Int. Med. In Press.

McGowan, C.M., and G. Riley. 2004. Long-term trilostane treatment for metabolic syndrome. In: Proc. BEVA Congress.

McIntosh, B., D. Kronfeld, R.J. Geor, W. Staniar, and J. Chatterton. 2007a. Circadian and seasonal patterns in forage nonstructural carbohydrate content. In: Proc. Equine Sci. Soc. 102-103.

McIntosh, B., D. Kronfeld, R.J. Geor, W. Staniar, and J. Chatterton. 2007b. Circadian and seasonal fluctuations of glucose and insulin concentrations in grazing horses. In: Proc Equine Sci. Soc. 100-101.

Millonovich, G.J., D.J. Trott, P.C. Burrell, E.L. Croser, R.A. Al Jassam, J.M. Morton, A.W. Van Eps, and C.C. Pollitt. 2007. Fluorescence in situ hybridization analysis of hindgut bacteria associated with the development of equine laminitis. Environ. Microbiol. 9:2090-2100.

Moore, R.M., S.C. Eades, and A.M. Stokes. 2004. Evidence for vascular and enzymatic events in the pathophysiology of acute laminitis: Which pathway is responsible for initiation of this process in horses? Equine Vet. J. 36:204-209.

Neville, R.F., T. Hollands, S.N. Collins and F.V. Keyte. 2004. Short communications: Evaluation of urinary TBARS in normal and chronic laminitic ponies. Equine Vet. J. 36:292-294.

Pagan, J.D., T.J. Lawrence, and L.A. Lawrence. 2007 Feeding protected sodium bicarbonate attenuates hindgut acidosis in horses fed a high grain ration. In: Proc. Amer. Assoc. Equine Pract. 53:530-533.

Parsons, C.S., J.A. Orsini, R. Krafty, L. Capewell, and R. Boston, R. 2007. Risk factors for development of acute laminitis in horses during hospitalization: 73 cases (1997-2004). J. Amer. Vet. Med. Assoc. 230:885-889.

Pass, M.A., S. Pollitt, and C.C. Pollitt. 1998. Decreased glucose metabolism causes separation of hoof lamellae in vitro: A trigger for laminitis? Equine Vet. J. 26:133-138.

Peroni, J.F., J.N. Moore, E. Noschka, M.E. Grafton, M. Aceves-Avila, S.J. Lewis, and T.P. Robertson. 2006. Predisposition for venoconstriction in the equine laminar dermis: Implications in equine laminitis. J. Appl. Physiol. 100:759-763.

Pollitt, C.C. 1996. Basement membrane pathology: A feature of acute laminitis. Equine Vet. J. 28:38-46.

Pollitt, C.C. 1999. Equine laminitis: Current concepts of inner hoof wall anatomy, physiology and pathophysiology. In: Large Anim. Proc. Ann. Amer. Coll. Vet. Surg. Symp. 175-180.

Pollitt, C.C. and M. Daradka. 1998. Equine laminitis basement membrane pathology: Loss of type IV collagen, type VII collagen and laminin immunostaining. The Equine Hoof: Equine Vet. J. Suppl. 27:139-144.

Pollitt, C.C., M.A. Pass, and S. Pollitt. 1998. Batimastat (BB-94) inhibits matrix metalloproteinases of equine laminitis. The Equine Hoof: Equine Vet. J. Suppl. 26:119-124.

Pollitt, C.C., and A.W. van Eps. 2002. Equine laminitis: A new induction model based on alimentary overload with fructan. In: Proc. Aust. Equine Vet. Assoc. 98-99.

Rattigan, S., C.T. Bussey, R.M. Ross, and S.M. Richards. 2007. Obesity, insulin resistance, and capillary recruitment. Microcirculation. 14:299-309.

Riggs, L.M., T. Franck, J.N. Moore, T.M. Krunkosky, D.J. Hurley, J.F. Peroni, G. de la Rebière, and D.A. Serteyn. 2007. Neutrophil myeloperoxidase measurements in plasma, laminar tissue, and skin of horses given black walnut extract. Amer. J. Vet. Res. 68:81-86.

Rodgerson, D.H., J.K. Belknap, J.N. Moore, and G.L. Fontaine. 2001. Investigation of mRNA expression of tumor necrosis factor-alpha, interleukin-1beta, and cyclooxygenase-2 in cultured equine digital artery smooth muscle cells after exposure to endotoxin. Amer. J. Vet. Res. 62:1957-1963.

Singer, G., and D.N. Granger. 2007. Inflammatory responses underlying the microvascular dysfunction associated with obesity and insulin resistance. Microcirculation. 14:375-387.

Souza, A.H., C.A.A. Valadão, S. Chirgwin, A.M. Stokes, and R.M. Moore. 2006. Transcription of MMP-2 and MMP-9 in horses with carbohydrate-induced laminitis treated with an intracecal buffering solution. In: Proc. Amer. Assoc. of Equine Practnr. 52:540-541.

Splan, R.K., D.S. Kronfeld, K.H. Treiber, T.M. Hess, and W.B. Staniar. 2005. Genetic predisposition for laminitis in ponies. In: Proc. Equine Sci. Soc. 219-220.

Treiber, K.H., R.A. Carter, L.A. Gay, C.A. Williams, and R.J. Geor. 2007. Oxidative stress and inflammatory markers in laminitis-prone ponies. In: Proc. Equine Sci. Soc. 142-143.

Treiber, K.H., D.S. Kronfeld, T.M. Hess, B.M. Byrd, R.K. Splan, and W.B. Stanier. 2006. Evaluation of genetic and metabolic predispositions and nutritional risk factors for pasture-associated laminitis in ponies. J. Amer. Vet. Med. Assoc. 228:1538-1541.

Treiber, K.H., D.S. Kronfeld, T.M. Hess, B.M. Byrd, and R.K. Splan. 2005. Pre-laminitic metabolic syndrome in genetically predisposed ponies involves compensated insulin resistance. J. Anim. Physiol. Anim. Nutr. 89:430-431.

USDA. 2000. Lameness and Laminitis in US Horses. USDA: APHIS: VS,CEAH, National Animal Health Monitoring System, Fort Collins, CO.

Van Eps, A.W., and C.C. Pollitt. 2004. Equine laminitis: Cryotherapy reduces the severity of the acute lesion. Equine Vet. J. 36:255-260.

Van Eps, A.W., and C.C. Pollitt. 2006a. Cryotherapy reduced the severity of laminitis evaluated seven days after induction with oligofructose. In: Proc. Amer. Assoc. Equine Practnr. 52:538-539.

Van Eps A.W., and C.C. Pollitt. 2006b. Equine laminitis induced with oligofructose. Equine Vet. J. 38:203-208.

Vervuert, I., M. Coenen, S. Dahlhoff, and W. Sommer. 2005. Fructan concentrations in grass, silages and hay. In: Proc. Equine Sci. Soc. 309-310.

Wattle, O., and C.C. Pollitt. 2004. Lamellar metabolism. In: Proc. Clin. Tech.Equine Pract. 13:22-33.

Willard, J.G., J.C. Willard, S.A. Wolfram, and J.P. Baker. 1977. Effect of diet on cecal pH and feeding behavior of horses. J. Anim. Sci. 45:87-93.

COLIC PREVALENCE, RISK FACTORS AND PREVENTION

NATHANIEL A. WHITE

Marion duPont Scott Equine Medical Center, Leesburg, Virginia

Introduction

Colic is one of the most difficult diseases to study with epidemiologic methods due to the large number of diseases that include colic (abdominal pain) as a clinical sign. Therefore, epidemiologic data related to colic are meaningful only if an accurate diagnosis of the primary disease process can be determined. Nevertheless, epidemiology has provided important information about incidence, mortality, and risk factors for colic, all of which may help the clinician make decisions about individual cases as well as herd problems.

Prevalence

Determining the incidence of colic can help to judge if the rate of colic on farms or in stables is excessive. Out of 100 horses in the general population, four to ten cases of colic are expected during an average year (Tinker et al., 1997a; Kaneene et al., 1997). The annual number of colic cases, however, may vary greatly between farms, ranging from 0 to 25 or 30 cases per 100 horses (Traub-Dargatz et al., 2001; Hillyer et al., 2001; Uhlinger, 1992). Approximately 10 to 15% of colic cases occur in horses that have experienced previous episodes of abdominal pain, with two to four colic episodes per year in some horses (Tinker et al., 1997a). Most colic, 80 to 85% of cases, can be designated as simple colic or ileus because no specific diagnosis is identified, and most horses respond to medical treatment or resolve spontaneously. In one cohort study, approximately 30% of horses with colic were reported by owners, but were never examined by a veterinarian because the colic was transient or resolved with owner treatment (Tinker et al., 1995). Studies of horses with colic that present to veterinary practices have also reported a predominance of simple obstruction or spasmodic colic, with impactions diagnosed in approximately 10% of affected horses (Proudman, 1992). Obstructing or strangulating diseases that require surgery represent only two to four percent of colic cases, though some risk factors in certain populations may increase this rate (White, 1990).

Colic mortality has decreased since the 1998 NAHMS study, when it was second only to old age as a cause of death in horses. In the 2005 NAHMS study, old age was still the most common cause of death while colic was third, almost equal to injuries, which ranked second. In the normal farm population, horse mortality from all types of colic was 0.7 deaths per 100 horse-years, with a colic case fatality rate of 6.7% (Tinker et al., 1997a). The predominant reasons for death were stomach rupture, strangulating lesions, or enteritis (Tinker et al., 1997a).

The true incidence of specific intestinal diseases causing colic in the general equine population is not known. Studies of horses presenting to veterinary teaching hospitals or practices for evaluation of colic rank simple colic and impaction colic as the most common diseases. When the segment of bowel involved can be determined, the large colon is the most commonly affected followed by the small intestine, cecum, and small colon, respectively (White, 1990). Large colon torsion is the most common cause of strangulation obstruction, with strangulating diseases of the small intestine causing the highest case fatality rate (White, 1990; Macdonald et al., 1989; Proudman et al., 2002).

In a study of colic in a population of 28,000 horses, loss of use due to colic averaged two to three days, less than that resulting from trauma, lameness, or neurological disease (Traub-Dargatz et al., 2001). The value of horses lost due to colic in the United States in 1998 and 1999 was estimated at $70 million, while the total cost of colic to the industry was estimated at $144 million. Based on smaller studies, anecdotal information from veterinary hospitals, and the total horse population in the United States (9.2 million), the number of abdominal surgeries performed on horses with colic in the United States could be as high as 24,000 annually, or possibly as many as 2.7 colic surgeries every hour.

General Risk Factors

Since only natural disease has been studied, determining the cause of different diseases that cause colic is problematic. In some cases, such as grain overload or enterolith presence, the proximate cause may be evident, but mechanism or the underlying problems often remain unknown. Determination of risk factors for specific types of colic may help identify the cause and lessen disease incidence by decreasing exposure to an incriminated risk.

The amount of risk is stated as the odds that the colic incidence will increase in a group of horses exposed to a particular factor compared to the colic incidence in a group that is not exposed to that factor. Horses that have had a previous episode of colic are three times more likely to have a second colic episode compared to a horse that has never had colic (Tinker et al., 1997b). Said another way, if the incidence of colic in a normal population of horses with no previous history of colic is 10 out of 100 horses in a year, the rate of colic in a population of horses with a history of previous colic would be 30 out of 100 horses per year. Colic risk may also be categorized into internal and external risks. Breed and enlarged inguinal rings are examples of internal risks, while diet and housing are considered external risks.

SIGNALMENT

While colic may affect horses of any breed, several studies suggest an increased incidence of disease in Arabian (Cohen et al., 1995) or Thoroughbred (Traub-Dargatz et al., 2001) horses. Standardbreds, gaited horses, and Warmblood stallions have an apparent increase in incidence of inguinal hernias due to the increased size of their inguinal rings (Schneider et al., 1982). Though rare, the recessive and lethal trait of aganglionosis, which occurs in American Paint Horse foals born to overo mares mated with overo stallions, is the only cause of colic that has been proven to date to have a genetic basis.

Younger (<2 years) and older (>10 years) horses appear to be at less risk for simple colic (Tinker et al., 1997b). Middle-aged horses are at higher risk of colic than older horses; however, older horses with colic are more likely to require surgery (Proudman, 1992). Weanling and yearling horses are more likely to have ileocecal intussusceptions and older horses (>12 years) are at increased risk of strangulating lipoma (Proudman, 1992).

Gender is an apparent risk for conditions such as inguinal hernia in stallions and large colon displacement/volvulus in periparturient mares. Male horses (geldings and stallions) and older horses appear to be at slightly higher risk of entrapment of the small intestine in the epiploic foramen. For the most part, male and female horses appear to be equally affected by simple colic, which is probably related to management or activity.

Recently increased height has been associated with an increased risk of epiploic foramen entrapment (Archer et al., 2008). Behavior and response to external environment appeared associated with an increased risk. This suggests that there is an innate risk for gastrointestinal dysfunction in some horses.

DIET

Feeds or feeding activity have long been associated with the incidence of colic, though information is still largely anecdotal. Coarse roughage with low digestibility or particularly coarse fiber is observed to be associated with impaction colic (White and Dabareiner, 1997). Poor dentition has been proposed to predispose to colic due to poor mastication of food, though this has not been confirmed (Hillyer et al., 2002). Grain overload increases the risk of colic and laminitis. Feeds such as lush clover and lush pasture have been implicated as causes of tympany. Horses fed poor-quality Bermuda grass hay have an increased risk of ileal impaction (Little and Blikslager, 2002) and some horses are reported to have more colic when fed alfalfa hay. Feeding hay from round bales is also associated with an increased risk of colic (Hudson et al., 2001).

Case control and cohort studies indicate that increased amounts of grain or changes in the type of hay and grain fed increase the odds of colic compared to horses without grain or changes in feed (Tinker et al., 1997b; Cohen et al., 1999). Daily feeding of concentrate at 2.5 to 5 kg/day and > 5 kg/day to adult horses increased the risk of colic 4.8 and 6.3 times, respectively, compared to horses fed no grain (Tinker et al., 1997b) (Figure 1). Horses fed grain in the form of pellets or sweet feeds had an increased risk of colic compared to horses that were not fed grain or were fed single-grain diets. Horses with duodenitis-proximal jejunitis were more likely to be fed grain and to have grazed pasture than control horses (Cohen et al., 2006).

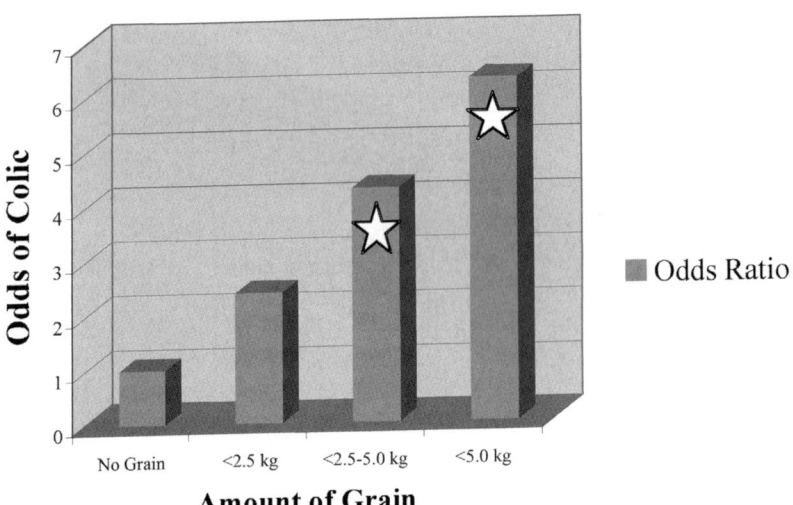

Figure 1. Odds of colic in horses fed concentrate (in kilograms) as part of their daily diet compared to horses fed no grain. The stars indicate a significant difference (P<0.05) for odds of having colic compared to no grain fed (White, 2006).

Grain diets decrease the water content of ingesta in the colon due to a decrease in fiber, which binds to water (Lopes et al., 2004). Grain in the diet also increases gas production and is more likely to create an intraluminal environment that favors gas production or altered motility leading to intestinal displacements.

Feeding small amounts of grain at frequent intervals reduces fluid shifts in the large colon as compared to fluid shifts that occur with twice-daily feeding of larger quantities of concentrate (Clarke et al., 1990). Though no relationship was found between feeding frequency in one study (Reeves et al., 1996), feeding more than twice daily increased the risk of colic in a Virginia-Maryland study (Tinker et al., 1997b). This increased risk was suspected to be due to an increased daily intake of grain rather than the frequency of feeding which would favor small amounts of starch reaching the large intestine and decrease the chance of hindgut acidosis (Geor and Harris, 2007).

ENVIRONMENT/MANAGEMENT

Housing and confinement on the farms in a Virginia-Maryland study were not risk factors for colic (Hillyer et al., 2001; Tinker et al., 1997b). However, other reports suggest there is an increased risk of cecal and large colon impaction in horses that have acute decreases in activity, such as curtailing regular exercise or changing from turn-out activity to strict stall confinement due to an injury or after surgery (Dabareiner and White, 1995). A case-control study in Texas found decreased colic risk with lower horse density on pasture and with access to a pond; these observations are supported by studies from the United Kingdom (Hillyer et al., 2002; Cohen et al., 1999). Turn-out in paddocks without water is associated with an increased risk of colic (Reeves et al., 1996). The type of activity is often related to the type of housing, possibly confounding interpretation of the results in some studies, and further investigations into the relationship between housing and type and frequency of exercise and their effect on the incidence of colic is needed.

Management factors are difficult to compare between farms, and changes in management are difficult to detect. The increased risk of colic associated with care by trainers and managers compared to care by owners is supported by two studies (Reeves et al., 1996; Hillyer et al., 2002). These findings suggest a difference either in the quality or frequency of observation between these two groups or better management by owners compared to trainers in horses with more intensive exercise.

It seems logical that housing, diet, and feeding routine are associated with a risk of colic. Anecdotal information from large breeding farms suggest that the routine of feeding horses grain after being brought in from pasture and then keeping them in stalls for part of the day increases the risk of colic, and specifically colon tympany and displacement of the large colon. By altering this daily routine, including keeping horses turned out after grain feeding, colic incidence is decreased. Similarly when hay is available to horses on lush pasture, the hay will be consumed as part of the diet, and incidence of colic is decreased in horses turned out 24 hours per day.

Specific causes of colic occur at differing frequencies in different regions of the world (White, 1990). Grass sickness is diagnosed in horses in the United Kingdom, Europe, and South America but not in North America. Ileal impactions are found predominantly in horses in the southeastern United States and Europe. Enteroliths are observed more frequently in horses in California, the Midwest, and Florida (White, 1990). Sand colic and impactions are seen where horses graze on pastures with sandy soils or where horses are forced to eat off ground consisting predominantly of sand or fine gravel.

Enteroliths appear to be related to diet and potentially mineral intake. Horses consuming hard water or alfalfa hay, and those with a higher pH and mineral concentrations of colonic ingesta, as well as horses living in California, are at higher risk for this problem (Cohen et al., 2000; Hassel et al., 2001; Hassel et al., 2004).

These diseases are not common causes of colic and their incidence may not be impacted by the same management, diet and environmental changes previously described (Tinker et al., 1997b; Cohen et al., 1999; Hillyer et al., 2002).

Event-Associated Colic Risk

PREVIOUS COLIC

Horses with a history of previous colic are at higher risk for future colic episodes (Cohen and Honnas, 1996; Tinker et al., 1997a). Horses with a prior history of abdominal surgery are at higher risk of repeat colic, which is often due to adhesions or bowel scarring with stricture (Cohen et al., 1995). Horses have a higher rate of repeat colic (one to two episodes) within the first two to three months after abdominal surgery; after that time, the incidence of colic decreases to near normal (Proudman et al., 2002). Horses with colon impactions have a high rate of repeat colic (Dabareiner and White, 1995). The reason for this increased risk is not known. Decreased numbers of neurons in the myenteric plexus of the pelvic flexure and right dorsal colon in horses with chronic colon obstruction may create alterations in bowel motility predisposing to future obstruction (Schusser and White, 1997).

PARASITES

Parasites (ascarids, tapeworms, strongyles) were associated with an increased risk of colic in several studies. Obstructions due to ascarids in foals, tapeworm infestation, and strongyle infestation have all been reported as causes of colic, usually based on small groups of cases. Uhlinger found a decrease in colic after controlling small strongyle infection on several farms with a high colic incidence. Tapeworm infestation is related to an increased frequency of colic, and specifically to colic associated with diseases of the ileum and cecum such as ileocecal intussusception or cecocecal intussusception (Proudman and Holdstock, 2000). Although there are no studies describing the incidence or prevalence of colic associated with thrombosis of the cranial mesenteric artery due to *Strongylus vulgaris* larva, the decrease in mesenteric artery thrombus formation observed in horses at surgery and necropsy appears to parallel the increased use of ivermectin in horses over the last 25 years.

CRIBBING

Recently cribbing, long associated with an increased risk of colic, was demonstrated to be associated with an increased risk of simple large colon obstruction and entrapment of the small intestine in the epiploic foramen (Archer et al., 2004; Archer et al., 2008). The act of aerophagia likely creates negative pressure in the abdomen leading to movement of bowel into the potential space within the lesser omental sac. The author

COLIC TREATMENT AND POST-COLIC NUTRITION

NATHANIEL A. WHITE
Marion duPont Scott Equine Medical Center, Leesburg, Virginia

Treatment of Colic

INTRODUCTION

The main goals for treating horses with colic include relieving pain, correcting physiologic imbalance, and stimulating or maintaining intestinal transit. Primary treatments are aimed at decompressing the gastrointestinal tract, treating dehydration or shock, correcting electrolyte imbalances, stimulating intestinal motility, and decreasing intestinal inflammation. When necessary, surgery is used to relieve strangulation or simple obstruction. However, treatment before and after surgery is often needed to address pain, ileus, or inflammation associated with obstructive disease.

Decompression

A primary method to alleviate abdominal pain is decompression of the distended stomach or intestine. Nasogastric intubation can help relieve gastric tympany or remove gastrointestinal reflux due to a small intestinal obstruction or ileus. The tube can be left in place for chronic decompression after surgery or in horses with proximal enteritis, but should be checked every 2 to 3 hours as stomach pressure may not force the fluid through the tube even with extreme distention (White, 1987). Horses with gastric dilatation can have stomach rupture, even after the recent passage of a stomach tube or with a stomach tube left in place for passive decompression. An attempt to start a siphon should be made in all cases by filling the tube with water and then lowering the end of the tube below the level of the stomach.

The other site at which distention from gas can be relieved is the cecum. Decompression (enterocentesis) can resolve a primary cecal tympany or help relieve gas buildup from a large colon or small colon obstruction. Decompression of the cecum is done in the right paralumbar fossa midway between the last rib and the ventral prominence of the tuber coxae. A 5- or 6-inch, 14-16 gauge needle or catheter over a needle is used. Suction is helpful for rapidly reducing cecal tympany. Concurrent palpation per rectum can help push gas into the cecal base and facilitate removing as much as possible. Once the gas is removed, saline or an antibiotic solution should be infused through the needle as it is pulled out of the cecum to avoid leaving a trail of contaminated material in the peritoneum or body wall.

Systemic Analgesics

Nonsteroidal anti-inflammatory drugs (NSAIDS): Some of the most useful drugs for relief of pain associated with either surgical or nonsurgical disease in horses are the nonsteroidal anti-inflammatory drugs (NSAIDs). They inhibit the enzyme cyclo-oxygenase, thereby decreasing the production of eicosanoids formed during degradation of arachidonic acid from cell membranes. The role of prostaglandins in equine intestinal disease is not fully understood. However, there is a favorable response during colic after administration of NSAIDs, which inhibit their formation. Different drugs produce varying levels of analgesia, possibly due to the different concentrations of the two types of cyclo-oxygenase, COX-1 and COX-2, in tissues (Morrow and Roberts, 2001). COX-1 regulates the production of prostaglandins necessary for normal organ and vascular function. COX-2 becomes active in response to cytokines, serum factors, or growth factors, and causes marked increases in prostaglandin production. COX-2 up-regulation by endotoxin is activated by p38 MAP kinase (Jones et al., 2005). Depending on their relative ability to inhibit COX-1 and COX-2, different NSAIDs provide different effects.

Prostaglandins have several effects on healing of the intestine. The constitutive prostaglandins, formed by COX-1, help regulate normal function such as motility and mucosal healing. PGE2 is needed to maintain the intestinal mucosa and glandular mucosa in the stomach. Excess use of nonselective COX inhibitors predisposes to gastric and intestinal ulceration. This creates a dilemma when treating horses for colic as the common NSAIDs—phenylbutazone, flunixin meglumine[i], ketoprofen[ii], and aspirin—inhibit COX-1 and COX-2, though apparently with different levels of effectiveness (Tomlinson and Blikslager, 2005).

Flunixin meglumine (flunixin) is the most effective of the NSAIDs used to treat acute abdominal disease in the horse. It blocks the production of prostaglandins, specifically thromboxane and prostacyclin, for 8 to 12 hours after a single dose (Semrad et al., 1985). In cases where a strangulated segment of intestine is suspected, the use of flunixin preoperatively can be helpful in diminishing the detrimental response due to the endotoxin release (6 to 8 hours) and return of borborygmi. The inability to eliminate pain with flunixin suggests a disease exists that requires more than simple medical treatment. For this reason, horses given flunixin should be observed carefully after its administration. If signs of colic return, particularly after a short period (1 to 2 hours), the horse should be immediately suspected of having more than a simple medical colic.

Clinical observation suggests phenylbutazone is not as good an analgesic for colic as flunixin. Its use appears to be more helpful for musculoskeletal problems than for visceral pain, perhaps because of differences in tissue concentrations. There is evidence that indicates phenylbutazone is more effective in reducing PGE2, thereby reversing ileus during endotoxemia (King and Gerring, 1989). The dosage response for this is not known, but 0.5 to 2 mg/kg has been used. The author has used a combination of flunixin (1.0 mg/kg IV, BID) and phenylbutazone (0.5-1.0 mg/kg IV, BID) by alternating administration of each drug every 6 hours. Whether this is more beneficial than either drug alone is unknown.

Ketoprofen has been used clinically for treatment of colic. It is effective in alleviating some clinical responses after experimental administration of endotoxin similar to flunixin. Gastric ulceration is also said to be less with this drug though at low doses this is not considered a problem with flunixin. Anecdotal reports suggest ketoprofen is less effective as an analgesic for colic than flunixin meglumine.

Eltenac[iii] has been tested in horses and has some adverse effects at 2 to 3 times the normal dose (Goodrich et al., 1998). Its effects in blocking the deleterious effects of endotoxemia are similar to those of flunixin (MacKay et al., 2000). Eltenac is reported to be less ulcerogenic than the commonly used NSAIDs in horses. This NSAID has not yet been used extensively for colic.

Disadvantages of the NSAIDs, particularly phenylbutazone, include the potential for adverse side effects such as mucosal ulceration of the gastrointestinal tract or renal damage (Collins and Tyler, 1984; Karcher et al., 1990; Meschter et al., 1990). This is particularly true if these drugs are administered orally, for long periods, during periods of dehydration and/or in combination with aminoglycoside antibiotics. Nonselective NSAIDs with COX-1 activity can decrease intestinal healing and, when used chronically, may alter intestinal motility (Blikslager et al., 1997; Van Hoogmoed et al., 2002). The administration of COX-2 inhibitors is limited to experimental use in horses (Morton et al., 2005; Tomlinson and Blikslager, 2005). Carprofen[iv] has been used as an anti-inflammatory after colic surgery (0.7 mg/kg SID or BID) because it is potentially less ulcerogenic, but its efficacy has not been clinically or scientifically proven. Meloxicam, currently available in Europe, is a selective COX-2 inhibitor that can be used for colic and does not inhibit healing of the intestinal mucosa after ischemia (Beretta et al., 2005).

Alpha-2 agonists: Several alpha-2 agonists are potent analgesics and cause muscle relaxation and sedation. This drug group includes xylazine[v], romifidine[vi], and detomidine[vii], which have been used for control of abdominal pain in horses. These drugs appear to act by stimulation of central alpha-2 adrenoreceptors, which modulates the release of norepinephrine and directly inhibits neuronal firing. This causes sedation, analgesia, bradycardia, and in the horse with colic, relief of pain (Muir and Robertson, 1985; Kohn and Muir, 1988; Merritt et al., 1998). The heart rate can be markedly reduced to less than 20 beats per minute by second-degree heart block. This causes a significant reduction in the cardiac output for a short period and thereby may have a detrimental effect on the horse that already has a critical reduction in circulating blood volume. Alpha-2 agonists reduce blood flow of obstructed large intestine and decrease intraluminal pressure (Muir and Robertson, 1985; Kohn and Muir, 1988). Similarly, in experimental small intestinal ischemia, xylazine reduced blood flow and increased oxygen utilization. There is a transient increase in urine production, which may complicate dehydration and circulatory shock (Stick et al., 1987).

Xylazine also has potent effects on intestinal motility. The jejunum and large intestine have less activity for up to 2 hours after a 1.1 mg/kg dose (Lowe et al., 1980; Adams et al., 1984; Roger and Ruckebusch, 1987; Mitchell et al., 2005). This is a profound effect giving relief from both somatic and visceral pain caused by distention or strangulation (Lowe et al., 1980; Muir and Robertson, 1985; Jochle et al., 1989; Dabareiner and White, 1995). Analgesia may last only 10 to 30 minutes or have minimal effect in horses with strangulating lesions such as large colon torsion. In horses with large or small colon impactions, xylazine appears beneficial in relieving the spasm of the intestine around the obstructing mass, thereby allowing passage of gas and rehydration of ingesta. This can often be accomplished with doses of 0.1 to 0.3 mg/kg intravenously and titrated to effect. If a prolonged effect is desired, xylazine can be administered intramuscularly at doses of 0.4 to 2 mg/kg.

Detomidine is an alpha-2 agonist like xylazine and is a potent sedative. It can produce complete cessation of colic for up to three hours, and during experimental cecal distention, it provided mean analgesia of 45 and 105 minutes at 20 µg/kg and 40 µg/kg respectively (Lowe and Hilfiger, 1986; Roger and Ruckebusch, 1987). Horses stand with their heads lowered and are reluctant to move. Second-degree heart blocks are common. Detomidine will reduce intestinal motility similar to xylazine, and it can obscure signs of pain that might help the clinician diagnose the cause of the colic. Because this is such a potent drug, any signs of colic observed within 30 to 60 minutes of administration are an indication that a severe disease is present and the horse may require surgery. The dosage can be titrated in 5-10 µg/kg increments (Dabareiner and White, 1995).

Opioids: The pure opioid agonists such as morphine and oxymorphone are potent analgesics, but they may cause excitation in the horse unless used in combination with drugs such as xylazine. Morphine reduces progressive motility of the small intestine and colon while potentially increasing mixing movements and increasing sphincter tone (Phaneuf et al., 1972; Senior et al., 2004). This can delay transit of ingesta. The disadvantages of morphine and oxymorphone in the horse with abdominal disease are sufficient to discourage their use. Epidural morphine (0.1 mg/kg qs to 30 cc of saline) can provide analgesia for 8 to 16 hours without CNS excitation.

Butorphanol[viii] is a partial agonist and antagonist, which gives the best pain relief with the least adverse effects of the opioids (Gingerich et al., 1985; Muir and Robertson, 1985; Kohn and Muir, 1988). It can be used in combination with xylazine or detomidine. The dosage can vary from 0.05 to 0.1 mg/kg, the high dosage being necessary for the most severe colic. Exceeding 0.2 mg/kg may cause an increase in heart rate, systolic blood pressure, and excitation in horses. Butorphanol can also be administered as a constant rate intravenous infusion at up to 23.7 µg/kg/hour. Butorphanol reduces small intestinal motility yet has minimal effect on pelvic flexure activity (Merritt et al., 1989; Merritt et al., 1998). Repeated use has the risk of delaying intestinal transit and causing impaction as seen with other opiate-like drugs. An overdose can be partially reversed with equal doses of naloxone[ix].

Spasmolytics: Spasmolytic drugs can indirectly provide analgesia by reducing spasms of the intestine. Increased frequency of intestinal contractions or spasms occurs with oral to intraluminal obstruction such as an impaction. Spasmolytic drugs include cholinergic blockers such as atropine. Because of the potential for prolonged intestinal stasis, use of atropine to treat equine acute abdomen is contraindicated.

The combination of hyoscine N-butylbromide and para-aminophenol derivative (dipyrone)[x] is popular in Europe for treatment of horses with colic, specifically spasmodic colic and impactions (Keller and Faulstich, 1985; Roelvink et al., 1991). Hyoscine has shorter-acting muscarinic cholinergic blocking effects compared to atropine and is effective in relaxing the bowel wall to prevent contraction. The drug can be detrimental in horses with ileus where inhibition of motility causes tympany and complicates the abdominal stasis that was already present (Keller, 1986). Hyoscine, by itself, is now available in the United States and is an effective antispasmodic. The drug is effective for treatment of spasmodic colic and impactions. Hyoscine gives excellent relaxation of the rectum facilitating examination per rectum. Lack of response to the drug suggests that there is a more serious problem that may require surgery or more aggressive treatment.

Lidocaine: Lidocaine has become popular as a prokinetic drug for use in the treatment of ileus (Malone and Turner, 1994; Cohen et al., 2004; Malone et al., 2006). Its effects appear to include both stimulation of gut motility and analgesic effects (Robertson et al., 2005). Lidocaine decreases inflammation by preserving microvascular integrity, preventing neutrophil migration and inhibiting cytokine production (Schmid et al., 1996; Takao et al., 1996; Lan et al., 2004a; Lan et al., 2004b). Lidocaine appears to be effective in treating pain for medical problems such as impactions and duodenitis-jejunitis as well as postoperative pain. An initial bolus of 1.3 mg/kg is followed by a constant-rate intravenous infusion at 0.05 mg/kg/min. Toxicity is exhibited as muscle fasciculation, erect hair, and weakness or recumbency (Malone and Turner, 1994). These signs quickly disappear after discontinuing the infusion.

Combating Ileus

Distention, endotoxemia, sympathetic stimulation, and bowel wall inflammation inhibit motility. The classic mechanisms of the sympathetic balanced with parasympathetic or cholinergic versus adrenergic stimulus no longer explains all the mechanisms controlling intestinal motility. The chief clinical problem is postoperative ileus involving the small intestine. Numerous drugs have been evaluated in normal horses. Few clinical trials have examined the efficacy of prokinetic drugs for treatment of equine postoperative ileus and those reporting success are limited to cisapride (Gerring and King, 1989), metoclopramide (Gerring and Hunt, 1986; Hunt and Gerring, 1986; Sojka et al., 1988), erythromycin (Nieto et al., 2000), and lidocaine (Malone and Turner, 1994; Malone et al., 2006). Recent research has supported the lack of usefulness of these compounds in horses with clinical disease (Nieto et al., 2000; Koenig and Cote, 2005). Inflammation from intestinal distention or ischemia potentially prevents the enteric nervous system or agents acting directly on muscle from stimulating progressive motility (Koenig and Cote, 2005). Only lidocaine appears to be of some value for treatment of postoperative ileus in horses with injured intestine, possibly due to its potential anti-inflammatory or analgesic effects rather than from direct stimulation of intestinal motility. New compounds that have yet to have reported for use in clinical cases include tegaserod[xi], a selective serotonin subtype 4 receptor agonist, and methylnaltrexone[xii], an opioid antagonist. Both stimulate pelvic flexure and jejunal motility in vitro (Delco et al., 2005; Van Hoogmoed et al., 2005).

Hydration

Hydration is usually accomplished with administration of balanced electrolyte solutions such as Ringer's, lactated Ringer's, or acetated Ringer's solutions. The greatest need is to replace total body water. Sodium replacement with the appropriate solution is needed to maintain water in the extracellular fluid (ECF) space without sacrificing potassium levels during long-term fluid administration. The level of dehydration is determined by evaluation of capillary refill, skin turgor, packed cell volume (PCV), and total protein (TP). The volume needed is calculated by estimating the water loss as a percent of the body weight or the percent of the blood or ECF change. An estimate can be calculated from the PCV and TP in the following formula:

Calculation for Initial Fluid Replacement

$$\frac{(\text{measured PCV or TP}) - (\text{normal PCV or TP}) \times 100}{(\text{normal PCV or TP})} = \text{percent change in the PCV or TP}$$

This percent change represents the change in the blood or the ECF volume from normal. The calculated percentage multiplied times the blood volume (7% of the body weight in kg = liters of blood) is the estimated amount of fluid which needs to be replaced immediately to provide an adequate circulatory volume. This estimate is critical for the horse requiring surgery. The same estimate calculated on the ECF volume (30% of the body weight in kg = liters of ECF) calculates the total replacement required for rehydration of the ECF space. Because the PCV can vary widely in horses during colic, calculations using total protein may give a better estimate.

Horses with slight intestinal distention and ileus with accompanying pain often respond immediately to fluid replacement. Intravenous fluid administration has also been helpful in increasing the available fluid for intestinal secretion. The constant secretion of the intestinal tract provides the needed water to soften an impacted food mass. This "overhydration" technique can be used as a primary treatment for pelvic flexure and cecal impactions. The fluid can be administered intravenously over a 24-hour period or as a bolus. By regulating intravenous fluid administration to maintain the plasma protein at 5.0 to 5.5 g/dl (normal 6.0-6.5 g/dl), a state of overhydration will be maintained with adequate fluid available to help intestinal secretion. This normally requires a fluid administration rate of 2 to 4 liters per hour, double or triple maintenance requirements. When a bolus of fluids is administered, 20 liters in 1 to 2 hours is usually sufficient to decrease the plasma protein concentration.

In horses with severe dehydration including horses with endotoxic shock, administration of hypertonic saline can be used as an emergency measure to restore circulating volume (Bertone et al., 1990). A 7.5% saline solution is administered at 4 to 5 ml/kg as rapidly as possible. This rapidly draws water from the extracellular and intracellular space into the vascular space. This will improve perfusion and lower heart rate, but it must be followed with adequate replacement fluids to help restore hydration. Hypertonic saline is very useful in resuscitating horses in severe shock, and its use should be reserved for those horses. Hypertonic saline (4 ml/kg) can also be combined with hetastarch[xiii] or pentastarch[xiv] (6-10 ml/kg) to provide colloid support in horses with decreased protein concentrations (Corley, 2006).

Electrolyte imbalances are not common in horses with acute simple colic. However, decreased serum calcium concentrations occur more frequently in horses with large colon displacements or small or large colon strangulations (Dart et al., 1992). Calcium gluconate or calcium borogluconate are commonly used to replace calcium at 0.2-1.0 ml/kg of a 20% solution (Corley, 2006). Hypomagnesemia is less commonly associated with colic and is most common in horses that are off feed without electrolyte supplementation. Depression, anorexia, and cardiac dysrhythmias are signs associated with hypomagnesemia. Intravenous administration of magnesium sulfate or magnesium chloride at 2 mg/kg/min should not exceed 50 mg at one time (Corley, 2006). Oral supplementation with magnesium oxide at 20-30 mg/kg/day may also be considered.

Treatment of Impactions

Impaction colic is the most frequent type of simple obstruction causing colic (Tinker et al., 1997; White and Dabareiner, 1997). Factors associated with impactions include poor dentition, lack of access to water, coarse feeds, acute cessation of routine exercise with confinement, and treatment for musculoskeletal diseases (Dabareiner and White, 1995; White and Lopes, 2003). Damage or dysfunction of the enteric nervous system may also cause alterations in motility leading to impaction. Intestinal adhesions, which are suspected to alter motility patterns at the pelvic flexure, are also known to cause colon impactions (Schusser and White, 1997).

The basic premise for treating colon impaction is relieving pain, softening the consistency of the impacted ingesta, and stimulating motility to increase fecal transit. Xylazine, detomidine, hyoscine/dipyrone, and flunixin meglumine are efficacious, at least in part, by reducing intestinal spasm at the obstruction (Dabareiner and White, 1995; White and Dabareiner, 1997; White and Lopes, 2003). In the author's experience, titration with xylazine or detomidine appears sufficient to relieve the pain and initiate transit without excessive decreases in motility seen with the alpha agonists. The combination of alpha agonists with flunixin also appears effective for managing impactions, which can take several days to soften and move from the colon (White and Lopes, 2003). If these drugs do not control pain, most likely the impaction is severe enough to require surgery or another surgical disease is present.

Though administration of mineral oil via nasogastric tube is widely recommended for treatment of impaction colic, there is evidence that administration of oral or intravenous fluids may be preferable when an impaction is resistant to routine analgesic and laxative therapy. Administration of intravenous fluids has been used to help "overhydrate" the circulatory system, thereby stimulating secretion into the dehydrated ingesta in the colon (White and Lopes, 2003). Beyond systemic hydration afforded by fluid administration, dilution of plasma protein in the vascular system reduces plasma osmotic pressure, allowing water diffusion into tissues and specifically in regions of distended bowel. However, fluid treatment administered at 10 ml/kg per hour for 12 hours did not significantly alter colon hydration in normal fistulated horses (Lopes et al., 2004)(Figure 1).

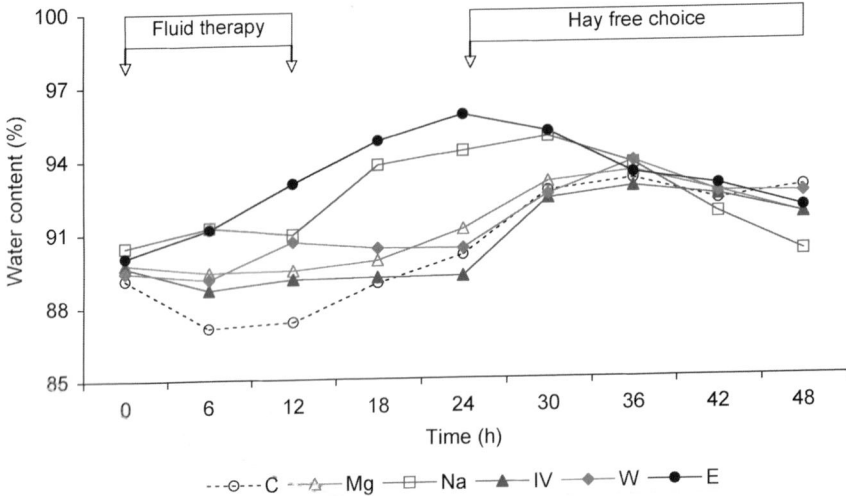

Figure 1. Water content of ingesta in the right dorsal colon increased significantly after enteral treatment with Na_2SO_4 (1.0 g/kg) and with 5 liters every hour for 12 hours of a balanced electrolyte solution. Enteral water, $MgSO_4$ (1.0 g/kg), and intravenous lactated Ringer's solution at 5 liters per hour for 12 hours did not affect water content in the colon in normal horses (Lopes et al., 2004).

Enteral administration of fluids is effective in increasing intestinal water (Lopes et al., 2004). Treatment of colon impactions with water administered via nasogastric tube

(10 liters every 30 to 60 minutes) until the impaction is resolved is effective; however, alterations in serum electrolytes can result from prolonged treatment (Lopes et al., 2002). Administration of $MgSO_4$ (1 g/kg in 1-2 liters of water via stomach tube) does not increase colon ingesta hydration but hydration of the feces did occur. Sodium sulfate (1 g/kg in 1-2 liters of water via stomach tube) significantly increases colon content hydration and created hypernatremia. Saline, originally prescribed for sand colic, increased colon water content but resulted in hypernatremia and hyperchloremia. Administration of a balanced electrolyte solution containing 5.37 g NaCl, .37 g KCl, and 3.78 g $NaHCO_3$ per liter is as effective as any laxative in hydrating colon contents without altering serum electrolyte values (Table 1). The balanced electrolyte solution is administered via a feeding tube at 5 to 10 liters per hour. This hydrates colon contents as well as restoring systemic hydration.

Table 1. Formula in grams with estimates using measuring teaspoons to make a balanced electrolyte solution for use as an enteral fluid to treat colon impactions. Administered at 5-10 liters per hour, this solution will soften impactions and provide systemic hydration.

Specific Ingredient	Grams/liter	Grams/5 liters
NaCl	5.37	26.85
KCl	0.37	1.85
$NaHCO_3$	3.78	18.9
Ingredient	Amount/5 liters	Total dose/5 liters
Salt	3 teaspoons	Equals 21 g NaCl
Litesalt®	1 teaspoon	Equals 3.5 g NaCl and 2 g KCl
Baking Soda	4 teaspoons	Equals 20 g $NaHCO_3$

Research suggests that colon hydration is increased when fasted horses are fed hay. Though feeding may increase motility and oral water intake, feeding horses with impactions should be delayed until there is evidence that the impaction is moving or is resolved (Dabareiner and White, 1995; White and Lopes, 2003). When initiating feeding after the impaction has moved out of the colon, a laxative diet without grain, such as grass or alfalfa hay, is preferred. Use of bran as a laxative is controversial. Though pure bran is high in fiber, most milled bran contains large amounts of carbohydrate, which reduces total fiber content and potentially decreases water content in the colon.

Equine Nutrition after Colic

INTRODUCTION

There is little research on how to feed horses after an episode of colic or after abdominal surgery. Veterinarians have adopted feeding protocols that have worked for the most common types of colic. This is likely because up to 80% of all colic episodes are considered simple colic with no specific diagnosis or known cause (Tinker et al., 1997). Spasmodic or gas colics make up about 8% of colic cases and rarely have a specific cause identified or specific dietary needs. Most of these simple types of colic episodes are easily treated and often there is no interruption in feed intake. Approximately 8-10% of colic episodes in the normal population result from impactions of the colon (Tinker et al., 1997). Though most are successfully treated with analgesics and a laxative, continued feeding is not recommended until transit of ingesta suggests that newly ingested feed will not add to the impaction (White and Dabareiner, 1997). Diseases that create ileus or complete obstruction are the most serious type of colic episodes and require a special feed type and timing of ingestion. Many of these serious diseases require surgery and treatment for shock or infection which complicate the nutritional needs of these horses. Currently, recommendations for nutrition have not been scientifically tested nor have specific types of diet been correlated with success in treating or preventing colic or specific type of obstruction of the horse's intestine.

Enteral Nutrition

The energy needs of horses after colic or abdominal surgery are not known. Because of the wide variation in the severity of colic, clinicians have assumed that there is no need for an increase in nutritional requirement after simple colic. In most cases horses are only off feed for a short period of time (12 to 48 hours), if at all, and there is no apparent clinical effect in these horses. Sixteen Mcal (32 kcal/kg), the energy requirement for maintenance for an adult horse on pasture, may not be needed for many horses that are stall-confined and considered to have basal metabolism. During the immediate postoperative period, less energy should be expended for digestion, possibly as much as a 15-20% decrease (Geor, 2007). The basal requirement for stall-confined horses postoperatively is likely sufficient unless they are challenged by a systemic inflammatory response syndrome due to peritonitis or endotoxemia. If the basal requirement is 70% of maintenance, the requirement for the stall-rested horse would be approximately 21 kcal/kg per day. Estimates for the increased energy requirement for horses due to abdominal surgery or shock are based on human information, which suggests an increase of 30-100% above maintenance, but this has not been substantiated in the horse. The protein requirement for maintenance is estimated at 1.25 g/kg per day providing 0.9 g/kg per day of available protein (Geor, 2007). Basal requirements for protein may also be decreased to 0.6-0.8 g/kg per day. Adequate energy from carbohydrates or fat is needed to prevent utilization of protein for energy during nutritional therapy. Though not currently recognized as the standard of care, horses that are not ingesting at least 50% of their maintenance requirement (15-18 kcal/kg per day) for 48 to 72 hours should have nutritional support (Dunkel and McKenzie, 2003; Magdesian, 2003).

Most hay or grass is not evaluated for nutrient content, so the daily energy and protein intake frequently is not known for horses during medical care. The use of pellet-formed feeds such as Equine Senior®[xv] allows calculation of energy and protein intake. Other total horse feeds supplied as pellets are usually made partially from grains, thereby increasing soluble carbohydrate concentrations. This may be appropriate for some horses after surgery, but this is dependent on concern for altering the flora in the cecum and colon. In some instances, this readily available source of carbohydrates may be an advantage. Nevertheless, feedstuffs such as bran are not recommended due to the high amount of carbohydrate often present after milling.

Horses suffering from simple colic rarely need alterations in their diet. Food and water should be withheld during the colic episode. Most horses can return to their normal diet after the pain is resolved and there is evidence of fecal transit. Since the cause of simple colic is rarely identified, clinical signs are used to determine whether normal feeding can be continued. In some cases, grain is withheld for several feedings to prevent excess gas production. However, there is no strict guideline as there is great variation in the severity of the colic and feeding practices in specific locales.

Impaction of the colon causes obstruction of the colon either at the pelvic flexure or the right dorsal colon (White and Dabareiner, 1997). The ingesta becomes dehydrated and forms a firm, large mass, which is resistant to moving aborally due to its size and contractions of colon around the mass. Continued feeding appears to prolong the process of clearing the mass from the intestine. In most cases impactions are successfully treated by administration of analgesics and a laxative such as mineral oil (White and Dabareiner, 1997). Impactions resistant to laxative treatment will most always resolve with hydration of the impacted mass using an intravenous or enteral balanced electrolyte administration (Lopes et al., 2002). During this treatment food is withheld until there is evidence of fecal transit and the impaction can no longer be identified by rectal examination. Resumption of feeding is best initiated with hay or pasture without grain until normal transit is established.

The best type of feed or feeding time for a horse after severe distention or abdominal surgery for obstruction or strangulation has not been scientifically determined. In most cases a forage diet of hay or fresh grass is chosen and fed as soon as medical judgment suggests ingested food can be tolerated. Alternatives include pellet-type feeds consisting of alfalfa or total diet feeds[xv]. Grains and sweet feed are avoided to decrease the risk of excess fermentation causing gas production and concern for abrupt changes in intestinal flora by providing too much soluble carbohydrate, thereby increasing the risk of diarrhea or laminitis.

After surgery for large colon disease, water can usually be offered immediately unless there is evidence of shock or lack of intestinal motility. After surgery for a large colon obstruction, grass hay, alfalfa hay, or fresh grass is routinely fed from 6 to 12 hours after surgery. Alfalfa hay is favored by many clinicians for its palatability, high energy and protein content, and laxative effect. Initially feeding 1 pound of hay every 3 hours allows monitoring of intake and response of intestinal motility. Ad lib feeding can usually be started 24 hours after the initial offering.

Water is not offered immediately after surgery for small intestinal disease until gastric reflux has ceased, there is evidence of intestinal motility, and absorption of fluid from the intestine can be documented by stabilization of vascular volume (PCV and TP) and overall hydration. Prior to feeding, the author recommends offering one liter every hour until the horse is no longer thirsty. Hay or a pellet feed is then offered at a rate of 0.5 to 1 pound every 3 hours increasing over 24 to 48 hours when ad lib hay or a specific amount of feed pellets equal to the basal energy requirements can be offered. Freeman and coworkers suggest feeding horses with small intestinal obstruction or strangulation including those with intestinal resection and anastomosis as soon as possible to stimulate normal motility (2000). Though feeding can be a stimulus for intestinal motility and is successful in many horses, early feeding can result in return of colic and accumulation of fluid in the stomach and small intestine. No methods have been established to predict which horses will not tolerate early feeding.

An increased risk of postoperative ileus is associated with an increased PCV and heart rate, prolonged surgery and anesthesia, and signs of endotoxemia prior to surgery (Blikslager et al., 1994; Roussel et al., 2001; Cohen et al., 2004). Other than intraluminal pressure measured at surgery, there is no measure of bowel inflammation or function that helps to predict when enteral feeding will be tolerated. The decision to feed a horse after small intestinal surgery remains a medical judgment without specific criteria to guide the clinician. Experience suggests that small amounts fed at frequently timed intervals prevents overload of the intestine and allows for early detection of problems such as ileus or obstruction.

Oral liquid diets made for humans have been used in horses but contain no fiber and increase the risk of colitis and laminitis (Buechner-Maxwell et al., 2003). Other diets consisting of alfalfa pellets, dextrose, vegetable oils, and amino acids maintained body condition of horses but also increased the risk of diarrhea and laminitis (Naylor et al., 1984). Development of an enteral energy/protein source, which is readily absorbed with minimal risk of disturbing motility or gut flora, is necessary for horses needing enteral nutrition during the initial postoperative period. Supplementation of glutamine has been suggested to help maintain or restore the intestinal epithelium, reduce the inflammatory response of the epithelium, and prevent bacterial translocation (Zhang et al., 1995; Blikslager et al., 1999; Liboni et al., 2005).

Parenteral Nutrition

Feeding horses intravenously, though shown to be possible, has not been proven to be necessary to improve horse survival after abdominal surgery (Lopes and White, 2002). In human medicine, there is no evidence that parenteral nutrition alters mortality of surgical or critical care patients, but there is evidence that complications are decreased particularly in patients that are malnourished (Heyland et al., 1998). A comparison of horses evaluated after abdominal surgery with or without supportive parenteral nutrition did not show a difference in outcome. Nevertheless, there was evidence of significantly decreased triglycerides, total bilirubin, albumin, and urea with significantly higher serum glucose and insulin in horses treated with parenteral nutrition after small intestinal resection and anatomosis (Durham et al., 2004). The treatment did not change time until enteral feeding, or time or cost of hospitalization.

Parenteral nutrition should be considered immediately if ileus, shock, or peritonitis is predicted to prevent oral ingestion of feed for more than a few days. Subjectively, it appears to the author that parenteral nutrition has been responsible for reducing convalescence time and cost for horses in shock and unable to tolerate enteral nutrition immediately after surgery.

Since total energy requirements may be decreased after surgery, partial parenteral nutrition may be sufficient for short-term nutrient supplementation. Use of glucose and amino acids without lipids appears to provide adequate calories. When endotoxemia and shock are present, the addition of lipids as a source of energy may be necessary as insulin resistance may be present in horses during endotoxemia (Lopes and White, 2002).

Addition of single or multiple trace elements as antioxidants (specifically selenium) during parenteral nutrition in human studies was associated with a significant decrease in mortality (Heyland et al., 2005). Since horses are not normally supported with parenteral nutrition for long periods, the benefit of vitamin and mineral supplementation is unknown.

Complications of parenteral nutrition include thrombophlebitis, hyperglycemia, hyperlipidemia, and electrolyte imbalance. Monitoring serum glucose is important during parenteral nutrition, particularly when initiating parenteral feeding. Glucose intolerance detected during the initial 24 to 48 hours requires reduction in the rate of administration or treatment with insulin. Normally the hyperglycemia is transient, but persistent hyperglycemia or hyperglycemia occurring after the initial period of accommodation may be an indicator of disease severity (Lopes and White, 2002).

Although enteral nutrition is always preferred, parenteral nutrition can provide long-term nutritional support. Horses have been kept on total parenteral nutrition for several weeks to one month and been able to maintain or gain weight.

Footnotes

[i] Banamine, Schering Plough Animal Health, Union, NJ 07083
[ii] Ketofen, Fort Dodge Animal Health, Overland Park, KS 66225
[iii] Eltenac, Schering Plough Animal Health, Union, NJ 07083
[iv] Rimadyl, Pfizer Animal Health, Exton, PA 19341
[v] Xylazine, Vedco, Inc., St. Joseph, MO 64507
[vi] Sedivet, Boerhinger Ingleheim, Vetmedica, Inc., St. Joseph, MO 64506
[vii] Dormosedan, Pfizer Animal Health, Exton PA 19341
[viii] Torbugesic, Fort Dodge Animal Health, Overland Park, KS 66225
[ix] Narcan, Endo Pharmaceuticals, Chadds Ford, PA 19317
[x] Buscopan, Boerhinger Ingleheim, Vetmedica, Inc., St. Joseph, MO 64506
[xi] Zelnorm, Novartis Pharmaceuticals, East Hanover, NJ 07936

xii Methylnaltrexone, Progenics Pharmaceuticals, Tarrytown, NY 10591
xiii Hetastarch, Baxter, Deerfield, IL 60015
xiv Pentastarch, Dupont Pharma, Wilmington, DE 19880
xv   Equine Senior®, Land 'O Lakes-Purina Feed, St. Louis, MO 63141

References

Adams, S.B., C.H. Lamar, and J. Masty. 1984. Motility of the distal portion of the jejunum and pelvic flexure in ponies: Effects of six drugs. Amer. J. Vet. Res. 45:795-799.

Beretta, C., G. Garavaglia, and M. Cavalli. 2005. COX-1 and COX-2 inhibition in horse blood by phenylbutazone, flunixin, carprofen and meloxicam: An in vitro analysis. Pharmacol. Res. 52:302-306.

Bertone, J.J., K.A. Gossett, K.E. Shoemaker, A.L. Bertone, and H.L. Schneiter. 1990. Effect of hypertonic vs. isotonic saline solution on responses to sublethal *Escherichia coli* endotoxemia in horses. Amer. J. Vet. Res. 51:999-1007.

Blikslager, A.T., K.F. Bowman, J.F. Levine, D.G. Bristol, and M.C. Roberts. 1994. Evaluation of factors associated with postoperative ileus in horses: 31 cases (1990-1992). J. Amer. Vet. Med. Assoc. 205:1748-1752.

Blikslager, A.T., J.M. Rhoads, D.G. Bristol, M.C. Roberts, and R.A. Argenzio. 1999. Glutamine and transforming growth factor-alpha stimulate extracellular regulated kinases and enhance recovery of villous surface area in porcine ischemic-injured intestine. Surgery 125:186-194.

Blikslager, A.T., M.C. Roberts, J.M. Rhoads, and R.A. Argenzio. 1997. Prostaglandins I2 and E2 have a synergistic role in rescuing epithelial barrier function in porcine ileum. J. Clin. Invest. 100:1928-1933.

Buechner-Maxwell, V.A., C.D. Elvinger, M.J. Murray, N.A. White, and D.K. Rooney. 2003. Physiologic response of normal adult horses to a low-residue liquid diet. J. Equine Vet. Sci. 23:310-317.

Cohen, N.D., G.D. Lester, L.C. Sanchez, A.M. Merritt, and A.J. Roussel, Jr. 2004. Evaluation of risk factors associated with development of postoperative ileus in horses. J. Amer. Vet. Med. Assoc. 225:1070-1078.

Collins, L.G., and D.E. Tyler. 1984. Phenylbutazone toxicosis in the horse: a clinical study. J. Amer. Vet. Med. Assoc. 184:699-703.

Corley, K.T. 2006. Treatment of shock. In: The Equine Acute Abdomen. N. White, J. Moore and M.T, Teton, ed. Jackson Hole. In press.

Dabareiner, D.M., and N.A. White. 1995. Large colon impaction in horses: 147 cases (1985-1991). J. Amer. Vet. Med. Assoc. 206:679-685.

Dart, A.J., J.R. Snyder, S.J. Spier, and K.E. Sullivan. 1992. Ionized calcium concentration in horses with surgically managed gastrointestinal disease: 147 cases (1988-1990). J. Amer. Vet. Med. Assoc. 201:1244-1248.

Delco, M., J. Nieto, A. Cragmill, S. Stanley, and J. Synder. 2005. Pharmacokinetics and in vitro effects of Tegaserod, a serotonin 5-hydroxytryptamine 4 (5HT4) receptor agonist with prokinetic activity in horses. In: Eighth International Equine Colic Research Symposium, AAEP, Quebec City. p. 71-72.

Dunkel, B., and H.C. McKenzie. 2003. Severe hypertriglyceridaemia in clinically ill horses: Diagnosis, treatment and outcome. Equine Vet. J. 35:590-595.

Durham, A.E., T.J. Phillips, J.P. Walmsley, and J.R. Newton. 2004. Nutritional and clinicopathological effects of post operative parenteral nutrition following small intestinal resection and anastomosis in the mature horse. Equine Vet. J. 36:390-396.

Freeman, D.E., P. Hammock, G.J. Baker, T. Goetz, J.H. Foreman, D.J. Schaeffer, R.A. Richter, O. Inoue, and J.H. Magid. 2000. Short- and long-term survival and prevalence of postoperative ileus after small intestinal surgery in the horse. Equine Vet. J. Suppl. 42-51.

Geor, R.J. 2007. How to feed horses recovering from colic. In: Proc. Amer. Assoc. Equine Practition. 52:196-201.

Gerring, E.E.L., and J.M. Hunt. 1986. Pathophysiology of equine postoperative ileus: Effect of adrenergic blockade, parasympathetic stimulation and metoclopramide in an experimental model. Equine Vet. J. 18:249-255.

Gerring, E.L., and J.N. King. 1989. Cisapride in the prophylaxis of equine postoperative ileus. Equine Vet. J. Suppl. 52-55.

Gingerich, D.A., J.E. Rourke, R.C. Chatfield, and P.W. Strom. 1985. Butorphanol tartrate: A new analgesic to relieve the pain of equine colic. Vet. Med. 80:74-77.

Goodrich, L.R., M.O. Furr, J.L. Robertson, and L.D. Warnick. 1998. A toxicity study of eltenac, a nonsteroidal anti-inflammatory drug, in horses. J. Vet. Pharmacol. Ther. 21:24-33.

Heyland, D.K., R. Dhaliwal, U. Suchner, and M.M. Berger. 2005. Antioxidant nutrients: A systematic review of trace elements and vitamins in the critically ill patient. Intensive Care Med. 31:327-337.

Heyland, D.K., S. MacDonald, L. Keefe, and J.W. Drover. 1998. Total parenteral nutrition in the critically ill patient: A meta-analysis. J. Amer. Med. Assoc. 280:2013-2019.

Hunt, J.M., and E.L. Gerring. 1986. A preliminary study of the effects of metoclopramide on equine gut activity. J. Vet. Pharmacol. Ther. 9:109-112.

Jochle, W., J.N. Moore, J. Brown, G.J. Baker, J.E. Lowe, S. Fubini, M.J. Reeves, J.P. Watkins, and N.A. White. 1989. Comparison of detomidine, butorphanol, flunixin meglumine and xylazine in clinical cases of equine colic. Equine Vet. J. 7:111-116.

Jones, S., J. Trujillo, R. Eckert, and Y. Sharief. 2005. Essential role of p38 MAPK in the mechanism of lipopolysaccharide-induced COX-2 gene expression in equine leukocytes. In: Eighth International Equine Colic Research Symposium, AAEP, Quebec City. p. 59.

Karcher, L.F., S.G. Dill, W.I. Anderson, and J.M. King. 1990. Right dorsal colitis. J.

Vet. Int. Med. 4:247-253.

Keller, H. 1986. Induction of intestinal paralysis by a large dose of Buscopan (scopolamine butylbromide) in the horse. Tierarztliche Umschau 41:266-268.

Keller, H., and A. Faulstich. 1985. Treatment of colic in the horse with Buscopan (hyoscine butylbromide with dipyrone). Tierarztliche Umschau 40:581-584.

King, J.N., and E.L. Gerring. 1989. Antagonism of endotoxin-induced disruption of equine bowel motility by flunixin and phenylbutazone. Equine Vet. J. 7:38-42.

Koenig, J., and N. Cote. 2005. The effect of inflammation of the equine jejunum on motilin receptors and binding of erythromycin lactobionate. In: Eighth International Equine Colic Research Symposium, AAEP, Quebec City. p. 80-81.

Kohn, C.W., and W.W. Muir. 1988. Selected aspects of the clinical pharmacology of visceral analgesics and gut motility modifying drugs in the horse. J. Vet. Int. Med. 2:85-91.

Lan, W., D. Harmon, J.H. Wang, K. Ghori, G. Shorten, and P. Redmond. 2004a. The effect of lidocaine on in vitro neutrophil and endothelial adhesion molecule expression induced by plasma obtained during tourniquet-induced ischaemia and reperfusion. Eur. J. Anaesthesiol. 21:892-897.

Lan, W., D. Harmon, J.H. Wang, K. Ghori, G. Shorten, and P. Redmond. 2004b. The effect of lidocaine on neutrophil CD11b/CD18 and endothelial ICAM-1 expression and IL-1beta concentrations induced by hypoxia-reoxygenation. Eur. J. Anaesthesiol. 21:967-972.

Liboni, K.C., N. Li, P.O. Scumpia, and J. Neu. 2005. Glutamine modulates LPS-induced IL-8 production through IkappaB/NF-kappaB in human fetal and adult intestinal epithelium. J. Nutr. 135:245-251.

Lopes, M.A., B.L. Walker, N.A. White, and D.L. Ward. 2002. Treatments to promote colonic hydration: Enteral fluid therapy versus intravenous fluid therapy and magnesium sulphate. Equine Vet. J. 34:505-509.

Lopes, M.A., and N.A. White. 2002. Parenteral nutrition for horses with gastrointestinal disease: A retrospective study of 79 cases. Equine Vet. J. 34:250-257.

Lopes, M.A., N.A. White, L. Donaldson, M.V. Crisman, and D.L. Ward. 2004. Effects of enteral and intravenous fluid therapy, magnesium sulfate, and sodium sulfate on colonic contents and feces in horses. Amer. J. Vet. Res. 65:695-704.

Lowe, J.E., and J. Hilfiger. 1986. Analgesic and sedative effects of detomidine compared to xylazine in a colic model using i.v. and i.m. routes of administration. Acta. Veterinaria Scandinavica 82:85-95.

Lowe, J.E., A.F. Sellers, and J. Brondum. 1980. Equine pelvic flexure impaction: A model used to evaluate motor events and compare drug response. Cornell Vet. 70:401-412.

MacKay, R.J., C.A. Daniels, H.F. Bleyaert, J.E. Bailey, K.D. Gillis, A.M. Merritt, T.L. Katz, J.C. Johnson, and K.C. Thompson. 2000. Effect of eltenac in horses with induced endotoxaemia. Equine Vet. J. Suppl. 26-31.

Magdesian, K.G. 2003. Nutrition for critical gastrointestinal illness: Feeding horses with diarrhea or colic. Vet. Clin. N. Amer. Equine Pract. 19:617-644.

Malone, E., J. Ensink, T. Turner, J. Wilson, F. Andrews, K. Keegan, and J. Lumsden. 2006. Intravenous continuous infusion of lidocaine for treatment of equine ileus. Vet. Surg. 35:60-66.

Malone, E.D., and E.D. Turner. 1994. Intravenous lidocaine for the treatment of ileus in the horse. In: Fifth Equine Colic Research Symposium, University of Georgia, Athens, Georgia. p. 39.

Merritt, A.M., J.A. Burrow, and C.S. Hartless. 1998. Effect of xylazine, detomidine, and a combination of xylazine and butorphanol on equine duodenal motility. Amer. J. Vet. Res. 59:619-623.

Merritt, A.M., M.L. Campbell Thompson, and S. Lowrey. 1989. Effect of butorphanol on equine antroduodenal motility. Equine Vet. J. 7:21-23.

Meschter, C.L., M. Gilbert, L. Krook, G. Maylin, and R. Corradino. 1990. The effects of phenylbutazone on the intestinal mucosa of the horse: A morphological, ultrastructural and biochemical study. Equine Vet. J. 22:255-263.

Mitchell, C.F., E.D. Malone, A.M. Sage, and K. Niksich. 2005. Evaluation of gastrointestinal activity patterns in healthy horses using B mode and Doppler ultrasonography. Can. Vet. J. 46:134-140.

Morrow, J., and L. Roberts. 2001. Lipid-derived autocoids. In: The pharmacological basis of therapeutics (10th ed.) J. Hardman, L. Limbird, and A.G. Gilman, ed. McGraw-Hill New York. p. 669-686.

Morton, A.J., N.B. Campbell, J.M. Gayle, W.R. Redding, and A.T. Blikslager. 2005. Preferential and nonselective cyclooxygenase inhibitors reduce inflammation during lipopolysaccharide-induced synovitis. Res. Vet. Sci. 78:189-192.

Muir, W.W., and J.T. Robertson. 1985. Visceral analgesia: Effects of xylazine, butorphanol, meperidine, and pentazocine in horses. Amer. J. Vet. Res. 46:2081-2084.

Naylor, J.M., D.E. Freeman, and D.S. Kronfeld. 1984. Alimentation of hypophagic horses. Comp. Cont. Educ. Pract. Vet. S93-S99.

Nieto, J.E., P.C. Rakestraw, J.R. Snyder, and N.J. Vatistas. 2000. In vitro effects of erythromycin, lidocaine, and metoclopramide on smooth muscle from the pyloric antrum, proximal portion of the duodenum, and middle portion of the jejunum of horses. Amer. J. Vet. Res. 61:413-419.

Phaneuf, L.P., M.L. Grivel, and Y. Ruckebusch. 1972. Electromyoenterography during normal gastrointestinal activity, painful or nonpainful colic and morphine analgesia in the horse. Can. J. Comp. Med. Vet. Sci. 36:138-144.

Robertson, S.A., L.C. Sanchez, A.M. Merritt, and T.J. Doherty. 2005. Effect of systemic lidocaine on visceral and somatic nociception in conscious horses. Equine Vet. J. 37:122-127.

Roelvink, M.E., L. Goossens, H.C. Kalsbeek, and T. Wensing. 1991. Analgesic and spasmolytic effects of dipyrone, hyoscine-N-butylbromide and a combination of the two in ponies. Vet. Rec. 129:378-380.

Roger, T., and Y. Ruckebusch. 1987. Colonic alpha-2-adrenoceptor-mediated responses in the pony. J. Vet. Pharmacol. Therap. 10:310-318.

Roussel, A.J., N.D. Cohen, R.N. Hooper, and P.C. Rakestraw. 2001. Risk factors associated with development of postoperative ileus in horses. J. Amer. Vet. Med. Assoc. 219:72-78.

Schmid, R.A., M. Yamashita, K. Ando, Y. Tanaka, J.D. Cooper, and G.A. Patterson. 1996. Lidocaine reduces reperfusion injury and neutrophil migration in canine lung allografts. Ann. Thorac. Surg. 61:949-955.

Schusser, G.E., and N.A. White. 1997. Morphologic and quantitative evaluation of the myenteric plexuses and neurons in the large colon of horses. J. Amer. Vet. Med. Assoc. 210:928-934.

Semrad, S.D., G.E. Hardee, M.M. Hardee, and J.N. Moore. 1985. Flunixin meglumine given in small doses: Pharmacokinetics and prostaglandin inhibition in healthy horses. Amer. J. Vet. Res. 46:2474-2479.

Senior, J.M., G.L. Pinchbeck, A.H. Dugdale, and P.D. Clegg. 2004. Retrospective study of the risk factors and prevalence of colic in horses after orthopaedic surgery. Vet. Rec. 155:321-325.

Sojka, J.E., S.B. Adams, C.H. Lamar, and L.L. Eller. 1988. Effect of butorphanol, pentazocine, meperidine, or metoclopramide on intestinal motility in female ponies. Amer. J. Vet. Res. 49:527-529.

Stick, J.A., C.C. Chou, F.J. Derksen, and W.A. Arden. 1987. Effects of xylazine on equine intestinal vascular resistance, motility, compliance, and oxygen consumption. Amer. J. Vet. Res. 48:198-203.

Takao, Y., K. Mikawa, K. Nishina, N. Maekawa, and H. Obara. 1996. Lidocaine attenuates hyperoxic lung injury in rabbits. Acta Anaesthesiol Scand. 40:318-325.

Tinker, M.K., N.A. White, P. Lessard, C.D. Thatcher, K.D. Pelzer, B. Davis, and D.K. Carmel. 1997. Prospective study of equine colic incidence and mortality. Equine Vet. J. 29:448-453.

Tomlinson, J.E., and A.T. Blikslager. 2005. Effects of cyclooxygenase inhibitors flunixin and deracoxib on permeability of ischaemic-injured equine jejunum. Equine Vet. J. 37:75-80.

Van Hoogmoed, L.M., P. Boscan, and J. Synder. 2005. In vitro evaluation of the effect of opioid antagonist, n-methylnaltrexone on motility in the equine jejunum and pelvic flexure and pharmacokinetics in normal horses. In: Eighth International Equine Colic Research Symposium, AAEP, Quebec City. p. 74-75.

Van Hoogmoed, L.M., J.R. Snyder, and F.A. Harmon. 2002. In vitro investigation of the effects of cyclooxygenase-2 inhibitors on contractile activity of the equine dorsal and ventral colon. Amer. J. Vet. Res. 63:1496-1500.

White, N.A. 1987. When equine colic calls for surgical intervention. Vet. Med. 82.

White, N.A., and R.M. Dabareiner. 1997. Treatment of impaction colics. Vet. Clin. N. Amer. Equine Pract. 13:243-259.

White, N., and M. Lopes. 2003. Large colon impaction. In: Current Therapy in Equine Medicine, by E. Robinson, ed. W.B.Saunders, Philadelphia. p. 131-135.

Zhang, W., W.L. Frankel, A. Bain, D. Choi, D.M. Klurfeld, and J.L. Rombeau. 1995. Glutamine reduces bacterial translocation after small bowel transplantation in cyclosporine-treated rats. J. Surg. Res. 58:159-164.

OVERVIEW OF GASTRIC AND COLONIC ULCERS

FRANK M. ANDREWS
The University of Tennessee, Knoxville, Tennessee

Introduction

Equine gastric ulcer syndrome (EGUS) and right dorsal colitis (RDC) are common in performance horses. Diagnoses are based on history, clinical signs, laboratory findings, gastroscopic examination, and response to altered diet and medical therapy. Effective treatment strategies for EGUS focus on increasing stomach pH by inhibiting or buffering gastric acid, which allows a permissive environment for ulcer healing, and environmental and dietary management. Effective treatment strategies for RDC focus on removing nonsteroidal anti-inflammatory drugs (NSAIDs), decreasing the bulk in the diet, reducing inflammation, coating and lubricating the colon, and decreasing environmental stress. Prevention of these conditions requires long-term dietary and environmental management.

Equine Gastric Ulcer Syndrome

Gastric ulcers are common in performance horses. The term "equine gastric ulcer syndrome" (EGUS) was coined to describe the condition of erosions and ulcerations occurring in the distal esophagus, nonglandular and glandular stomach, and proximal duodenum of horses (Andrews et al., 1999). EGUS is caused by many factors including anatomy of the stomach, exercise, restricted feed intake, diet, environmental stress (stall or transport), and the use of nonsteroidal anti-inflammatory agents (Buchanan and Andrews, 2002). Diagnosis of EGUS is based on history, clinical signs, endoscopic examination, and response to treatment. All ages and breeds of horses are susceptible to EGUS, and current therapeutic strategies focus on blocking gastric acid secretion and raising stomach pH to ≥ 4.0. To date there is only one Federal Drug Administration (FDA) approved pharmacologic agent for treatment of EGUS: GastroGard® (Merial Limited, Duluth, GA). However, a more comprehensive approach to EGUS diagnosis and treatment includes determining and correcting the underlying cause, environmental management, dietary manipulation, and pharmacologic intervention.

DIAGNOSIS

The approach to diagnosis of EGUS requires a thorough history, physical examination, and a minimum database (Figure 1). Identifying risk factors and clinical signs is

348 Overview of Gastric and Colonic Ulcers

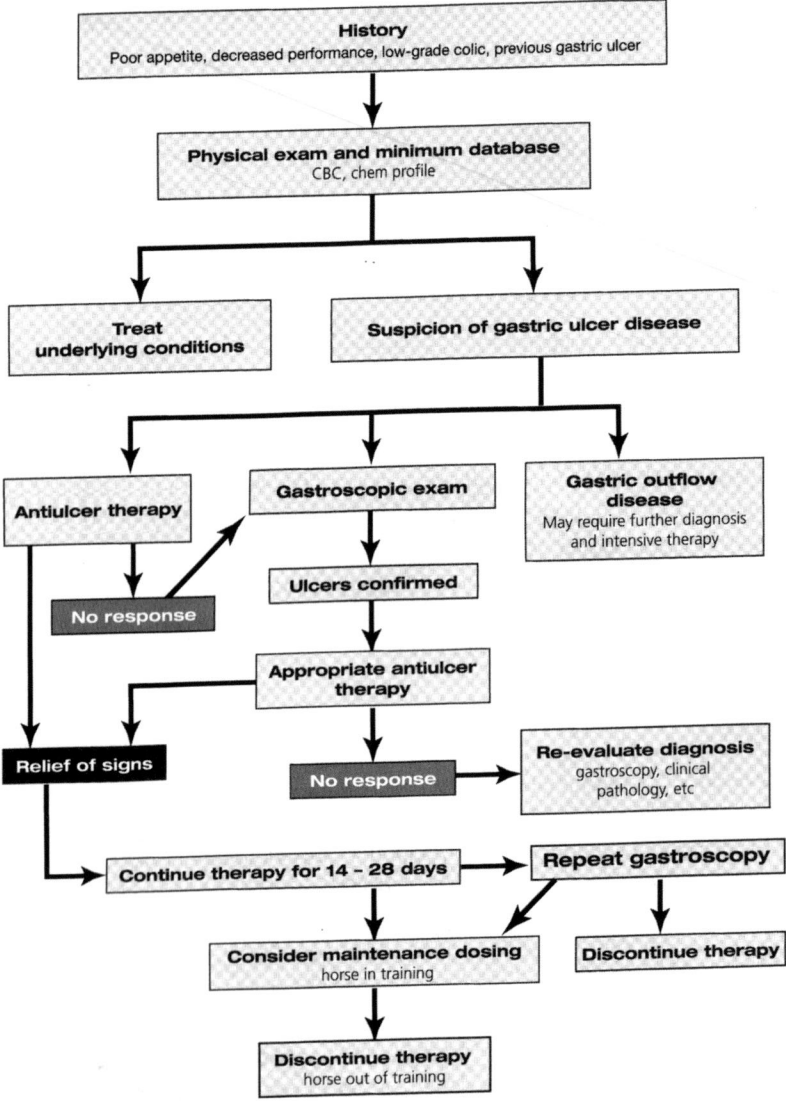

Figure 1. Diagnosis and treatment of EGUS.

helpful in diagnosing EGUS (Table 1). However, gastroscopy is the only definitive diagnostic technique currently available. The procedure for gastroscopy has been described in detail elsewhere, but requires at least a 2-meter endoscope to visualize the nonglandular mucosa and margo plicatus and a 2.5- to 3-meter endoscope to visualize the pyloric antrum and proximal duodenum in most adult horses. Once visualized, ulcers should be rated using a scoring system developed for horses (Andrews et al.,

Table 1. Commonly used antiulcer medications and recommended does.

Drug	Dosage	Route of Administration	Dosing Interval
Omeprazole	0.5-1.0 mg/kg	Intravenously	Q 24 hrs
Omeprazole (GastroGard™)	4 mg/kg (Treatment of ulcers)	Orally	Q 24 hrs
Omeprazole (GastroGard™)	2 mg/kg (Prevention of recurrence)		
Omeprazole (UlcerGard™)	1 mg/kg (Prevention of ulcers)	Orally	Q 24 hrs
Ranitidine	1.5 mg/kg	Intravenously	Q 6 hrs
Ranitidine	6.6 mg/kg	Orally	Q 8 hrs
Ranitidine	11.0 mg/kg	Orally	Q 12 hrs
Misoprostol	5 mcg/kg	Orally	Q 8 hrs
Sucralfate	20-40 mg/kg	Orally	Q 8 hrs
AlOH/MgOH antacids	30g AlOH/15 g MgOH	Orally	Q 2 hrs
Bethanecol	0.025 - 0.30 mg/kg	Subcutaneous	Q 3-4 hrs
Bethanecol	0.3 - 0.45 mg/kg	Orally	Q 6-8 hrs

1999). Use of a scoring system allows the clinician to compare gastroscopic findings and monitor healing of ulcers to evaluate efficacy of treatment. Currently there are no hematologic or biochemical markers to diagnose EGUS. However, a recent report showed that horses with gastric ulcers had lower RBC counts and hemoglobins than horses that did not have gastric ulcers (McClure et al., 1999). Some horses with EGUS may be slightly anemic or hypoproteinemic, but in my experience the RBC or hemoglobin values are rarely out of the normal range.

O'Connor et al. (2004) recently evaluated the potential of a sucrose permeability test to diagnose gastric ulcers. Urine sucrose concentrations were significantly higher for horses with gastric ulcer scores >1. Using a urine sucrose concentration cutoff value of 0.7 mg/ml or higher revealed an apparent sensitivity of 83% and specificity of 90% to detect ulcers in horses tested using the sucrose permeability test. Thus, this test may provide a simple, noninvasive way to detect and monitor gastric ulcers. Because of the lack of any additional laboratory diagnosis, in situations where ulcers are strongly suspected but gastroscopy is not available, it may be worthwhile to start empirical treatment and observe for resolution of clinical signs. If the horse does not respond to treatment within several days, referral to a facility for gastroscopic examination is indicated (Figure 1).

TREATMENT

The goals of EGUS therapy are to relieve pain, eliminate clinical signs, promote healing, prevent secondary complications, and prevent recurrence. The mainstay of EGUS treatment is to increase stomach pH by suppressing stomach HCl acid secretion. Pharmacologic therapy is popular and several agents have proven helpful in EGUS treatment, but the only FDA-approved drug for treatment and prevention of recurrence of gastric ulcers in horses is GastroGard®. Because of the high recurrence rate, effective acid control should be followed by altered management strategies and/or long-term treatment to prevent ulcer recurrence. Recently, UlcerGard® (Merial LTD, Duluth, GA), a low-dose omeprazole paste, was approved as a nonprescription medication for prevention of gastric ulcers in horses. Many feed additives and nutraceutical agents claim efficacy, but to the author's knowledge there are no published scientific data on the efficacy of these compounds in the treatment or prevention of EGUS. A short time ago we tested an equine supplement (SeaBuck® Complete Liquid, SeaBuck Equine, LLC) containing seabuckthorn berry extract. This compound was effective in preventing increased gastric ulcer scores in horses that were stressed. Therefore, this compound may be helpful in preventing recurrence once ulcers have healed.

Compounded formulations of omeprazole lack the stringent efficacy and safety studies that are required for FDA approval and have little chance of efficacy. Also, the chemical properties of omeprazole make it difficult to compound while maintaining efficacy and potency. Many compounded forms of omeprazole are inactivated in the bottle prior to administration and two recent studies confirmed that compounded omeprazole suspensions were ineffective in healing gastric ulcers in racehorses in training (Nieto et al., 2002; Orsini et al., 2003).

ANTIBIOTICS (*HELICOBACTER* SPP.)

Helicobacter has not been cultured from the horse stomach, but DNA from a *Helicobacter*-like bacteria was found in the stomach mucosa of horses using a polymer chain reaction test (PCR) (Scott et al., 2001; Contreras et al., 2007). Although *Helicobacter* has not been cultured from horses, there are some horses that do not respond to conventional acid suppressive therapy. In horses with chronic nonresponsive EGUS, bacteria (primarily *E. coli* and *Streptococcus* sp.) may colonize the ulcer bed and prevent healing. Bacterial colonization of the nonglandular mucosa and gastric ulcer has been shown to occur in horses (Yuki et al., 2000). The use of antibiotics may decrease the bacterial population in these ulcers and allow healing. In horses with gastric ulcers that do not respond to conventional therapy, I recommend combination therapy consisting of omeprazole (4 mg/kg, orally, q 24 h) or ranitidine (6.6 mg/kg, orally, q 8 h), metronidazole (15 mg/kg, orally, q 6-8 h) and/or trimethoprim/sulfa (15 to 25 mg/kg, orally, q 12 h), and bismuth subsalicylate (3.8 mg/kg, orally, q 6 h). An initial 14-day treatment period is prescribed, which should be followed by gastroscopy.

Some horses may require longer treatment. Omeprazole therapy should be continued for the full 28 days if needed.

DIETARY MANAGEMENT

In conjunction with pharmacological therapy, environmental and dietary management may be helpful to facilitate ulcer healing. Limited fasting periods, limited feeding of high-soluble-carbohydrate diets (not to exceed 0.5 kg grain/220 kg body weight) (Andrews et al., 2006) and providing good-quality alfalfa or alfalfa-mix hay can help buffer stomach contents and reduce gastric acidity. Alfalfa hay has been shown to buffer gastric contents and decrease gastric ulcer severity in horses housed in stalls and exercising (Nadeau et al., 2000; Lybbert et al., 2007). Also, pasture turnout when possible can help reduce stress and prevent gastric ulcers.

Right Dorsal Colitis (Colonic Ulcers)

Unlike EGUS, colonic ulcers and right dorsal colitis (RDC) occur less frequently, but may lead to hypoproteinemia and more severe clinical signs. In a necroscopic study of 545 horses, 44% of the nonperformance horses and 65% of the performance horses had colonic ulcers (Pellegrini, 2005). Colonic ulcers are probably associated with inhibition of prostaglandins by stress-induced release of endogenous corticosteroids or the administration of NSAIDs. Early in the condition, horses present with nonspecific signs of mild intermittent or recurring colic episodes, lethargy, and partial anorexia. However, as the condition worsens, clinical signs may include complete anorexia, fever, and diarrhea. Progression of RDC may lead to dehydration, ventral edema, and weight loss. Differential diagnoses for this condition include EGUS, large colon displacement and/or impaction, infectious causes of diarrhea (salmonellosis, Potomac horse fever, *Clostridium*), granulomatous enteritis, eosinophilic enterocolitis, and intestinal neoplasia.

DIAGNOSIS

A presumptive diagnosis of RDC can be made on history, clinical signs, changes on CBC (mild anemia, toxic changes in PMNs, left shift), hyperfibrinogenemia, hypoalbuminemia, and hypocalcemia. Peritoneal fluid analysis may show a mild increase in WBC count and increase in total protein concentration. In a recent study, a guaiac-based fecal occult blood test was shown to have a good positive predictive value (72%) and a poor negative predictive value (51%) in the diagnosis of RDC (Pellegrini, 2005). In that study, many horses that had gastric or colonic ulcers had negative tests (i.e., false negatives). Gastroscopic examination of the stomach, if negative, may help diagnose RDC in horses showing typical clinical signs, especially if there is concurrent hypoproteinemia. Abdominal ultrasonography of the right dorsal colon may show mural thickening (normal = < 4 mm) (Jones et al., 2003). The peripheral wall of the right dorsal colon can be scanned percutaneously through intercostal spaces 11 to 15, ventral to the ventral margin of the right lung field.

Every effort should be made to rule out infectious causes of diarrhea such as salmonellosis and Potomac horse fever (PHF) in horses with diarrhea. Fecal cultures and PHF serology and PCR can be helpful in ruling out these conditions. Horses with salmonellosis will have signs similar to RDC and these diseases may occur together.

TREATMENT

The principal components of treatment for RDC include discontinuing use of NSAIDs, decreasing gut fill to allow the colon to rest, and offering frequent feedings. These steps should lead to reduced inflammation and restoration of normal colon absorptive function (Cohen et al., 1995). Reduction in gut fill can be accomplished by decreasing or eliminating dry hay from the diet and replacing with frequent feeding of alfalfa-based pelleted complete feeds with at least 30% dietary fiber (Purina Senior™, Purina Mills, St. Louis, MO). This reduces gut fill and decreases the mechanical load on the colon. The horse can be allowed to graze small amounts of fresh grass (10- to 15-minute intervals, four to six times daily) to help maintain body weight. The switch to a complete feed diet should be made over several days to a week to allow the gastrointestinal tract time to acclimatize to the feed change. The complete feed diet should be continued for three to four months, at which time hypoproteinemia and hypoalbuminemia should have resolved.

Psyllium mucilloid (Equisyl Advantage™, Animal Heath Care Products) or psyllium hydrophilic mucilloid (Metamucil®, Proctor & Gamble, Cincinnati, OH) can be added to the diet to shorten transit time for ingesta and increase water content of the gastrointestinal tract. Also, psyllium increases the concentration of short-chain fatty acids, an effect which has been shown in other species to reduce inflammation, and thus may reduce inflammation in the equine colon also. Furthermore, safflower oil (1 cup, added to feed, q 12 h) can be added to the complete feed to increase omega-3 fatty acids. Omega-3 fatty acids competitively inhibit the activity of the cyclooxygenase enzyme necessary for eicosanoid production. A diet rich in omega-3 fatty acids may reduce the eicosanoid production, thereby decreasing inflammation.

The use of medications routinely used for gastric ulcer treatment (antacids, omeprazole, or ranitidine) would not be expected to be effective in treatment of RDC. However, sucralfate (22 mg/kg, orally, q 6-8 h), a sucrose octasulfate and polyaluminum hydroxide complex, has been used for treatment of RDC. This compound has a strong affinity to bind to gastrointestinal mucosa. It has a greater affinity to bind to ulcer craters when compared to intact epithelial cells. In man, sucralfate is more adherent to duodenal ulcers than gastric ulcers despite the duodenal pH >4.0. Thus, sucralfate may bind to ulcer craters in the colons of horses, forming a proteinacous bandage. Furthermore, sucralfate, once bound to the ulcer crater, may stimulate local prostaglandin production, which may exert a "cytoprotective"effect on the colon mucosa.

Minimizing physiologic and environmental stresses can also be helpful in controlling RDC. Stall rest, reduction of strenuous exercise or training, and reduction in transport are ways to decrease stress. Horses should always have adequate amounts of clean, fresh water and should be provided a mineral/salt mix to ensure adequate water intake (Cohen et al., 1995).

References

Andrews, F.M., W. Bernard, D. Byars, N. Cohen, T. Divers, C. MacAllister, A. McGladdery, M. Murray, J. Orsini, J. Snyder, and N. Vastistas. 1999. Recommendations for the diagnosis and treatment of equine gastric ulcer syndrome (EGUS). Eq.Vet. Educ. 1:122-134.

Buchanan, B.R., and F.M. Andrews. 2002. Treatment and prevention of equine gastric ulcer syndrome. Vet. Clin. N. Am. Eq. Pract. 19:575-579.

Cohen, N.D, G.K. Carter, R.H. Mealey, and T.S. Taylor. 1995. Medical management of right dorsal colitis in 5 horses: A retrospective study (1987-1993). J.Vet. Int. Med. 9:272-276.

Contreras, M., A. Morales, M.A. Garcia-Amado, M. De Vera, V. Bermúdez, and P. Gueneau. 2007. Detection of *Helicobacter*-like DNA in the gastric mucosa of Thoroughbred horses. Lett. Appl. Microbiol. 45:553-557.

Jones, S.L., J. Davis, and K. Rowlingson. 2003. Ultrasonographic findings in horses with right dorsal colitis: Five cases (2000-2001). J. Am. Vet. Med. Assoc. 222:1248-1251.

Lybbert, T., P. Gibbs, N. Cohen, B. Scott, and D. Sigler. 2007. Feeding alfalfa hay to exercising horses reduces the severity of gastric squamous mucosal ulceration. In: Proc. Amer. Assoc. Eq. Practnr. 53:525-526.

Nadeau, J.A., F.M. Andrews, and A.G. Matthew. 2000. Evaluation of diet as a cause of gastric ulcers in horses. Am. J. Vet. Res. 61:784-790.

Nieto, J.E., S. Spier, F.S. Pipers, S. Stanley, M.R. Aleman, D.C. Smith, and J.R. Snyder. 2002. Comparison of paste and suspension formulations of omeprazole in the healing of gastric ulcers in racehorses in active training. J. Am. Vet. Med. Assoc. 221:1139-1143.

O'Connor, M.S., J.M. Steiner, A.J. Roussel, D.A. Williams, J.B. Meddings, F. Pipers, and N.D. Cohen. 2004. Evaluation of urine sucrose concentration for detection of gastric ulcers in horses. Am. J. Vet. Res. 65:31-39.

Orsini, J.A., M. Haddock, L. Stine, E.K. Sullivan, T.S. Rabuffo, and G. Smith. 2003. Odds of moderate or severe gastric ulceration in racehorses receiving antiulcer medications. J. Am. Vet. Med. Assoc. 223:336-339.

Pellegrini, F.L. 2005. Results of a large-scale necroscopic study of equine colonic ulcers. J. Eq. Vet. Sci. 25:113-117.

Scott, D.R., E.A. Marcus, S.S.P. Shirazi-Beechey, and M. Murray. 2001. Evidence of *Helicobacter* infection in the horse. In: Proc. Amer. Soc. Microbiologists 287 (Abstract).

Yuki, N., T. Shimazaki, A. Kushiro, K. Watanabe, K. Uchida, T. Yuyama, and M. Morotomi. 2000. Colonization of the stratified squamous epithelium of the nonsecreting area of horse stomach by *Lactobacilli*. Appl. Environ. Micro. 66: 5030-5034.

INSULIN RESISTANCE – WHAT IS IT AND HOW DO WE MEASURE IT?

STEPHANIE VALBERG AND ANNA FIRSHMAN
University of Minnesota, St. Paul, Minnesota

Introduction

Insulin resistance is defined as the diminished ability of cells to respond to the action of insulin in transporting glucose (sugar) from the bloodstream into muscle and other tissues. In humans, insulin resistance typically develops with obesity and heralds the onset of type 2 (non-insulin-dependent) diabetes (Shepherd and Kahn, 1999). In horses, insulin resistance is commonly associated with equine metabolic syndrome (Johnson, 2002; Powell et al., 2002; Hoffman et al., 2003b; Vick et al., 2006), Cushing's disease (pituitary pars intermedia dysfunction) (Garcia and Beech, 1986; McGowan et al., 2004), and some forms of laminitis (Kronfeld et al., 2006; Treiber et al., 2006c; Bailey et al., 2007). In addition, insulin resistance is thought to potentially play a role in other diseases such as hyperlipemia (Forhead, 1994), endotoxemia (Tóth et al., 2008), and osteochondritis dissecans (Henson et al., 1997; Ralston, 1996) in horses. An understanding of insulin resistance requires a brief review of the mechanism of glucose transport into the two major insulin-sensitive tissues, muscle and fat (adipose tissue). Much of this information is derived from humans and animal species other than the horse. This is followed by a review of the tests currently available to assess insulin resistance in horses.

Glucose Transport Into Muscle and Adipose Cells

INSULIN-MEDIATED GLUCOSE TRANSPORT

Ingestion of meals containing starches and blood sugar produces a rise in blood glucose which triggers the secretion of insulin by the pancreas. Insulin acts to increase glucose transport, metabolism, and storage in skeletal muscle, the largest glucose sink, followed by adipose tissue (Gould, 1993). Insulin also both inhibits glucagon secretion and lowers serum free-fatty-acid concentrations, contributing to a sharp decline in liver glucose production (Shepherd and Kahn, 1999). Prolonged elevation of blood glucose concentrations has toxic effects on cells (Yki-Jarvinen, 1992). Low blood glucose concentrations result in seizures. Therefore, blood glucose concentrations need to be maintained within narrow limits by finely tuned hormonal regulation.

Glucose transport is the rate-controlling step in skeletal muscle glucose metabolism. The lipid bilayers in cell membranes are naturally impermeable to glucose and therefore a special transport system is required for glucose to enter cells. Facilitated diffusion down glucose-concentration gradients is mediated by transmembrane proteins, GLUT-1, 2, 3, 4, and 5, that are encoded by distinct genes (Gould, 1993). In skeletal muscle and adipocytes GLUT-1 is constantly present in muscle and fat cell membranes and provides basal levels of glucose uptake not influenced by insulin. In contrast, 90 percent of GLUT-4 is sequestered intracellularly and only translocates to the cell membrane under the influence of either insulin or exercise (Holman and Kasuga, 1997). Translocation of GLUT-4 to the cell membrane occurs via a complex process that is initiated when insulin binds to its receptor in the plasma membrane. This results in phosphorylation of the receptor and insulin-receptor substrates. These substrates form complexes with docking proteins, which eventually results in activation of phosphoinositide-3 kinase, a major pathway involved in the mediation of insulin-stimulated glucose transport and metabolism (Shepherd et al., 1998). The functionally important targets further downstream in the phosphoinositide- 3-kinase signaling cascade have not been identified, but they may be proteins that regulate the docking of GLUT-4-containing vesicles at the plasma membrane and their fusion with it (Rea and James, 1997).

NON–INSULIN-MEDIATED GLUCOSE UPTAKE

Although insulin is the chief acute stimulus for glucose uptake into cells, other stimuli, such as thyroid hormone and leptin, can also activate translocation of GLUT-4 into muscle and fat cells membranes. Exercise stimulates glucose transport by pathways that are independent of phosphoinositide-3 kinase and that may involve 5'-AMP–activated kinase (Shepherd and Kahn, 1999). Thyroid hormone increases both basal and insulin-stimulated glucose uptake into muscle and adipocytes, at least partly as a result of increases in GLUT-4 expression (Abel et al., 1996; Kahn, 1992). In horses, levothyroxine improves insulin sensitivity and decreases blood lipid concentrations (Frank et al., 2005). Leptin is secreted by adipocytes and signals the brain in response to changes in energy stores (Berti et al., 1997). Concentrations have been assessed in obese horses (Waller et al., 2006). Administration of leptin improves glucose uptake indirectly, possibly via leptin-induced increases in fatty acid oxidation (Muoio et al., 1997) or via changes in physical activity and thermogenesis mediated by the brain and sympathetic nervous system (Kamohara et al., 1997).

Mechanisms of Insulin Resistance

In horses, a number of factors such as age, breed, state of fasting, diet, access to pasture, exercise, and training all affect the degree of response of the pancreas to blood glucose concentrations and/or the rate of clearance of glucose from the bloodstream into muscle cells (Jacobs and Bolton, 1982; Garcia and Beech et al., 1986; Jeffcott and Field, 1986; June et al., 1992; Murphy et al., 1997; Williams et al., 2001; Powell et al., 2002; Hoffman et al., 2003a; Hoffman et al., 2003b; de Graaf-Roelfsema, 2006; Pratt et al., 2006; Stewart-Hunt et al., 2006; Treiber et al., 2006b; Bailey et al., 2007). These factors are often adaptive and reversibly affect insulin sensitivity. However, at some point, many horses become resistant to the effects of insulin, resulting in chronic disease. Resistance to the stimulatory effect of insulin on glucose utilization is a key pathogenic feature of obesity, metabolic syndrome, and most human forms of type 2 diabetes (Shepherd and Kahn, 1999). It is also known to be a factor in equine metabolic syndrome (Johnson, 2002; Hoffman et al., 2003b), and Cushing's disease in horses (Garcia and Beech, 1986) as well as a potential cause of some forms of laminitis (Treiber et al., 2006a; Treiber et al., 2006c; Bailey et al., 2007). The precise mechanisms that cause insulin resistance are not known in either humans or horses. Several mechanisms detailed below may possibly be involved.

1. *Changes in GLUT-4 expression or production.* Although mutations in GLUT-4 are theoretically possible causes of insulin resistance, they have not been linked to type 2 diabetes in humans. Further, reduced expression of GLUT-4 has not been found in skeletal muscle of type 2 diabetics (Abel et al., 1996; Kahn, 1992). Thus, in humans at least, a decrease in the production of GLUT-4 does not explain the impairment of whole-body insulin sensitivity.

2. *Defects in the intracellular translocation of GLUT-4 and signaling pathways.* The reduction in insulin-stimulated glucose uptake in skeletal muscle in obese humans is associated with impairment in insulin-stimulated movement of GLUT-4 from intracellular vesicles to the plasma membrane and in reduced activation of phosphoinositide-3 kinase by insulin in muscle (Zierath et al., 1996). To date the precise part of the complex pathway regulating glucose uptake that is impaired with most cases of type 2 diabetes and obesity in humans as well as obese horses is not known.

3. *Impairment of Insulin-stimulated glucose transport by circulating or paracrine factors.* The cytokine tumor necrosis factor alpha (TNF-α) has potent inhibitory effects on insulin signaling in isolated muscle and adipose tissue (Hotamisligil and Spiegelman, 1994). TNF-α is released in response to endotoxin, and in horses IV administration of endotoxin has been shown to impair insulin sensitivity for up to 24 hours (Tóth et al., 2008). Chronic elevation of serum free-fatty-acid concentrations, such as that which occurs in many humans with obesity or diabetes and horses with Cushing's or metabolic syndrome, may also contribute to the decreased uptake of glucose into peripheral tissues. In humans this has been shown to be mediated by a loss of the ability of insulin to stimulate phosphoinositide-3 kinase activity (Boden, 1997). Increased circulating cortisol (which occurs in Cushing's disease) also has a direct effect in impairing insulin sensitivity (Firshman et al., 2005; Tiley et al., 2008). Corticosteroids impair phosphorylation of insulin receptors (Coderre, 1992) and cause a large reduction in insulin-stimulated translocation of GLUT-4 (Dimitriadis, 1997).

4. *Hexosamine pathway.* Hyperglycemia itself has detrimental effects on insulin secretion and on the action of insulin in peripheral tissues (McClain and Crook, 1996). The mechanism of glucose toxicity in muscle may involve the hexosamine pathway, in which the enzyme glutamine:fructose-6-phosphate amidotransferase diverts glucose from the glycolytic pathway at the level of fructose-6-phosphate, resulting in the production of glucosamine-6-phosphate and, subsequently, other hexosamine products. Exposure of muscle to glucosamine at very high concentrations reduces stimulation by insulin of glucose transport and GLUT-4 translocation (Baron et al., 1995).

Effects of Chronic Hyperglycemia

Glucose in chronic excess causes toxic effects on structure and function of many organs, including the pancreatic islet (Yki-Jarvinen, 1992). One potential central mechanism for glucose toxicity is the formation of excess reactive oxygen species that over time cause chronic oxidative stress, defective insulin gene expression, and impaired insulin secretion (Robertson, 2004). In humans, tissues that are particularly susceptible to glucose toxicity include the pancreas, vascular epithelium, retina, and kidneys (Shepherd and Kahn, 1999). The propensity of horses with Cushing's disease and metabolic syndrome to develop laminitis and the ability to induce laminitis with prolonged supraphysiologic infusion of insulin (Asplin et al., 2007) suggest that the laminae in the hooves may have a particular sensitivity to the damaging effects of chronically elevated blood glucose or insulin concentrations. Another consequence of chronic peripheral insulin resistance in humans is damage or exhaustion of the pancreas leading to reduced secretion of insulin and exacerbation of hyperglycemia. It also has been proposed that pancreatic damage or exhaustion may develop in equine metabolic syndrome (Kronfeld et al., 2006).

Measuring Insulin Resistance in Horses

Because both the amount of insulin secreted by the pancreas in response to glucose and the insulin sensitivity of skeletal muscle and adipose tissue affect whole body insulin resistance, both need to be assessed to accurately measure insulin resistance (Firshman and Valberg, 2007). Several procedures have been developed to accomplish this task. The procedures themselves are not particularly difficult to perform. The biggest barrier to their use is the adequacy of normal ranges for each test that accounts for varying ages, breeds, fitness levels, and dietary regimes of horses.

BASAL GLUCOSE AND INSULIN MEASUREMENT

Single fasting glucose and insulin measurements have been used in the field to identify horses with suspected insulin resistance (Kronfeld, 2005b; Treiber, 2006a).

The accuracy of this simple measurement has been questioned because both insulin and glucose concentrations can vary widely in an individual in a short time period (Treiber, 2005; Treiber, 2006a). In addition, it has been suggested that in the later stages of insulin resistance in horses, pancreatic compensation becomes inadequate and hyperinsulinemia may not be detected (Kronfeld, 2006). Therefore more accurate assessments of measuring insulin sensitivity in the horse have been developed.

PROXIES AND REFERENCE QUINTILES FOR BASAL GLUCOSE AND INSULIN

Two proxies for assessing insulin sensitivity and pancreatic beta-cell response have been developed using minimal model testing of healthy horses (Treiber et al., 2005). Insulin sensitivity (SI) is estimated from the reciprocal of basal insulin concentration:

$$SI = (7.93(1/(\sqrt{[insulin]})) - 1.03$$

The acute pancreatic ß cell response to glucose (AIR_g) is estimated from a function of basal glucose with the reciprocal of basal insulin concentration:

$$AIR_g = (70.1 \, (MIRG)) - 13.8$$
$$[\text{where } MIRG = (800-0.30[insulin - 50]^2) / (glucose - 30)]$$

The combined use of both proxies is suggested to distinguish normal (normal SI and AIR_g), compensatory insulin secretion in normoglycemic insulin resistance (normal or reduced SI and increased AIR_g), and compensatory failure of insulin secretion in hyperglycemic insulin resistance (reduced SI and normal to reduced AIR_g). These proxies have also been used to document insulin resistance in ponies and predict their likelihood of developing laminitis (Treiber, 2006c). Limitations of such proxies include the fact that the reference quintiles developed are not likely universal and should be established to match the type of population of horses or ponies that will be assessed for insulin resistance.

ORAL GLUCOSE TOLERANCE TEST (OGTT)

The OGTT assesses small intestinal absorption of glucose, hepatic glucose uptake, and to an extent the endocrine function of the pancreas and peripheral insulin resistance (Roberts, 1973; Breukink, 1974; Jacobs et al., 1982; June et al., 1992). The test requires an overnight fast, 1 g/kg bodyweight of glucose is administered via a nasogastric tube, and blood glucose is then measured at 0, 30, 60, 90, 120, 180, 240, 300, and 360 minutes after administration. A peak in blood glucose level occurs 90 to 120 minutes hours after administration of the glucose, and blood glucose concentrations should return to normal after 4 to 6 hours (Roberts, 1973; Kaneko, 1989; Ralston, 2002). An increased glucose response in comparison to normal might suggest reduced pancreatic function or insulin resistance (Ralston, 2002). However, the test is affected by the length of previous fasting, and the age and diet of horses/ponies prior to testing (Breukink, 1974; Jacobs et al., 1982; June et al., 1992; Murphy et al., 1997). In addition, the test may be affected by the stress of nasogastric intubation and variable rates of glucose administration, gastric emptying, and intestinal absorption (Kronfeld et al., 2005a).

INTRAVENOUS GLUCOSE TOLERANCE TEST (IVGTT)

Diet, disease states, and breed of horse, pony or donkey also affect the IVGTT (Argenzio et al., 1970; Garcia and Beech, 1986). However, it avoids the variable absorption of glucose by the intestinal tract inherent with the OGTT (Kronfeld et al., 2005a). Horses must be kept off feed for 12 to 24 hours after which 0.5 g glucose/kg bodyweight is infused via an intravenous catheter over about 10 minutes. Blood glucose and insulin concentrations are determined at 0, 5, 15, 30, 60, and 90 minutes and then hourly for 5 to 6 hours after injection. Measures of half-life of glucose disposal and the fractional turnover rate, which is a measure of glucose utilization and thus peripheral insulin resistance, are calculated (Kaneko, 1989). Normal horses usually show an immediate rise in blood glucose concentration and a return to normal levels within one hour. The insulin response curve should parallel the glucose response curve with a peak at around 30 minutes post injection of glucose (Garcia and Beech, 1986; Ralston, 2002). Insulin resistance would potentially produce a higher peak in blood glucose and a consistent delay in return to baseline of > 2 hours. Insulin concentrations must also be measured in order to determine whether this is due to an impairment of insulin secretion from the pancreas or from impairment of insulin-stimulated glucose disposal. If a horse has impaired pancreatic beta cell function, a delayed glucose curve might be observed and the insulin response may be blunted or delayed. However, the IVGTT is not a sensitive means to measure diminished pancreatic response (Firshman and Valberg, 2007).

INSULIN TOLERANCE TEST (ITT)

The ITT measures the blood glucose response to an injection of insulin. It is a direct measure of the sensitivity of tissues to the test dose of insulin, which is highly variable but may range from 0.2 IU/kg to 0.6 IU/kg and also assesses the response of the animal to the insulin-induced hypoglycemia. Normally, depending upon the dose of insulin used, the blood glucose levels drop to 50% of the original value within 20 to 30 minutes and return to the fasting level within 1.5 to 2 hours (Kaneko, 1989; Ribeiro et al., 2004). Typically when the ITT is performed in an animal that is resistant to insulin, blood glucose levels will not fall as dramatically and will return to normal levels more quickly compared to a normal individual. It should be emphasized, however, that the response to this test depends on a number of factors such as, but not limited to, age, diet, stress, and others.

FREQUENTLY SAMPLED GLUCOSE INSULIN TOLERANCE TEST (FSGIT)

A combined IV glucose and insulin tolerance test has recently been developed as a means to assess both pancreatic insulin secretion as well as peripheral insulin resistance (Treiber et al., 2005; Pratt et al., 2005). Horses are not fasted, 300 mg/kg of glucose solution is administered rapidly IV, and blood is drawn via a catheter prior to administration of and at 0,1, 2, 3, 4, 5, 6, 7, 8, 10, 12, 14, 16, and 19 minutes afterward. At 20 minutes after glucose administration, a small IV dose of insulin (20 mU/kg) is given and blood is collected at 22, 23, 24, 25, 27, 30, 35, 40, 50, 60, 70, 80, 90, 100, 120, 150, and 180 minutes after glucose administration. Glucose and insulin dynamics are assessed via minimal model analysis. This test is designed to assess both the pancreatic response to elevated blood glucose and peripheral tissue sensitivity to insulin. Normal values for horses of similar breed, age, diet, and fitness are required for its interpretation.

HYPERGLYCEMIC AND HYPERINSULINEMIC CLAMPING

The disadvantage of the previously described tests is that endogenous insulin secretion cannot be controlled and any potential fluctuations during the test alter glucose homeostasis (Firshman and Valberg, 2007). To break the endogenous glucose-insulin negative feedback loop, two types of glucose clamp techniques have been used in horses (DeFronzo et al., 1979; Rijnen and van der Kolk, 2003; Annandale et al., 2004; Firshman et al., 2005). The hyperglycemic clamp fixes plasma glucose at an acutely elevated level for two hours, thus suppressing endogenous hepatic glucose production. The glucose infusion rate becomes a measure of pancreatic insulin secretion and therefore the technique allows quantification of the sensitivity of the pancreatic beta cells to glucose. Hyperinsulinemic euglycemic clamping provides supra-maximal steady state insulin concentrations during which the rate of glucose infusion required to maintain euglycemia during the clamp serves as a measure of the insulin sensitivity of muscle and adipose tissues. Arguments against the clamping technique have centered on the nonphysiological nature of the test and technical difficulties performing the test. However, it remains one of the most accurate means to assess sensitivity of tissues to hyperglycemia and hyperinsulinemia (Firshman and Valberg, 2007).

Conclusion

Insulin resistance is an important component of many equine diseases including Cushing's disease, metabolic syndrome and forms of laminitis. In advanced cases, clinical signs are often sufficient to establish a diagnosis of these diseases. However, in the prodromal stages of disease, diagnosis of insulin resistance may be an aid to identifying susceptibility to these disorders and instituting early treatment. The tests described may become a useful clinical means to assess the degree of insulin resistance in horses and responses to treatments. However, it is clear that at present there is not one ideal test that is both practical and accurate. To interpret results of insulin sensitivity testing, normal values need to be established for various breeds and ages of horses as well as for varying stages of fitness and diets ranging from pasture to concentrates.

References

Abel, E.D., P.R. Shepherd, and B.B. Kahn. 1996. Glucose transporters and pathophysiologic states. In: D. Le Roith, S.I. Taylor, and J.M. Olefsky (Eds). Diabetes mellitus: A fundamental and clinical text. Philadelphia:Lippincott-Raven p. 530-543.

Annandale, E.J., S.J. Valberg, J.R. Mickelson, and E.R. Seaquist. 2004. Insulin sensitivity and skeletal muscle glucose transport in horses with equine polysaccharide storage myopathy. Neuromuscul. Disord. 14:666-674.

Argenzio, R.A., and H.F. Hintz. 1970. Glucose tolerance and effect of volatile fatty acid on plasma glucose concentrations in ponies. J. Anim. Sci. 30:514-518.

Asplin, K.E., M.N. Sillence, C.C. Pollitt, and C.M. McGowan. 2007. Induction of laminitis by prolonged hyperinsulinaemia in clinically normal ponies.Vet. J. 74:530-535.

Bailey, S.R., N.J. Menzies-Gow, P.A. Harris, J.L. Habershon-Butcher, C. Crawford, Y. Berhane, R.C. Boston, and J. Elliott. 2007. Effect of dietary fructans and dexamethasone administration on the insulin response of ponies predisposed to laminitis. J. Amer. Vet. Med. Assoc. 231:1365-1373.

Baron, A.D., J.S. Zhu, H. Weldon, L. Maianu, and W.T. Garvey. 1995. Glucosamine induces insulin resistance in vivo by affecting GLUT 4 translocation in skeletal muscle: Implications for glucose toxicity. J. Clin. Invest. 96:2792-2801.

Berti, L., M. Kellerer, E. Capp, and H.U. Haring. 1997. Leptin stimulates glucose transport and glycogen synthesis in C2C12 myotubes: Evidence for a P3-kinase mediated effect. Diabetologia 40:606-609.

Boden G. 1997. Role of fatty acids in the pathogenesis of insulin resistance and NIDDM. Diabetes 46:3-10.

Breukink, H.J. 1974. Oral mono- and disaccharide tolerance tests in ponies. Amer. J. Vet. Res. 35:1523-1527.

Coderre, L., A.K. Srivastava, and J.L. Chiasson. 1992. Effect of hypercorticism on regulation of skeletal muscle glycogen metabolism by insulin. Amer. J. Physiol. 262:E427–E433.

DeFronzo, R.A., J.D. Tobin, and R. Andres. 1979. Glucose clamp technique: A method for quantifying insulin secretion and resistance. Amer. J. Physiol. 237: E214–E223.

de Graaf-Roelfsema, E., M.E. van Ginneken, E. van Breda, I.D. Wijnberg, H.A. Keizer, and J.H. van der Kolk. 2006. The effect of long-term exercise on glucose metabolism and peripheral insulin sensitivity in Standardbred horses. Equine Vet. J., Suppl. 36:221-225.

Dimitriadis, G., B. Leighton, M. Parry-Billings, S. Sasson, M. Young, U. Krause, S. Bevan, T. Piva, G. Wegener, and E.A. Newsholme. 1997. Effects of glucocorticoids excess on the sensitivity of glucose transport and metabolism to insulin in rat skeletal muscle. Biochem. J. 321:707–712.

Firshman, A.M., and S.J. Valberg. 2007. Factors affecting assessment of insulin sensitivity in horses. Equine Vet. J. 39:567-575.

Firshman, A.M., S.J. Valberg, T.L. Karges, L.E. Benedict, E.J. Annandale, and E.R. Seaquist. 2005. Serum creatine kinase response to exercise during dexamethasone-induced insulin resistance in Quarter Horses with polysaccharide storage myopathy. Amer. J. Vet. Res. 66:1718-1723.

Forhead, A.J. 1994. Relationship between plasma insulin and triglyceride concentrations in hypertriglyceridaemic donkeys. Res. Vet. Sci. 56:389-392.

Frank, N., C.S. Sommardahl, H. Eiler, L.L. Webb, J.W. Denhart, and R.C. Boston. 2005. Effects of oral administration of levothyroxine sodium on concentrations of plasma lipids, concentration and composition of very-low-density lipoproteins, and glucose dynamics in healthy adult mares. Amer. J. Vet. Res. 66:1032-1038.

Garcia, M.C., and J. Beech. 1986. Equine intravenous glucose tolerance test: Glucose and insulin responses of healthy horses fed grain or hay and of horses with pituitary adenoma. Amer. J. Vet. Res. 47:570-572.

Gould, G.W., and G.D. Holman. 1993. The glucose transporter family: Structure, function, and tissue-specific expression. Biochem. J. 295:329-341.

Henson, F.M., C. Davenport, L. Butler, I. Moran, W.D. Shingleton, L.B. Jeffcott, and P.N. Schofield. 1997. Effects of insulin and insulin-like growth factors I and II on the growth of equine fetal and neonatal chondrocytes. Equine Vet. J. 29:441-447.

Hoffman, R.M., R.C. Boston, D. Stefanovski, D.S. Kronfeld and P.A. Harris. 2003b. Obesity and diet affect glucose dynamics and insulin sensitivity in Thoroughbred geldings. J. Anim. Sci. 81:2333-2342.

Hoffman, R.M., D.S. Kronfeld, W.L. Cooper, and P.A. Harris. 2003a. Glucose clearance in grazing mares is affected by diet, pregnancy, and lactation. J. Anim. Sci. 81:1764-1771.

Holman, G.D., and M. Kasuga. 1997. From receptor to transporter: Insulin signaling to glucose transport. Diabetologia 40:991-1003.

Hotamisligil, G.S., and B.M. Spiegelman. 1994. Tumor necrosis factor alpha: A key component of the obesity/diabetes link. Diabetes 43:1271-1278.

Jacobs, K.A., and J.R. Bolton. 1982. Effect of diet on the oral glucose tolerance test in the horse. J. Amer. Vet. Med. Assoc.180:884-886.

Jeffcott, L.B., and J.R. Field. 1986. Glucose tolerance and insulin sensitivity in ponies and Standardbred horses. Equine. Vet. J. 18:97-101.

Johnson, P.J. 2002. The equine metabolic syndrome peripheral Cushing's syndrome. Vet. Clin. N. Amer. Equine Pract. 18:271-293.

June, V., V. Soderholm, H.F. Hintz, and W.R. Butler. 1992. Glucose tolerance in the horse, pony and donkey. Equine Vet. Sci. 12:103-105.

Kahn, B.B. 1992. Facilitative glucose transporters: Regulatory mechanisms and dysregulation in diabetes. J. Clin. Invest. 89:1367-1374.

Kamohara, S., R. Burcelin, J.L. Halaas, J.M. Friedman, and M.J. Charron. 1997. Acute stimulation of glucose metabolism in mice by leptin treatment. Nature 389:374-377.

Kaneko, J.J. 1989. Carbohydrate metabolism and its diseases. In: J.J. Kaneko, J.W. Harvey, and M.L. Bruss (Eds.). Clinical Biochemistry of Domestic Animals, 4th ed. Academic Press Inc., San Diego. p. 44-81.

Kronfeld, D.S., K.H. Treiber, and R.J. Geor. 2005a. Comparison of nonspecific indications and quantitative methods for the assessment of insulin resistance in horses and ponies. J. Amer. Vet. Med. Assoc. 226:712-719.

Kronfeld, D.S., K.H. Treiber, T.M. Hess, and R.C. Boston. 2005b. Insulin resistance in the horse: Definition, detection and dietetics. J. Anim. Sci. 83:E22-E31.

Kronfeld, D.S., K.H. Treiber, T.M. Hess, R.K. Splan, B.M. Byrd, W.B. Staniar, and N.W. White. 2006. Metabolic syndrome in healthy ponies facilitates nutritional countermeasures against pasture laminitis. J. Nutr. 136:2090S-2093S.

McClain, D.A., and E.D. Crook. 1996. Hexosamines and insulin resistance. Diabetes 45:1003-1009.

McGowan, CM., R. Frost, D.U. Pfeiffer, and R. Neiger. 2004. Serum insulin concentrations in horses with equine Cushing's syndrome: Response to a cortisol inhibitor and prognostic value. Equine Vet J. 36:295-298.

Muoio, D.M., G.L. Dohm, F.T. Fiedorek, E.B. Tapscott, and R.A. Coleman. 1997. Leptin directly alters lipid partitioning in skeletal muscle. Diabetes 46:1360-1363.

Murphy, D., S.W.J. Reid, and S. Love. 1997. The effect of age and diet on the oral glucose tolerance test in ponies. Equine Vet. J. 29:467-470.

Powell, D.M., S.E. Reedy, D.R. Sessions, and B.P. Fitzgerald. 2002. Effect of short-term exercise training on insulin sensitivity in obese and lean mares. Equine Vet. J. Suppl. 34:81-84.

Pratt, S.E., R.J. Geor, and L.J. McCutcheon. 2005. Repeatability of two methods for assessment of insulin sensitivity and glucose dynamics in horses. J. Vet. Intern. Med. 19:883-888.

Pratt, S.E., R.J. Geor, and L.J. McCutcheon. 2006. Effects of dietary energy source and physical conditioning on insulin sensitivity and glucose tolerance in Standardbred horses. Equine Vet. J. Suppl. 36:579-584.

Ralston, S.L. 1996. Hyperglycemia/hyperinsulinemia after feeding a meal of grain to young horses with osteochondrosis dissecans (OCD) lesions. Pferdeheilkunde 12:320-322.

Ralston, S.L. 2002. Insulin and glucose regulation. Vet. Clin. N. Amer. Equine Pract. 18:295-304.

Rea, S., and D.E. James. 1997. Moving GLUT4: The biogenesis and trafficking of GLUT4 storage vesicles. Diabetes 46:1667-1677.

Ribeiro, W., S.J. Valberg, J.D. Pagan, and B. Essen Gustavsson. 2004. The effect of varying dietary starch and fat content on creatine kinase activity and substrate availability in equine polysaccharide storage myopathy J. Vet. Int. Med.18:887-894.

Rijnen, K.E., and J.H. van der Kolk. 2003. Determination of reference range values indicative of glucose metabolism and insulin resistance by use of glucose clamp techniques in horses and ponies. Amer. J. Vet. Res. 64:1260-1264.

Roberts, M.C., and F.W.G. Hill. 1973. The oral glucose tolerance test in the horse. Equine Vet. J. 5:171-173.

Robertson, R.P. 2004. Chronic oxidative stress as a central mechanism for glucose toxicity in pancreatic islet beta cells in diabetes. Biol. Chem. 279:42351-42354.

Shepherd, P.R., and B.B. Kahn. 1999. Glucose transporters and insulin action: Implications for insulin resistance and diabetes mellitus. N. Engl. J. Med. 341(4):248-257.

Shepherd, P.R., D.J.Withers, and K. Siddle. 1998. Phosphoinositide 3-kinase: The key switch mechanism in insulin signalling. Biochem. J. 333:471-490.

Stewart-Hunt, L., R.J. Geor, and L.J. McCutcheon. 2006. Effects of short-term training on insulin sensitivity and skeletal muscle glucose metabolism in Standardbred horses. Equine Vet. J. Suppl. 36:226-232.

Tiley, H.A., R.J. Geor, and L.J. McCutcheon. 2008. Effects of dexamethasone administration on insulin resistance and components of insulin signaling and glucose metabolism in equine skeletal muscle. Amer. J. Vet. Res. 69:51-58.

Tóth, F., N. Frank, S.B. Elliott, R.J. Geor and R.C. Boston. 2008. Effects of an intravenous endotoxin challenge on glucose and insulin dynamics in horses. Amer. J. Vet. Res. 69:82-88.

Treiber, K.H., D.S. Kronfeld, T.M. Hess, R.C. Boston, and P.A. Harris. 2005. Use of proxies and reference quintiles obtained from minimal model analysis for determination of insulin sensitivity and pancreatic beta-cell responsiveness in horses. Amer. J. Vet. Res. 66:2114-2121.

Treiber, K.H., D.S. Kronfeld, and R.J. Geor. 2006a. Insulin resistance in equids: Possible role in laminitis. J. Nutr. 136:2094S-2098S.

Treiber, K.H., T.M. Hess, D.S. Kronfeld, R.C. Boston, R.J. Geor, M. Friere, A.M. Silva, and P.A. Harris. 2006b. Glucose dynamics during exercise: Dietary energy sources affect minimal model parameters in trained Arabian geldings during endurance exercise. Equine Vet. J. Suppl. 36:631-636.

Treiber, K.H., D.S. Kronfeld, T.M. Hess, B.M. Byrd, R.K. Splan, and W.B. Staniar. 2006c. Evaluation of genetic and metabolic predispositions and nutritional risk factors for pasture-associated laminitis in ponies. J. Amer. Vet. Med. Assoc. 228:1538-1545.

Vick, M.M., D.R. Sessions, B.A. Murphy, E.L. Kennedy, S.E. Reedy, and B.P. Fitzgerald. 2006. Obesity is associated with altered metabolic and reproductive activity in the mare: Effects of metformin on insulin sensitivity and reproductive cyclicity. Reprod. Fertil. Dev. 18:609-617.

Waller, C.A., D.L. Thompson, J.A. Cartmill, W.A. Storer, and N.K. Huff. 2006. Reproduction in high body condition mares with high versus low leptin concentrations. Theriogenology 66:923-928.

Williams, C.A., D.S. Kronfeld, W.B. Staniar, and P.A. Harris. 2001. Plasma glucose and insulin responses of Thoroughbred mares fed a meal high in starch and sugar or fat and fiber. J. Anim. Sci. 79:2196-2201.

Yki-Jarvinen, H. 1992. Glucose toxicity. Endocr. Rev. 3:415-431.

Zierath JR, L. He, A. Guma, E.O. Wahlstrom, A. Klip, and H. Wallberg-Henriksson. 1996. Insulin action on glucose transport and plasma membrane GLUT4 content in skeletal muscle from patients with NIDDM. Diabetologia 39:1180-1189.

EXERCISE-INDUCED PULMONARY HEMORRHAGE

KENNETH W. HINCHCLIFF
The Ohio State University, Columbus, Ohio

Epidemiology

Exercise-induced pulmonary hemorrhage (EIPH) occurs in horses that race at high speeds, such as Thoroughbred and Standardbred racehorses. The disease is almost unknown in endurance horses or draft breeds. As a general rule, the more intense the exercise or higher the speed attained, the greater the proportion of horses with EIPH.

The prevalence of EIPH varies with the method used to detect it and the frequency with which horses are examined. Almost all Thoroughbred racehorses in active training have hemosiderophages in bronchoalveolar lavage fluid, indicating that all have some degree of EIPH (McKane et al., 1993). The prevalence of EIPH decreases when diagnosis is based on endoscopic examination of horses after exercise or racing.

EIPH is very common in Thoroughbred racehorses with estimates of prevalence, based on a single endoscopic examination of the trachea and bronchi, of 43 to 75% (Pascoe et al., 1981a; Raphel and Soma, 1982; Mason et al., 1983). The prevalence increases with the frequency of examination, with over 80% of horses having evidence of EIPH on at least one occasion after three consecutive races (Sweeney et al., 1990). When examined after each of three races, 87% of Standardbred racehorses have evidence of EIPH on at least one occasion (Lapointe et al., 1994), suggesting that EIPH is as common in Standardbred racehorses as it is in Thoroughbred racehorses.

History and Presenting Complaint

Poor athletic performance or epistaxis (bleeding from the nostrils) are the most common presenting complaints for horses with EIPH. Epistaxis due to EIPH occurs during or shortly after exercise and is usually first noticed at the end of a race, particularly when the horse is returned to the paddock or winner's circle and is allowed to lower its head.

Failure of racehorses to perform to the expected standard (poor performance) is often attributed to EIPH. Many horses with poor performance have cytologic evidence of EIPH on microscopic examination of tracheobronchial aspirates or bronchoalveolar lavage fluid or have blood evident on endoscopic examination of the tracheobronchial tree performed 30 to 90 minutes after strenuous exercise or racing (McKane et al.,

1993; Martin et al., 1999). Severe EIPH undoubtedly results in poor performance and, on rare occasions, death of Thoroughbred racehorses (Gunson et al., 1988).

We recently completed a study of Thoroughbred horses racing in Melbourne, Australia. The study involved endoscopic examination of 744 horses after racing. There was a clear association between presence and severity of EIPH and performance; horses with any more than a fleck of blood in the airway had poorer performances than unaffected horses. These horses were not racing after administration of furosemide (Lasix, Salix) as use of this drug is not permitted on race day in Australia. However, it is important to recognize that EIPH is very common in racehorses and it should be considered the cause of poor performance only after other causes have been eliminated.

Diagnosis of EIPH

There are a variety of techniques available for determining the presence and severity of EIPH including direct visualization of the airways through a flexible endoscope or examination of bronchial lavage fluid or tracheal aspirates for evidence of hemorrhage. The utility of these diagnostic tests varies and choice of examination technique depends on the time between the horse racing and the examination, and the desired sensitivity of the test. For instance, tracheobronchoscopic examination is most appropriate if a horse is examined within 1-2 hours of exercise, whereas examination of airway washings is most appropriate if the examination is days to a week after strenuous exercise. Radiography, pulmonary scintigraphy, and lung function tests are useful in eliminating other respiratory diseases as a cause of poor performance, but are minimally useful in confirming a diagnosis of EIPH or in determining the severity of hemorrhage.

Observation of blood in the trachea or large bronchi of horses 30-120 minutes after racing or strenuous exercise provides a definitive diagnosis of EIPH. The amount of blood in the large airways varies from a few small specks on the airway walls to abundant blood covering the tracheal surface. Blood may also be present in the larynx and nasopharynx. If there is a strong suspicion of EIPH and blood is not present on a single examination conducted soon after exercise, the examination should be repeated 60-90 minutes later. Some horses with EIPH do not have blood present in the rostral airways immediately after exercise, but do so when examined 1-2 hours later. Blood is detectable by tracheobronchoscopic examination for 1-3 days in most horses, with some horses having blood detectable for up to 7 days.

A grading system can be used to estimate the severity of EIPH following bronchoscopic examination (Pascoe et al., 1981b; Mason et al., 1983; Pascoe et al., 1985; Lapointe et al., 1994). A commonly used grading system has four levels from 0 (no hemorrhage visible) to 3 (streak of blood >5 mm wide).

The presence of red cells or macrophages containing either effete red cells or the breakdown products of hemoglobin (hemosiderophages) in tracheal or bronchoalveolar lavage fluid provides evidence of EIPH. Detection of red cells or hemosiderophages in tracheal aspirates or bronchoalveolar lavage fluid is believed to be both sensitive and specific in the diagnosis of EIPH (Fogarty and Buckley, 1991; McKane et al., 1993). Examination of airway fluids indicates the presence of EIPH in a greater proportion of horses than does tracheobronchoscopic examination after strenuous exercise or racing. The greater sensitivity of examination of airway fluid is likely attributable to the ability of this examination to detect the presence of small amounts of blood or its residual products and the longevity of these products in the airways. Recent studies have reported on the use of red cell numbers in bronchoalveolar lavage fluid as a quantitative indicator of EIPH (Meyer et al., 1998; Langsetmo et al., 2000; Geor et al., 2001; Kindig et al., 2001). However, this indicator of EIPH severity has not been validated or demonstrated to be more reliable or repeatable than tracheobronchoscopic examination and visual scoring.

Pathophysiology and Etiology

Ultimately, the cause of EIPH is rupture of alveolar capillary membranes with subsequent leakage of blood into interstitial and alveolar spaces (West et al., 1993). The source of blood in such instances is the pulmonary circulation. Bleeding from bronchial circulation during exercise has been suggested based on histologic evidence of bronchial angiogenesis in horses that have experienced previous episodes of EIPH (Pascoe, 1996). Whether there is a contribution of the bronchial circulation to EIPH has not been determined. Hemorrhage into the interstitial space and alveoli, with subsequent rostral movement of blood into the airways, results in blood in the trachea and bronchi and, infrequently, epistaxis.

Rupture of alveolar capillaries occurs secondary to an exercise-induced increase in transmural pressure (pressure difference between the inside of the capillary and the alveolar lumen). If the transmural stress exceeds the tensile strength of the capillary wall, the capillary ruptures (West and Mathieu-Costello, 1994). The proximate cause of alveolar capillary rupture is the high transmural pressure generated by positive intracapillary pressures (largely attributable to capillary blood pressure) and the lower intraalveolar pressure (generated by the negative pleural pressures associated with inspiration). During exercise, the absolute magnitudes of both pulmonary capillary pressure and alveolar pressure increase, with a consequent increase in transmural pressure (West and Mathieu-Costello, 1994; Ducharme et al., 1999). Other theories of the pathogenesis of EIPH include small airway disease, upper airway obstruction, hemostatic abnormalities, changes in blood viscosity and erythrocyte shape, intrathoracic shear forces associated with gait, and bronchial artery angiogenesis (Pascoe, 1996; Schroter et al., 1998). It is likely that the pathogenesis of EIPH involves several processes, including pulmonary hypertension, lower alveolar pressure, and changes in lung structure, that summate to induce stress failure of pulmonary capillaries.

Regardless of the cause, rupture of pulmonary capillaries and subsequent hemorrhage into airways and interstitium cause inflammation of both airways and interstitium with subsequent development of fibrosis and alteration of tissue compliance. Heterogeneity of compliance within the lungs, and particularly at the junction of normal and diseased tissue, results in development of abnormal shear stress with subsequent tissue damage. These changes are exacerbated by inflammation and obstruction of small airways with resulting uneven inflation of the lungs (Robinson and Derksen, 1980). The structural abnormalities, combined with pulmonary hypertension and the large intrathoracic forces associated with respiration during strenuous exercise, cause repetitive damage at the boundary of normal and diseased tissue with further hemorrhage and inflammation. The process continues for as long as the horse performs strenuous exercise (Pascoe, 1996).

Treatment and Prognosis

Therapy for EIPH is controversial in that many treatments are used but none are backed by conclusive evidence of efficacy in horses under field conditions (i.e., racing). Therapy for EIPH is usually a combination of attempts to reduce the severity of subsequent hemorrhage and efforts to minimize the effect of recent hemorrhage.

Treatment of EIPH is problematic for a number of reasons. Firstly, the pathogenesis of EIPH has not been determined, although the available evidence supports a role for stress failure of pulmonary capillaries secondary to exercise-induced pulmonary hypertension (see below).

Secondly, there is a lack of information using large numbers of horses under field conditions that demonstrates an effect of any medication or management practice (with the exception of bedding) on EIPH. There are numerous studies of small numbers of horses (<~40) under experimental conditions, but these studies often lacked the statistical power to detect treatment effects, and the relevance of studies conducted on a treadmill to horses racing competitively is questionable. Treatments for EIPH are usually intended to address a specific aspect of the pathogenesis of the disease and will be discussed in that context.

PREVENTION OF STRESS FAILURE OF THE PULMONARY CAPILLARIES

Stress failure of pulmonary capillaries, and subsequent hemorrhage, is believed to occur as a result of the high transmural pressures in pulmonary capillaries that develop in the lungs of horses during strenuous exercise. Consequently, there is interest in reducing the pressure difference across the pulmonary capillary membrane in an effort to reduce EIPH. Theoretically, this can be achieved by reducing the pressure within the capillary or increasing (making less negative) the pressure within the intrathoracic airways and alveolus.

FUROSEMIDE (LASIX, SALIX)

Furosemide administration as prophylaxis of EIPH is permitted in a number of racing jurisdictions worldwide (Anonymous, 2002). Within the United States and Canada, almost all Thoroughbred, Standardbred, and Quarter Horse racing jurisdictions permit administration of furosemide before racing. Approximately 85% of all Thoroughbred racehorses in the United States and Canada receive furosemide at some stage in their careers, and on average, 75% of horses in a race receive furosemide (Gross et al., 1999). Although accurate numbers are not available, it appears that a smaller proportion of Standardbred and Quarter Horse racehorses receive furosemide before racing. Furosemide is administered to 22-32% of Standardbred racehorses and 19% of racing Quarter Horses in two racing jurisdictions (Sime et al., 1994; Soma et al., 1996; Soma et al., 2000).

The efficacy of furosemide in treatment of EIPH is uncertain. While field studies of large numbers of horses do not demonstrate an effect of furosemide on the prevalence of EIPH (Sweeney et al., 1990; Birks et al., 2002), studies of Thoroughbred horses running on a treadmill provide evidence that furosemide reduces the severity of EIPH (Geor et al., 2001; Kindig et al., 2001). Under field conditions, based on tracheobronchoscopic evaluation of the severity of bleeding, furosemide has been reported to reduce or have no influence on the severity of bleeding (Pascoe et al., 1985; Birks et al., 2002). This apparent inconsistency may be attributable to measurement of red blood cell counts in bronchoalveolar lavage fluid of horses that have run on a treadmill not being representative of effects of furosemide under field conditions. The weight of evidence from field studies does not support a role for furosemide in preventing or reducing the severity of EIPH.

Furosemide is associated with superior performance in both Thoroughbred and Standardbred racehorses (Gross et al., 1999; Soma et al., 2000). Thoroughbred horses treated with furosemide were 1.4 times as likely to win a race and earn more money, and had a standardized 6-furlong race time 0.56 to 1.09 seconds less than untreated horses (Gross et al., 1999). Similarly, furosemide reduced one-mile race times of Standardbred pacers by 0.31 to 0.74 seconds (Soma et al., 2000).

NITRIC OXIDE

Nitric oxide is a potent vasodilator in many vascular beds. Administration of nitroglycerin (a nitric oxide donor) reduces pulmonary artery pressure of standing horses but does not affect pulmonary artery pressure of horses during intense exercise (Manohar and Goetz, 1999). L-arginine is a nitric oxide donor with no demonstrated efficacy in reducing pulmonary capillary pressure or EIPH in horses. Sildenafil, a phosphodiesterase inhibitor that accentuates the effect of nitric oxide and is used in the treatment of erectile dysfunction in men, has been administered to horses in an apparent attempt to reduce EIPH. However, its efficacy in preventing EIPH or reducing pulmonary capillary pressure has not been demonstrated.

INCREASING ALVEOLAR INSPIRATORY PRESSURE

Recently, the role of the nares in contributing to upper airway resistance, and hence lowering inspiratory intrapleural pressure during intense exercise, has attracted the attention of some investigators. Application of nasal dilator bands (Flair® strips) reduces nasal resistance by dilating the nasal valve (Holcombe et al., 2002), and reduces red cell count of bronchoalveolar lavage fluid collected from horses after intense exercise on a treadmill (Geor et al., 2001; Kindig et al., 2001). However, the effect of this intervention in horses racing competitively has not been demonstrated.

The role of small airway inflammation and bronchoconstriction in the pathogenesis of EIPH is unclear. However, horses with EIPH are often treated with drugs intended to decrease lower airway inflammation and relieve bronchoconstriction. Beta-adrenergic bronchodilatory drugs such as clenbuterol and albuterol are effective in inducing bronchodilation in horses with bronchoconstriction, but their efficacy in preventing EIPH is either unknown or, in very small studies, is not evident. Clenbuterol does not alter the hemodynamic responses of horses to exertion or attenuate exercise-induced arterial hypoxemia in normal horses (Slocombe et al., 1992; Manohar et al., 2000). Ipratropium, a parasympatholytic drug administered by inhalation, showed promised in a very small study (2 horses) of preventing EIPH (Sweeney et al., 1984). Corticosteroids, including dexamethasone, fluticasone, and beclomethasone administered by inhalation, parenterally, or enterally, reduce airway inflammation and obstruction, but have no demonstrated efficacy in preventing EIPH. Cromolyn sodium (sodium cromoglycate) has no efficacy in preventing EIPH (Hillidge et al., 1987).

Reducing Inflammation

Hemorrhage into interstitial tissues induces inflammation with subsequent development of fibrosis and bronchial artery angiogenesis (O'Callaghan et al., 1987; McKane and Slocombe, 1999; McKane and Slocombe, 2002). The role of these changes in perpetuating EIPH in horses is unclear but likely is of some importance. Treatments to reduce inflammation and promote healing with minimal fibrosis have been proposed. Rest is an obvious recommendation and many racing jurisdictions have rules regarding enforced rest for horses with epistaxis. While the recommendation for rest is intuitive, there is no information that rest reduces the severity or incidence of EIPH in horses with prior evidence of this disorder.

Similarly, corticosteroids are often administered, either by inhalation, enterally or parenterally, in an attempt to reduce pulmonary inflammation and minimize fibrosis. Again, the efficacy of this intervention in preventing or minimizing severity of EIPH has not been documented.

Excessive Bleeding

These is no evidence that horses with EIPH have defective coagulation or increased fibrinolysis (Bayly et al., 1983; Johnstone et al., 1991). Regardless, aminocaproic acid, a potent inhibitor of fibrin degradation, has been administered to horses to prevent EIPH. The efficacy of aminocaproic acid in preventing EIPH has not been demonstrated. Similarly, estrogens are given to horses with the expectation of improving hemostasis although effect of estrogens on coagulation in any species is unclear. There is no evidence that estrogens prevent EIPH in horses.

Vitamin K is administered to horses with EIPH presumably with the expectation that it will decrease coagulation times. However, as EIPH is not associated with prolonged bleeding times, it is unlikely that this intervention will affect the prevalence or severity of EIPH.

PLATELET FUNCTION

Aspirin inhibits platelet aggregation in horses and increases bleeding time (Kopp et al., 1985). Seemingly paradoxically, aspirin is sometimes administered to horses with EIPH because of concerns that increased platelet aggregation contributes to EIPH (Mahony et al., 1992). There is no evidence that aspirin exacerbates or prevents EIPH.

CAPILLARY INTEGRITY

Capillary fragility increases the risk of hemorrhage in many species. Various bioflavinoids have been suggested to increase capillary integrity and prevent bleeding. However, hesperidin and citrus bioflavinoids have no efficacy in prevention of EIPH in horses (Sweeney and Soma, 1984). Similarly, vitamin C is administered to horses with EIPH without scientific evidence of any beneficial effect.

Overview of Treatment

Selection of therapy for horses with EIPH is problematic. Given that most horses have some degree of pulmonary hemorrhage during most bouts of intense exercise, the decision must be made not only as to the type of treatment and its timing but also which horses to treat. Moreover, the apparent progressive nature of the disease with continued work highlights the importance of early and effective prophylaxis and emphasizes the need for studying factors, such as air quality and respiratory infections, that incite the disorder.

The currently favored treatment for EIPH is administration of furosemide before intense exercise. Its use is permitted in racehorses in a number of countries. Increasingly persuasive laboratory evidence of an effect of furosemide to reduce red cell count in bronchoalveolar lavage fluid collected from horses soon after intense exercise supports the contention that furosemide is effective in reducing the severity of EIPH in racehorses. However, it should be borne in mind that neither the relationship between severity of EIPH and red cell count in bronchoalveolar lavage fluid nor the efficacy of furosemide in reducing severity of EIPH in racehorses in the field have been demonstrated. In fact, there is strong evidence that furosemide does not reduce the prevalence of EIPH and other evidence that it does not reduce the severity of EIPH under field conditions. The association between furosemide administration and superior performance in Standardbred and Thoroughbred racehorses should be considered when recommending use of this drug.

Rest is an obvious recommendation for horses with EIPH, but the hemorrhage is likely to recur when the horse is next strenuously exercised. The duration of rest and the optimal exercise program to return horses to racing after EIPH is unknown, although some jurisdictions require exercise no more intense than trotting for 2 months. Firm recommendations cannot be made on duration of rest because of a lack of objective information.

Although a role for lower airway disease (either infectious or allergic) in the genesis of EIPH has not been demonstrated, control of infectious diseases and minimization of noninfectious lower airway inflammation appears prudent.

Prognosis

The prognosis for racing for horses with clinically significant EIPH is guarded because of the progressive nature of the disease. Horses that have experienced severe EIPH on one occasion are likely to do so again regardless of treatment. However, the risk of horses experiencing a repeated bout of severe hemorrhage and the effect of EIPH on career longevity are unknown.

Further Reading

Couetil L., and K.W. Hinchcliff. 2004. Non-infectious diseases of the lungs. In: Hinchcliff K.W., A.J. Kaneps, and R.J. Geor (Eds.) Equine Sports Medicine and Surgery: Basic and Clinical Sciences of the Equine Athlete. Elsevier Science, London.

References

Anonymous. 2002. International agreement on breeding and racing and appendices, International Federation of Horse Racing Authorities.
Bayly, W.M., K.M. Meyers, and M.T. Keck. 1983. Effects of furosemide on exercise-induced alterations in haemostasis in Thoroughbred horses exhibiting post-exercise epistaxis. In: D.H. Snow, S.G.B. Persson, and R.J. Rose (Eds.) Equine Exercise Physiology. pp. 64-70. Granta Editions, Cambridge.
Birks, E.K., K.M. Shuler, L.R. Soma, B.B. Martin, L. Marconato, Jr., F. Del Piero, D.C. Teleis, D. Schar, A.E. Hessinger, and C.E. Uboh. 2002. EIPH: Postrace endoscopic evaluation of Standardbreds amd Thoroughbreds. Equine Vet. J. Suppl. 34:375-378.
Ducharme, N.G., R.P. Hackett, R.D. Gleed, D.M. Ainsworth, H.N. Erb, L.M. Mitchell,

and L.V. Soderholm. 1999. Pulmonary capillary pressure in horses undergoing alteration of pleural pressure by imposition of various airway resistive loads. Equine Vet. J. Suppl. 30:27-33.

Fogarty, U., and T. Buckley. 1991. Bronchoalveolar lavage findings in horses with exercise intolerance. Equine Vet. J. 23: 434-437.

Geor, R.J., L. Ommundson, G. Fenton, and J.D. Pagan. 2001. Effects of an external nasal strip and frusemide on pulmonary haemorrhage in Thoroughbreds following high-intensity exercise. Equine Vet. J. 33: 577-584.

Gross, D.K., P.S. Morley, K.W. Hinchcliff, and T.E. Wittum. 1999. Effect of furosemide on performance of Thoroughbreds racing in the United States and Canada. J. Amer. Vet. Med. Assn. 215:670-675.

Gunson, D.E., C.R. Sweeney, and L.R. Soma. 1988. Sudden death attributable to exercise-induced pulmonary hemorrhage in racehorses: Nine cases (1981-1983). J. Amer. Vet. Med. Assoc. 193:102-106.

Hillidge, C., T. Whitlock, and T. Lane. 1987. Failure of inhaled disodium cromoglycate aerosol to prevent exercise-induced pulmonary hemorrhage in racing Quarter Horses. J. Vet. Pharmacol. Ther. 10:257-260.

Holcombe, S.J., C. Berney, C.J. Cornelisse, F.J. Derksen, and N.E. Robinson. 2002. Effect of commercially available nasal strips on airway resistance in exercising horses. Amer. J. Vet. Res. 63:1101-1105.

Johnstone, I.B., L. Viel, S. Crane, and T. Whiting. 1991. Hemostatic studies in racing standardbred horses with exercise-induced pulmonary hemorrhage. Hemostatic parameters at rest and after moderate exercise. Can. J. Vet. Res. 55:101-106.

Kindig, C.A., P. McDonough, G. Fenton, D.C. Poole, and H.H. Erickson. 2001. Efficacy of nasal strip and furosemide in mitigating EIPH in Thoroughbred horses. J. Appl. Physiol. 91:1396-1400.

Kopp, K., J. Moore, T. Byars, and P. Brooks. 1985. Template bleeding time and thromboxane generation in the horse: Effects of three non-steroidal anti-inflammatory drugs. Equine Vet. J. 17:322-324.

Langsetmo, I., M.R. Meyer, and H.H. Erickson. 2000. Relationship of pulmonary arterial pressure to pulmonary haemorrhage in exercising horses. Equine Vet. J. 32:379-384.

Lapointe, J.M., A. Vrins, and E. McCarvill. 1994. A survey of exercise-induced pulmonary haemorrhage in Quebec standardbred racehorses. Equine Vet. J. 26:482-485.

Mahony, C., N.W. Rantanen, J.A. DeMichael, and B. Kincaid. 1992. Spontaneous echocardiographic contrast in the Thoroughbred: High prevalence in racehorses and a characteristic abnormality in bleeders. Equine Vet. J. 24:129-133.

Manohar, M., and T.E. Goetz. 1999. Pulmonary vascular pressures of strenuously exercising Thoroughbreds during intravenous infusion of nitroglycerin. Amer. J. Vet. Res. 60:1436-1440.

Manohar, M., T.E. Goetz, P. Rothenbaum, and S. Humphrey. 2000. Clenbuterol administration does not attenuate the exercise-induced pulmonary arterial,

capillary or venous hypertension in strenuously exercising Thoroughbred horses. Equine Vet. J. 32:546-550.
Martin, Jr., B.B., J. Beech, and E.J. Parente. 1999. Cytologic examination of specimens obtained by means of tracheal washes performed before and after high-speed treadmill exercise in horses with a history of poor performance. J. Amer. Vet. Med. Assoc. 214:673-677.
Mason, D.K., E.A. Collins, and K.L. Watkins. 1983. Exercise-induced pulmonary haemorrhage in horses. In: D.H. Snow, S.G.B. Persson, and R.J. Rose (Eds.) Equine Exercise Physiology. pp. 57-63. Granta Editions, Cambridge.
McKane, S., and R. Slocombe. 1999. Sequential changes in bronchoalveolar cytology after autologous blood inoculation. Equine Vet. J. Suppl. 30:126-130.
McKane, S.A., P.J. Canfield, and R.J. Rose. 1993. Equine bronchoalveolar lavage cytology: Survey of Thoroughbred racehorses in training. Aust. Vet. J. 70:401-404.
McKane, S.A., and R.F. Slocombe. 2002. Alveolar fibrosis and changes in lung morphometry in response to intrapulmonary blood. Equine Vet. J. Suppl. 34:451-458.
Meyer, T.S., M.R. Fedde, E.M. Gaughan, I. Langsetmo, and H.H. Erickson. 1998. Quantification of exercise-induced pulmonary haemorrhage with bronchoalveolar lavage. Equine Vet. J. 30:284-288.
O'Callaghan, M.W., J.R. Pascoe, W.S. Tyler, and D.K. Mason. 1987. Exercise-induced pulmonary haemorrhage in the horse: Results of a detailed clinical, post-mortem and imaging study. III. Subgross findings in lungs subjected to latex perfusions of the bronchial and pulmonary arteries. Equine Vet. J. 19:394-404.
Pascoe, J., G. Ferraro, J. Cannon, R. Arthur, and J. Wheat. 1981a. Exercise-induced pulmonary hemorrhage in racing Thoroughbreds: A preliminary study. Amer. J. Vet. Res. 42:703-707.
Pascoe, J.R. 1996. Exercise-induced pulmonary hemorrhage: A unifying concept. In: Proc. 45th Amer. Assoc. Equine Practit. pp. 220-226.
Pascoe, J.R., G.L. Ferraro, J.H. Cannon, R.M. Arthur, and J.D. Wheat. 1981b. Exercise-induced pulmonary hemorrhage in racing Thoroughbreds: A preliminary study. Amer. J. Vet. Res. 42:703-707.
Pascoe, J.R., A.F. McCabe, C.F. Franti, and R.M. Arthur. 1985. Efficacy of furosemide in the treatment of exercise-induced pulmonary hemorrhage in Thoroughbred racehorses. Amer. J. Vet. Res. 46:2000-2003.
Raphel, C.F., and L.R. Soma. 1982. Exercise-induced pulmonary hemorrhage in Thoroughbreds after racing and breezing. Amer. J. Vet. Res. 43:1123-1127.
Robinson, N.E., and F.J. Derksen. 1980. Small airway obstruction as a cause of exercise-associated pulmonary hemorrhage. In: Proc. 26th Amer. Assoc. Equine Practit. pp. 421-430.
Schroter, R.C., D.J. Marlin, and E. Denny. 1998. Exercise-induced pulmonary haemorrhage (EIPH) in horses results from locomotory impact induced trauma—a novel, unifying concept. Equine Vet. J. 30:186-192.

Sime, D., R. Engen, and P. Miller-Graber. 1994. Frequency and use of medications in horses racing in Prairie Meadows. Iowa State Univ. Vet. 54.

Slocombe, R., G. Covelli, and W. Bayly. 1992. Respiratory mechanics of horses during stepwise treadmill exercise tests, and the effect of clenbuterol pretreatment on them. Aust. Vet. J. 69:221-225.

Soma, L.R., F.K. Birks, C.E. Uboh, L. May, D. Teleis, and J. Martini. 2000. The effects of frusemide on racing times of Standardbred pacers. Equine Vet. J. 32:334-340.

Soma, L.R., C.E. Uboh, and L. Nann. 1996. Prerace venous blood acid-base values in Standardbred horses. Equine Vet. J. 28:390-396.

Sweeney, C.R., and L.R. Soma. 1984. Exercise-induced pulmonary hemorrhage in Thoroughbred horses: Response to furosemide or hesperidin-citrus bioflavinoids. J. Amer. Vet. Med. Assoc. 185:195-197.

Sweeney, C.R., L.R. Soma, C.A. Bucan, and S.G. Ray. 1984. Exercise-induced pulmonary hemorrhage in exercising Thoroughbreds: Preliminary results with pre-exercise medication. Cornell Vet. 74:263-268.

Sweeney, C.R., L.R. Soma, A.D. Maxson, J.E. Thompson, S.J. Holcombe, and P.A. Spencer. 1990. Effects of furosemide on the racing times of Thoroughbreds. Amer. J. Vet. Res. 51:772-778.

West, J.B., and O. Mathieu-Costello. 1994. Stress failure of pulmonary capillaries as a mechanism for exercise induced pulmonary haemorrhage in the horse. Equine Vet. J. 26:441-447.

West, J.B., O. Mathieu-Costello, J.H. Jones, E.K. Birks, R.B. Logemann, J.R. Pascoe, and W.S. Tyler. 1993. Stress failure of pulmonary capillaries in racehorses with exercise-induced pulmonary hemorrhage. J. Appli. Physiol. 75:1097-1109.

FOOD ALLERGY IN THE HORSE: A DERMATOLOGIST'S VIEW

DAWN LOGAS
Veterinary Dermatology Center, Maitland, Florida

Definition

Food allergy is an uncommon and poorly understood disease in the horse. Symptoms can be gastrointestinal, dermatologic, or both. The terminology itself is confusing. The term food allergy implies an immunologic reaction to an ingested substance. Not all food allergies are truly allergic in nature. A better term for the condition would be "adverse reactions to food." This designation includes immunologic and nonimmunologic reactions to food substances. Nonimmunologic food sensitivities include metabolic, pharmacologic, and idiosyncratic reactions. An example of this would be pruritus resulting from the histamine content of a food (e.g., mackerel or tuna), instead of from an allergic reaction to the food itself. Fortunately, clinical symptoms and treatment of immunologic and nonimmunologic food reactions are identical. Therefore, for the sake of simplicity, most clinicians use the term food allergy to indicate adverse reactions to food.

Pathogenesis

Very little is known about the pathogenesis of food allergy in the horse. Most of the research into food allergy has concentrated on human food hypersensitivities, particularly in children. True food allergies in humans have been classified as type I hypersensitivity reactions for the most part, but type III and IV hypersensitivity reactions are also suspected. Type I reactions (immediate type hypersensitivity) encompass all IgE-mediated reactions such as pruritus, erythema, and urticaria. Type III (arthus) hypersensitivities typically cause vasculitic lesions. Type IV reactions (delayed type hypersensitivity) usually cause a papular eruption. All three types of clinical reactions have been observed in the food-allergic horse, but detailed information about the pathogenesis of each type of reaction is lacking. Unfortunately, at this time much of the information known about food allergy in the horse is case-based and anecdotal.

The first stage of any hypersensitivity reaction is the sensitization phase. During sensitization, the antigen is repeatedly presented to T lymphocytes and an abnormal hypersensitivity response occurs instead of tolerance. For a food allergy to occur, an allergen must breach the intestinal mucosal barrier in order to be exposed to the immune system. Normally, the intestinal tract has various mechanisms to prevent the absorption of potentially allergenic substances. Intestinal enzymes break down large molecules into smaller, less antigenic ones. The mucous coating and tight junctions of the intestinal epithelium do not allow larger, more antigenic macromolecules to pass the intestinal barrier and reach the immune system. Secretory IgA binds to smaller antigenic molecules, thereby preventing their penetration of the mucosa. Intestinal peristalsis also helps by moving large molecules through the intestinal tract at a relatively rapid rate.

Hypersensitivity can result when there is a break in intestinal barrier function and an abnormal immune response to a presented antigen. This can occur in young animals whose intestinal mucosal barrier is not fully developed, in old animals whose intestinal mucosal barrier has begun to degenerate, and in animals with gastrointestinal illnesses that have damaged the intestinal barrier. In these cases, macromolecules (>12 kilodaltons) are able to pass through the mucosal barrier and reach the immune system. Under normal circumstances, especially in the young animal, a CD8 positive T cell response occurs and results in tolerance/anergy. However, if Th2 lymphocytes are activated, a type I hypersensitivity reaction can develop. The reason this abnormal immunologic response occurs in some individuals is still unknown. It may be genetically determined, or may occur secondary to another event such as a heavy parasite load. Parasite antigens cause activation of many T helper cells, some of which may inadvertently react to food antigens instead of parasite antigens. Another possibility is the formation of a hapten-antigen complex. This can occur when a small, theoretically nonantigenic molecule is easily absorbed through the mucosal barrier, then combines with a hapten to form a complex that is now large enough to elicit an immunologic response.

In the diet, water-soluble glycoproteins are thought to act as the base of many of these antigens. These glycoproteins can be found in fresh or prepared foods, supplements, or other additives. Unfortunately, what is not known is which glycoprotein(s) in a particular food item is important, or what part of each particular glycoprotein is antigenic.

Incidence

The true incidence of adverse food reactions in the horse is not known. It is assumed to be uncommon; however, it can be difficult to rule out, so many food-allergic horses may not be properly diagnosed. It is also possible that the condition is recognized and corrected by an owner prior to seeking veterinary attention, so we have no knowledge of these cases. Diet items reported to cause adverse food reactions in horses include alfalfa, barley, beet pulp, bran, buckwheat, chicory, clover, malt, oats, potatoes, St. John's wort, wheat, feed additives, and feed supplements.

History

Obtaining a good history, while sometimes difficult, is crucial for the diagnosis and management of food allergy. The person who is responsible for the day-to-day care, feeding, and grooming of the patient must be interviewed. This is not necessarily the owner of the horse. Important historical information to ascertain includes the patient's age at onset, time of year of onset of condition, seasonality, environmental conditions, and changes in environment and their effect on symptoms. Gather as much information as possible about the horse's past and current diet. Commercial feeds, hay types, pasture, treats, and supplements/additives must be recorded. It is also important to note if the horse's diet is consistent throughout the year. Other information that should be obtained includes previous treatments and response (if any), current treatment and response, insect control measures, intestinal parasite control measures, and any other current/past illnesses.

Food allergies can start at any age (1 year to 10 years). Symptoms of food allergy are usually nonseasonal and do not vary with changes in environment (provided the diet is not changed).

Clinical Signs

Clinical signs of food allergy are extremely variable both in the horse and other species. Food allergy is usually pruritic, but nonpruritic urticaria is also reported. Other dermatologic signs seen with adverse food reactions include angioedema, papules, excoriations, erythema, crusts, alopecia, and vasculitic lesions. Gastrointestinal symptoms may also be present. Since the signs of food allergy are not unique, other dermatologic diseases must be eliminated from the differential diagnosis list before the diagnosis of food allergy is made.

Various mites (sarcoptic, psoroptic, chorioptic) can cause a typically nonseasonal pruritic dermatosis. Most of these parasites can be found on skin scraping. Trial therapy with ivermectin can also be helpful in ruling out parasitic infections. Dermatophytosis, bacterial folliculitis, and dermatophilosis can all cause a severe, nonseasonal pruritic dermatitis that can look identical to food allergy. Fungal culture, bacterial culture, skin surface cytology, and skin biopsy can be used to diagnose these infections.

Food allergy must also be differentiated from other allergic diseases such as insect bite allergy, contact allergy, and atopy. Contact allergic reactions almost always have a primary eruption (papules, pustules, erythematous macules, wheals, erythematous plaques). The eruption may be seasonal (if plant related) or nonseasonal (topical medications, shampoos, tack cleaners). The distribution of lesions can often give clues to the presence of a contact reaction. Insect bite allergy (*Culicoides* hypersensitivity, other biting flies) typically results in a severely pruritic, papular dermatitis that is most often seasonal. Atopy (inhalant allergic dermatitis) can cause mild to severe pruritus.

A primary eruption (papules, pustules, erythematous macules, erythematous plaques) is not always present, and pruritus varies from mild to severe. Atopy can be seasonal or nonseasonal, depending on geographic location.

Diagnosis

The only reliable way to confirm a diagnosis of food allergy is with an elimination diet. Both intradermal allergen testing and serum testing have been shown to be unreliable for identifying food allergies. These diagnostic tests have been investigated in other species, and were found to produce an unacceptable number of false positives and false negatives. Intradermal allergen testing is useful for identifying important allergens in atopic individuals. The diagnosis of atopy is made by history, clinical signs, and exclusion of other pruritic dermatoses. The diagnosis of atopy is not made by intradermal allergen testing. Some of the pollens on an intradermal testing panel are from grasses that are used for hay. A positive reaction on an intradermal test does not mean this grass is a food allergen for this individual. However, most hay will contain pollen from the grass, as well as a variety of other pollens, dust, etc. For this reason, a change in the type of hay being fed may be recommended. At the very least, the hay should be fed on the ground and lightly misted with water to minimize dust.

A good elimination diet consists of a single protein source and carbohydrate source to which the patient has had no previous exposure. Finding a novel protein and carbohydrate source can be particularly difficult in the equine patient. In addition, all supplements and dietary additives must be discontinued. Limiting the diet to fresh hay from a different grass (e.g., timothy to alfalfa) and offering a single-ingredient pelleted diet is often the best option available. Dietary manipulation can be difficult to impossible in performance horses.

The food trial should be continued for 8 to 12 weeks to see maximal improvement. Most food allergic individuals show improvement in clinical signs in 4 to 6 weeks. If clinical improvement is noted, the patient can be challenged with items from its previous diet. One new item should be introduced every week. This allows the offending diet items to be identified.

Management

The only effective treatment for food allergies is avoidance of the offending allergen. Antihistamines and glucocorticoid therapy can be tried, but are not particularly effective. The lack of readily available, prepared feeds that consist of a limited number of ingredients makes management of food allergic horses difficult. A variety of single-ingredient feeds designed for the various life stages and activities of horses would make diagnosing and managing equine food allergies much easier.

References

Logas, D.B., G. Kunkle, M. Calderwood-Mays, and L. Frank. 1992. Cholinergic pruritus in a horse. J. Am. Vet. Med. Ass. 201:90-91.

Logas, D.B., and J. Barbet. 1999. Diseases characterized by wheals, papules or small nodules. In: Colohan, P.T., A.M. Merritt, J.N. Moore, and J.G. Mayhew (Eds.). Equine Medicine and Surgery (5th Ed.). pp. 1868-1946. Mosby Inc, St. Louis.

Scott, D.W. 2003. Equine Dermatology. pp. 453-458. WB Saunders Company, Harcourt Brace Jovanovich, Inc. Philadelphia.

BEYOND THE X-RAY: THE LATEST METHODS TO DETECT AND PREDICT SKELETAL DAMAGE

C. WAYNE MCILWRAITH
Colorado State University, Fort Collins, Colorado

Introduction

While osteochondral fragmentation, fractures, subchondral bone disease, and osteoarthritis are common in the horse, diagnosis of these diseases usually occurs only after the disease has become established. The detection of early or subtle disease in the past has been poor, but the situation is improving. Clinical examination and radiographic imaging are still the most commonly used techniques for diagnosis of osteochondral disease, yet osteochondral damage seen during arthroscopic surgery is usually more severe than that seen on radiographs. It is the author's subjective opinion that there is commonly a good correlation between the severity of clinical symptoms (principally lameness and synovial effusion) and the amount of damage or disease found at arthroscopy of joints. However, it has been reported in humans that, while the most common complaint of the patient with osteoarthritis (OA) is pain, only about half of the patients with radiographic OA have symptoms (Hochberg et al., 1989). The reason that half the patients with radiographic OA have pain is not always clear since only some of the causes of pain have been researched (Altman and Dean, 1989). It is recognized that there is no "diagnostic test" for OA in man (Altman, 1997), but focus on MRI and biomarkers has occurred in recent years.

Human clinical trials are now very specific about the recording of outcome measures. Outcome variables in OA clinical trials need to be selected on the basis of the therapeutic objective and are a critical part of assessing the results of medication. In a workshop of the World Health Organization and the American Academy for Orthopedic Surgeons, the methods to assess progression of OA of the hip and knee were reviewed (Dieppe et al., 1994). In addition, the European Group for the Respect of Ethics and Excellence in Science (GREES) has made recommendations on methods for registration of drugs for OA (1996). We are equally in need of objective outcome parameters in assessing the results of various treatments for musculoskeletal disease in general and joint disease in particular in the horse.

It has been proposed that to completely characterize joint disease in the horse, the following measurements are necessary: 1) mechanical inputs into the joint; 2) tissue architecture and geometry; 3) tissue matrix properties, including measurement of material and biochemical matrix properties; and 4) the level of inflammation within the joint (Kawcak, 2001). The current state of diagnostic capabilities for horses will

Measurement of Mechanical Inputs

CLINICAL EXAMINATION

Assessment of joint effusion, range of motion, joint capsule thickening, and pain with flexion are currently used and subjectively graded by veterinarians doing lameness examinations. The lameness grading guidelines set up by the American Association of Equine Practitioners are used frequently (AAEP, 1991). While flexion tests are commonly used in humans, the reliability of such tests is controversial. Confounding factors make this objective evaluation of an individual for pain difficult. The principal ones are differences in observer scores and differences in a particular subject's tolerance to pain. The same is true for a horse. Motion analysis has been employed as a research tool. The characteristics of limb movement and force can be determined. Abnormalities in these parameters can be characterized in patients with disease (Craik and Otis, 1995). As an example, it has been found in humans that impulsive loading often leads to osteoarthritis (Radin and Rose, 1986). Because data analysis involves sophisticated, expensive equipment and is often labor intensive, most gait analysis in veterinary medicine occurs in the research field.

Motion analysis systems that combine data from force plates, EMG analysis and muscle forces, and kinematics can provide sensitive information about an individual's movement (Radin and Rose, 1986). These systems have been extensively studied in humans and are used clinically to evaluate an individual's gait. Limb use and muscle forces play a large role in joint loading (Bassey et al., 1997), and recent work from our laboratory in the horse has shown this. For instance, in measuring contact forces across the carpus at the trot, the peak ground reaction force is 1,350 pounds, whereas the peak muscle forces are 2,700 pounds, leading to a total joint force of 4,050 pounds. In other words, muscle forces are two times ground forces (Brown et al., 2003a; Brown et al., 2003b). Diagnostic techniques that describe kinematics and muscle forces are research tools that allow clinicians to identify those individuals with potential problems related to movement.

We have also evaluated the use of thin-film sensor systems to evaluate limb loading in horses. The system was attractive because a sensor could be attached to the bottom of a horse's hoof to measure force distribution throughout the sole surface (Judy et al., 2001), or it could be used like a force plate for jogging horses across. Evaluation of the force plate system for accuracy and durability has shown it to be inadequate.[a] Preliminary results indicate, however, that using an "in-shoe" system for the sensor film deploys results similar to the force plate.[b]

COMPUTER MODELS

Computer models of joint loading have been studied in both humans and animals. Modeling is the computer-based mathematical representation of the skeleton, ligaments, and muscles used to calculate forces in muscles and joints. The principle is to develop the model based on kinematic parameters and compare that model to those developed from imaging techniques such as computed tomography (CT) and magnetic resonance imaging (MRI). Muscle, tendon, ligament, and ground reaction forces in tissue properties can be inserted into the model. Once developed, imaging-based modeling can be performed so that subtle changes in joint geometry and loading can be detected with the ultimate goal to develop long-term models in which data can be continually added. The clinical goal is to develop patient-specific models in which abnormalities in loading and tissue response can be detected (Pandy et al., 1998).

Researchers in the Equine Orthopedic Research Laboratory at Colorado State University (CSU), in collaboration with the Orthopedic Research Laboratory at Columbia University and Steadman Hawkins Sports Medicine Foundation, have performed a kinematic and MRI study to develop a model of the equine carpus. This study has determined the center of force of the joint surfaces in the carpus, and these data have been correlated with those obtained from MRI scans. At the moment this is certainly a research tool, but ultimately we hope the subtle irregularities in joint loading can be determined in clinical patients using MRI and CT.

Measurement of Tissue Architecture and Geometry

RADIOGRAPHY

Radiography is still the most widely used imaging technique for the diagnosis of osteochondral disease, but it is an insensitive method of diagnosis. Articular cartilage cannot be viewed radiographically except when there is extensive loss and decreased joint space, and 30-40% change in bone mineral density is required before bone changes can be appreciated (Greenfield, 1986). In addition, multiple images are required for evaluation of a three-dimensional structure. Disease is often recognized after significant damage has occurred. This lack of sensitivity can prevent early and accurate diagnosis. Measuring joint space is fraught with error (Adams and Wallace, 1991). The significance of osteophytes is frequently unrelated to intra-articular pathological change and considerable change in bone density is necessary to identify sclerosis and erosion. In a study correlating radiographic and histologic changes in the tarsi of horses, Laverty and coworkers found that radiographs were insensitive for detecting subchondral bone sclerosis and erosion when compared to histology (1991). It has also been pointed out that superimposition of osteophytes may appear as sclerosis (Widmar and Blevins, 1994).

COMPUTED TOMOGRAPHY

Computed tomography (CT) has had increasing use in the horse, both as a research tool and a clinical tool. Benefits of CT are visualization of the area of interest in three dimensions (which alleviates superimposition) and the ability to determine density patterns.

Density patterns of bone can be determined by three-dimensional modeling of CT images (computed tomography osteoabsorptiometry or CTO). CTO allows three-dimensional evaluation of the joint in any plane. Hounsfield units, which are the CT measure of bone density, are determined and coordinated into ranges and then the ranges of density are represented by colors. This color map is then superimposed over a three-dimensional image of the joint surface to show a representation of the relative subchondral density (Figure 1).

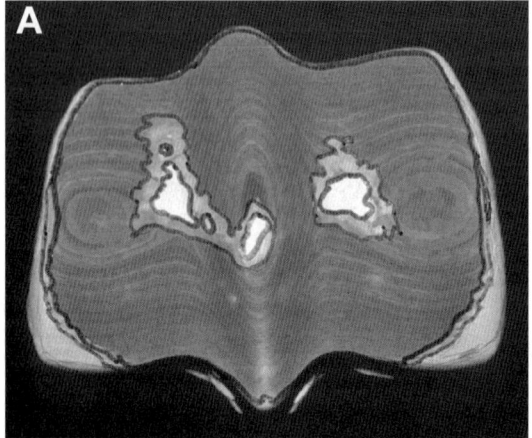

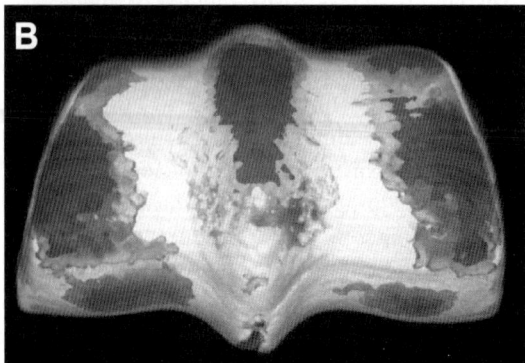

Figure 1. Computed tomography osteoabsorptiometry (CTO), a three-dimensional evaluation of the surface of the third metacarpal condyles of a horse exercised on a treadmill (A) and a hand-walked horse (B). Notice the increased density of subchondral bone (black areas) in the treadmill-exercised horse compared with the hand-walked horse (reprinted from Kawcak et al., 2000. Amer. J. Vet. Res.).

The use of a density phantom has allowed for objective measures of density to be determined. Since it has been shown that stress distribution within an osteochondral section is related to the density pattern, it can be concluded that the subchondral density pattern is the representation of the loading history of the joint (Muller-Gerbl et al., 1989). Considerable work has been done in our laboratory by Kawcak. Initially the subchondral density patterns of bones in equine carpal and metacarpophalangeal joints were established. Since that time the effects of exercise in young horses where exercise was commenced in foals at three weeks have been followed and compared to those in pasture-reared horses. In addition, we have evaluated the changes in bone density patterns with age.[c]

Riggs and coworkers identified substantial density gradients between the denser subchondral bone of the condyles and the subchondral bone of the sagittal groove in the distal MCIII and MTIII with a view to explaining the etiology of distal condylar fractures (1999). These density gradients were shown to equate to anatomical differences in loading intensity and locomotion, and it was hypothesized that such difference in bone density results in stress concentration at the palmar/plantar aspect of the condylar groove, which may be predisposed to fracture (Riggs et al., 1999a). In a companion paper, linear defects in mineralized articular cartilage and subchondral bone were found in the palmar/plantar aspects of the condylar groove, adjacent to the sagittal ridge (Riggs et al., 1999b). These were closely related to the pattern of densification of subchondral bone and were associated with intense focal remodeling of the immediate subjacent bone. Parasagittal fractures of the condyles originated in similar defects. This work and subsequent examination of CTs in our laboratory have demonstrated a potential to diagnose incipient condylar fractures in the racehorse.

MRI

Results from human studies have shown that MRI is a sensitive and specific imaging tool for examination of hard and soft tissues in joints and that it is as good as, if not better than, arthroscopy for detecting subchondral lesions (Reeve et al., 1992). MRI is the best measure of articular geometry, and more recently an ability to quantify articular cartilage matrix properties using contrast enhancement has been demonstrated (Bashir et al., 1997). Postmortem MRI, as well as other imaging modalities including clinical examination, radiographs, nuclear scintrigraphy, and arthroscopy, was used to evaluate an osteoarthritic metacarpophalangeal joint in a horse (Martinelli et al., 1996). Kawcak and coworkers have also used this technique to evaluate the effects of exercise on subchondral bone of horses and found that it could image osteochondral damage, including small fragments (Figure 2) (Kawcak et al., 2001).

More recently there have been reports of the clinical use of MRI (high-field strength) in anesthetized horses to diagnose specific changes in the distal limb and a paper on the use of a low-field strength standing MRI to image the distal limb has been reported (Dyson et al., 2005; Mair et al., 2005).

390 Beyond the X-ray: The Latest Methods

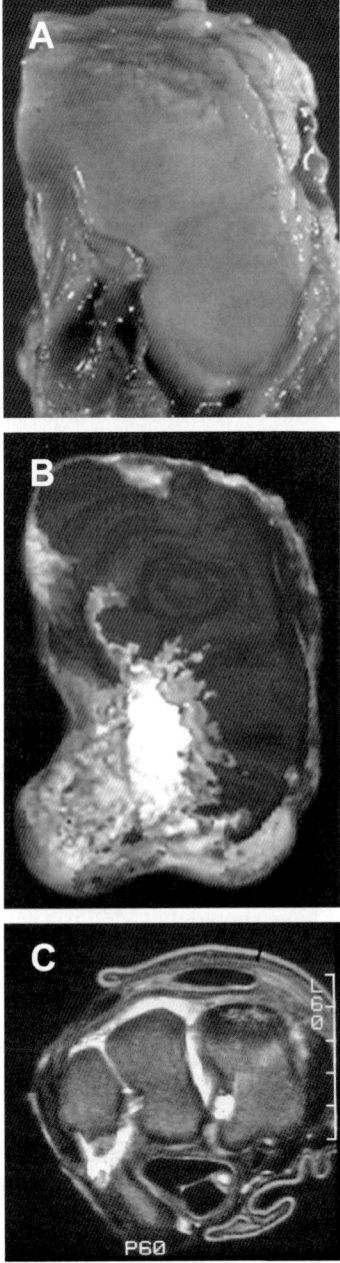

Figure 2. Imaging of an osteochondral fragment on the distal aspect of the radial carpal bone: (A) gross photographic view; (B) a CTO image; and (C) an MR image of the distal aspect of the radial carpal bone showing the fragment (reproduced with permission from C.E. Kawcak, 2001. Proc. Amer. Assoc. Equine Practnr.).

We have had a high-field strength MRI at CSU for a year, and it is being used effectively on clinical patients to diagnose problems from the tarsus and carpus down. Changes in the joint capsule and ligaments associated with joints can be diagnosed equally well as those in articular cartilage and bone (Figure 3).

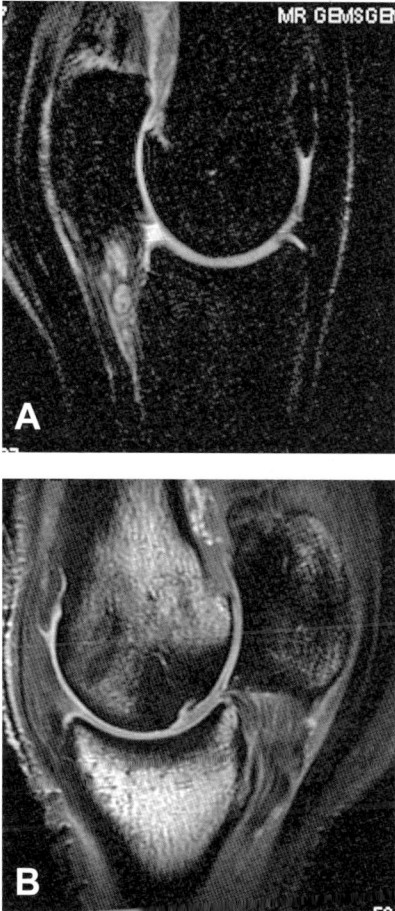

Figure 3. (A) MRI of tearing of the oblique distal sesamoidean ligament (STIR sequence). (B) MRI of bone edema and sclerosis with defect in distal metacarpus (T1-weighted spin echo sequence). Both images are from racehorses (courtesy of Dr. N. Werpy).

ULTRASONOGRAPHIC EXAMINATION

Ultrasonographic examination of joints was pioneered by Denoix (1996). The technique can be used to evaluate soft tissues associated with the joint, including collateral ligaments, joint capsule, other associated ligaments, and menisci (Marks et al., 1992). The use of ultrasonography to image the medial palmar intercarpal ligament in the carpus has also recently been described (Driver et al., 2004).

Measurement of Tissue Matrix Properties, Including Measurement of Material and Biochemical Matrix Properties

NUCLEAR SCINTIGRAPHY

Nuclear scintigraphy has been extremely helpful in detecting cortical bone disease and, in particular, stress fractures in horses. Its most significant use, in my opinion, has been in detecting stress fractures of the pelvis, tibia, femur, and humerus prior to their becoming complete fractures. A nuclear scintigraphic image shows the physiologic distribution of radioisotope throughout the bone and therefore is more sensitive than radiographs in detecting early osteoarthritis in human knees (McCrae et al., 1992). In humans, nuclear scintigraphy has been the best early predictor of joint space narrowing in knees, and in some cases has been more sensitive than arthroscopy and MRI for detecting early and subtle subchondral bone pathology (Marks et al., 1992; Dieppe et al., 1993). One problem, however, is the inability of nuclear scintigraphy to distinguish stress response due to subchondral bone adaptation from osteochondral damage. Osteochondral fragments show up as discrete focal areas of increased radioisotope uptake, but any remodeling change due to stress will also show increased uptake of radioisotope (Chambers et al., 1995; Parks et al., 1996). Because of these, mild to moderate increases in uptake of radioisotope in the joints of horses, especially young exercising horses, can lead to confusion. However, scintigraphy can be used as a screening tool, but it needs to be recognized that, while sensitive, it is not sensitive enough to demonstrate a specific anatomical problem.

More objective means of assessment have been used to eliminate some of the subjectivity with nuclear scintigraphy. Using computer programs, areas of particular interest can be highlighted, the counts per pixel determined for that area, and normalized to the counts per pixel for a reference area within the same limb (Wittbjer et al., 1982). This is of particular benefit because the distribution of radioisotope within an area varies between animals and between different regions within the same animal. If we outline an area of interest such as the distal condyles of the third metacarpus, and then normalize the count to a reference area such as the cortical area of the first phalanx, it is possible to eliminate the influence of individual horse uptake in assessing this area (Figure 4).

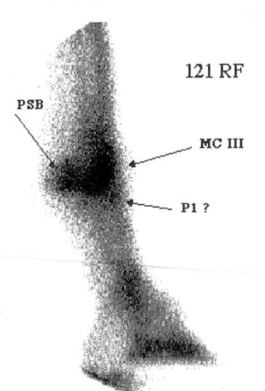

Figure 4. Nuclear scintigraphic view of a metacarpophalangeal joint of a healthy horse. PSB, proximal sesamoid bone; MCIII, third metacarpal condyle; P1?, presumed proximal phalanx (reproduced with permission from Kawcak et al. 2000. Amer. J. Vet. Res.).

Care needs to be taken to ensure the reference area is normal and has no increased uptake compared to the surrounding bone. This technique takes into account the regional limb response to exercise and therefore potentially reduces the effect of exercise-induced increases.

Material properties of subchondral tissues can be inferred from the CT examination. The densities of subchondral and cortical bone have shown to be proportional to their strengths; therefore, a measure of bone density can give the clinical impression of bone strength (Wachter et al., 2001). This is commonly used in an outpatient setting for humans in which peripheral quantitative CT (pQCT) is used for diagnosis and to monitor therapy for osteoporosis. However, unlike cortical bone, there is a maximum density at which subchondral bone can be damaging to articular cartilage (Radin and Rose, 1986). From this it can be insinuated that there exists an appropriate density range at which subchondral bone must be maintained in order to avoid joint damage, a range which we have not yet determined (Kawcak, 2001).

Histologic properties of osteochondral tissues can be assessed using optical coherence tomography, and this has been likened by Kawcak to an in vivo form of biopsy (Herrmann et al., 1999; Kawcak, 2001). In humans, optical coherence tomography has shown a fairly good correlation between images and histologic change (Herrmann et al., 1999).

SYNOVIAL AND SERUM BIOMARKERS

Conventional synovial fluid analysis will not provide a specific diagnosis, but it will give an indication of degree of synovitis and metabolic derangement within the joint. It will not define the degree of articular cartilage damage, but merely the degree of synovitis. Previous attempts at techniques such as synovial sediment analysis have also not solved this problem. Over the past 10-15 years, researchers have developed biochemical and immunologic biomarkers to quantitate breakdown products of the articular cartilage, and the use of this technique in the horse has been the subject of reviews (Ray et al., 1996; McIlwraith et al., 2001).

The terms biomarker, biochemical marker, and molecular marker have all been used to describe either direct or indirect indicators of musculoskeletal turnover (McIlwraith et al., 2001). These markers are often molecules that are normal products and by-products of the metabolic process occurring within the musculoskeletal system. Disease alterations occur between the anabolic and catabolic processes within the skeletal tissues, and consequently, concentration of biomarkers may increase or decrease. In joint disease these molecules can be released into the synovial fluid when the source is articular cartilage, menisci, ligament, or synovial membrane. If the underlying subchondral bone is involved, molecules from osseous tissue will usually be delivered into the bloodstream. Biomarkers potentially can be used to 1) clarify pathobiological processes in the joint; 2) differentiate diagnostically between affected and nonaffected joints and distinguish the degree of degradation in articular cartilage; and 3) monitor the response to therapy.

Direct biomarkers originate principally from cartilaginous structures and provide specific information about alterations in cartilage matrix, anabolism, or catabolism (Thonar et al., 1999). On the other hand, indirect biomarkers are not derived principally from cartilage but have the potential to influence the metabolism of chondrocytes or the integrity of the matrix. These include proteolytic enzymes and their inhibitors, growth factors, pro-inflammatory cytokines, and other molecules from noncartilaginous sources that can provide information, including MMPs, aggrecanase, TIMP, IGF-I, IL-1, IL-6, TNFα, HA, and C-reactive protein (CRP). Indirect markers used in the horse have been recently reviewed (McIlwraith, 2005).

Individual Direct Biomarkers of Cartilage Metabolism

BIOMARKERS OF ANABOLIC PROCESSES

The carboxypropeptide of type II collagen (CPII) is a useful measure of type II collagen synthesis. Although CPII concentrations were not significantly higher in synovial fluid samples of joints with osteochondral fragmentation, their levels were significantly higher in the serum of horses with osteochondral fragmentation (Frisbie et al., 1999). In the same study with horses, another synthetic marker, chondroitin sulfate 846 (CS-846), was significantly higher in the synovial fluid of joints with osteochondral fragmentation compared to control joints, and serum levels were also significantly higher (Frisbie et al., 1999). CS-846 and CPII concentrations were not linearly related to greater fragmentation but were significantly higher with grades I and II. Discriminate analysis using a combination of serum CS-846 and CPII concentrations allowed for 79% of horses to be correctly classified as having osteochondral damage.

BIOMARKERS OF CATABOLIC PROCESSES

Measuring the degradation of type II collagen with biomarkers has proven to be a benefit in monitoring OA as well as OCD in the horse. Antibodies have been developed to identify type II collagen fragments that have been cleaved and/or denatured, exposing previously inaccessible regions (neo-epitopes) of the molecule. Using these antibodies, significant elevations in levels of degraded type II collagen have been demonstrated in synovial fluid and serum samples from horses, dogs, and rabbits with experimental OA (Billinghurst et al., 1997). Initially the Col-2-3/4$_{short}$ immunoassay for detecting collagenase-cleaved collagen fragments (able to detect both type I and II collagen degradation) was developed. This assay had been used in the author's laboratory for monitoring collagenase-induced collagen degradation and to measure the inhibitory effect of a synthetic MMP inhibitor on IL-1-induced degradation of equine articular cartilage explants (Billinghurst et al., 1999). More recently a collagen degradation immunoassay that is specific for equine type II collagen degradation was developed (Billinghurst et al., 2001). The antibody in this assay is designated as 234CEQ.

In a recent study of skeletal markers in osteochondrosis in foals, a combination of significantly higher serum levels of CPII, higher levels of Col-2-3/4$_{short}$ and lower levels of 234CEQ correlated with high osteochondrosis (OC) scores (radiographically) (Billinghurst et al., 2004). This study suggests that there is increased collagen turnover in OC, and by measuring the serum levels of specific biomarkers of collagen metabolism, it is possible to identify horses with OC (Billinghurst et al., 2004). An earlier study in cases of OC found that there were significantly higher levels of CPII and lower levels of CS-846 and KS epitopes in synovial fluids of affected compared to normal joints (Laverty et al., 2000).

Other biomarkers that have been measured in the horse include keratin sulfate (KS) and cartilage oligomeric protein (COMP), but up until now these have proven less useful. On the other hand, the development of monoclonal antibodies that distinguish the two different sites of aggrecan degradation can help identify which is the most responsible for aggrecan degradation in the horse (Caterson et al., 2000). At present it appears that aggrecanase is much more important that stromelysin in this degradation process.

Individual Direct Biomarkers of Bone Metabolism

BIOMARKERS OF ANABOLIC PROCESSES

During normal type I collagen synthesis, as with type II collagen, cleavage of carboxy and amino terminal propeptides (PICP and PINP respectively) of the procollagen molecule occurs and these cleaved propeptide fragments can be exploited as markers reflective of bone formation. In a preliminary study PICP was shown to have potential value as a molecular marker for monitoring changes in matrix turnover following tendon injury (Jackson et al., 2003), and increases in PICP with age and exercise have been demonstrated (Price et al., 1995; Price et al., 2001).

Osteocalcin is a small, noncollagenous protein associated with bone assembly and turnover, and levels in the horse appear to vary with age or administration of corticosteroids, as well as general anesthesia. In a study in our laboratory where various serum markers were used to differentiate changes with exercise from pathologic change in joints, concentrations of osteocalcin as well as CS-846 provided the best correlation to the modified Mankin score (r2=0.72) and clinical degree of pain (r2=0.70) using multivariate linear regression (stepwise model selection) (Frisbie et al., 2003).

Bone-specific alkaline phosphatase (BAP) is expressed at high levels in the cell surface in the bone-forming osteoblasts. In a study with treadmill exercise in young horses, serum BAP levels were not different between exercise and control groups, although previously there had been a suggestion that there was a correlation between levels of BAP and the amount of arthroscopically defined joint damage (Fuller et al., 2001).

BIOMARKERS OF CATABOLIC PROCESSES

The release of a fragment of the type I collagen nonhelical telopeptide (ICTP), which includes the collagen cross-linking region, has been evaluated as a marker of bone resorption in humans (Cortet et al., 1997; Garnero et al., 1999). Levels of ICTP in the horse have not been of value in detecting pathological processes (Price et al., 1995; Jackson et al., 2003).

A relatively new set of antibodies recognizing type I collagen C-telopeptides (CTX) has proven to be useful markers of specific bone resorption based on clinical data from cases of human joint disease (Bonde et al., 1997). In the same study from our laboratory evaluating the ability of serum markers to differentiate exercise from pathology and correlate biomarkers to clinical parameters of pain in an osteoarthritic model, CTX was less useful than CS-846, CPII and GAG biomarker levels in predicting if serum was from either a control, exercised, or an osteoarthritic horse (Frisbie et al., 2003). Other work in our laboratory has identified CPII and CTX-1 as potential serum indicators of the exercise effects on the developing skeletal system in young horses. There were higher serum levels of CTX-1 and lower levels of CPII in trained foals compared to other groups, but these differences later disappeared during an additional six months of identical exercise (Billinghurst et al., 2003).

One of the principal aims of biomarker research is to diagnose early subchondral bone disease and thereby potentially predict fracture. This was the basis of a study funded by the Grayson-Jockey Club Foundation and carried out with racing Thoroughbreds in southern California.

Gene Chip Microarray

Gene chip microarray is the latest advance in biomarkers and represents a molecular approach to defining a disease process. The principle is to have an array of a large number of gene sequences (cDNAs) on a computer chip. The entire human genome is currently available on a computer chip (Affymetrics) and the same company, in corroboration with the Australian company Genetraks®, has produced an equine gene chip containing over 3,000 sequences. The production of this chip facilitates the simultaneous relative quantitation of multiple mRNAs and allows for comprehensive assessment of expression levels.

In recent work from our laboratory (Frisbie et al., unpublished data), the potential usefulness of gene chip microarray as a diagnostic tool in osteoarthritis has been explored. Blood samples were taken during the development of experimental OA (using the carpal chip fragment-exercise model) in the horse, and we were able to identify significant upregulation of 18 different genes in the osteoarthritis group compared to the controls. This change in gene expression started very early in the development of the osteoarthritic disease process. It is envisioned that this ability will be combined with conventional immunologic biomarkers (previously discussed) to provide a diagnostic platform for osteoarthritis as well as other diseases.

Summary

We are progressing towards the ability to diagnose cartilage and bone disease in an individual with a single sample using biomarkers. We are not there yet, but we are at the stage where we can monitor disease process with regular sampling.

Footnotes

[a] Perino, V. 2003. M.S. thesis, Colorado State University, Ft. Collins, CO.
[b] Perino, V., C.E. Kawcak, D.D. Frisbie, et al. 2005. Unpublished data.
[c] Shearin, M. 2005. Ph.D. dissertation; Colorado State University, Ft. Collins, CO.

References

Adams, M.E., and C.J. Wallace. 1991. Quantitative imaging of osteoarthritis. Semin. Arthritis Rheum. 20:26-39.

Altman, R.D. 1997. The syndrome of osteoarthritis. J. Rheumatol. 24:766-767.

Altman, R.D., and D.D. Dean. 1989. Introduction and overview: Pain and osteoarthritis. Semin. Arthritis Rheum. (Suppl. 2) 18:1-3.

American Association of Equine Practitioners. 1991. Guide for Veterinary Services and Judging of Equestrian Events. 19.

Bashir, A., M.L. Gray, R.D. Boutin, and D. Burstein. 1997. Glycosaminoglycan in articular cartilage: In vivo assessment with delayed Gd(DTPA)(2-)-enhanced MR imaging. Radiology 205:551-558.

Bassey, E.J., J.J. Littlewood, and S.J. Taylor. 1997. Relations between compressive axial forces in an instrumented massive femoral implant, ground reaction forces, and integrated electromyographs from vastus lateralis during various 'osteogenic' exercises. J. Biomech. 30:213-223.

Billinghurst, R.C., P.A. Brama, P.R. van Weeran, M.S. Knowlton, and C.W. McIlwraith. 2003. Significant exercise-related changes in the serum levels of two biomarkers of collagen metabolism in young horses. Osteoarthritis and Cartilage 11:760-769.

Billinghurst, R.C., P.A. Brama, P.R. van Weeren, M.S. Knowlton, and C.W. McIlwraith. 2004. Evaluation of serum concentrations of biomarkers of skeletal metabolism and results of radiography as indicators of severity of osteochondrosis in foals. Amer. J. Vet. Res. 65:143-150.

Billinghurst, R.C., E.M. Buxton, M.G. Edwards, M.S. McGraw, and C.W. McIlwraith. 2001. Use of an anti-neoepitope antibody for identification of type-II collagen degradation in equine articular cartilage. Amer. J. Vet. Res. 62:1031-1039.

Billinghurst, R.C., L. Dahlberg, M. Ionescu, A. Reiner, R. Bourne, C. Rorabeck, P. Mitchell, J. Hambor, O. Diekmann, H. Tschesche, J. Chen, H. van Ward, and A.R. Poole. 1997. Enhanced cleavage of type II collagen by collagenases in

osteoarthritic articular cartilage. J. Clin. Invest. 99:1534-1545.
Billinghurst, R.C., K. O'Brien, R.A. Poole, and C.W. McIlwraith. 1999. Inhibition of articular cartilage degradation in culture by a novel nonpeptidic matrix metalloproteinase inhibitor. Ann. NY Acad. Sci. 878:594-597.
Brown, N.A.T., C.E. Kawcak, N.G. Pandy, and C.W. McIlwraith. 2003a. Moment arms of muscles about the carpal and metacarpophalangeal joints in the equine forelimb. Amer. J. Vet. Res. 64:357-358.
Bonde, M., P. Garnero, C. Fledelius, et al. 1997. Measurement of bone degradation products in serum using antibodies reactive with an isomerized form of an 8-amino acid sequence of the C-telopeptide of type I collagen. J. Bone Miner. Res. 12:1028-1034.
Brown, N.A.T., C.E. Kawcak, N.G. Pandy, and C.W. McIlwraith. 2003b. Force and moment-generating capacities of muscles in the distal forelimb of the horse. J. Anat. 203:101.113.
Caterson, B., C.R. Flannery, C.E. Hughes, and C.B. Little. 2000. Mechanisms involved in cartilage proteoglycan catabolism. Matrix Bio. 19:333-344.
Chambers, M.D., M.J. Martinelli, G.J. Baker, et al. 1995. Nuclear medicine for diagnosis of lameness in horses. J. Amer. Vet. Med. Assoc. 206:792-796.
Cortet, B., R.M. Flipo, P. Pigny P, et al. 1997. How useful are bone turnover markers in rheumatoid arthritis? Influence of disease activity in corticosteroid therapy. Rev. Rheum. Engl. Ed. 64:153-159.
Craik, R., and C.A. Otis. 1995. Gait analysis: Theory and application. Mosby, St. Louis.
Denoix J-M. 1996. Ultrasonographic examination in the diagnosis of joint disease. In: C.W. McIlwraith and G.W. Trotter (Eds). Joint Disease in the Horse. WB Saunders Co., Philadelphia. 165-202.
Dieppe, P., R.D. Altman, J.A. Buckwalter, et al. 1994. Standardization of methods used to assess the progression of osteoarthritis of the hip or knee joints. In: K.E. Kuettner and V.M. Goldberg (Eds). Osteoarthritis Disorders. Rosemont, IL. Amer. Acad. Ortho. Surg. Symp. 481-496.
Dieppe, P., J. Cushnaghan, P. Young, and J. Kirwan. 1993. Prediction of the progression of joint space narrowing in osteoarthritis of the knee by bone scintigraphy. Ann. Rheum. Dis. 52:557-563.
Driver, A.J., F.J. Barr, C.J. Fuller, et al. 2004. Ultrasonography of the medial palmar intercarpal ligament in the Thoroughbred: Technique and normal appearance. Equine Vet. J. 36:402-408.
Dyson, S., R. Murray, M. Schramme, et al. 2005. Lameness associated with magnetic resonance imaging in 199 horses (January 2001-December 2005). Equine Vet. J. 37:113-121.
Frisbie, D.D., F. Al-Sobayil, R.C. Billinghurst, and C.W. McIlwraith. 2003. Serum biomarkers distinguish exercise from osteoarthritic pathology. In: Proc. Amer. Assoc. Equine Practnr. 49:116-117.

Frisbie, D.D., C.S. Ray, M. Ionescu, A.R. Poole AR, P.L. Chapman, and C.W. McIlwraith. 1999. Measurement of the 846 epitope of chondroitin sulfate and of carboxy propeptides of type II procollagen for diagnosis of osteochondral fragmentation in horses. Amer. J. Vet. Res. 60:306-309.

Fuller, C.J., A.R. Barr, M. Sharif, et al. 2001. Cross-sectional comparison of synovial fluid biochemical markers in equine osteoarthritis and the correlation of these markers with articular cartilage damage. Osteoarthritis Cartilage 9:49-55.

Garnero, P., P. Jouvenne, N. Buchs et al. 1999. Uncoupling of bone metabolism in rheumatoid arthritis patients with or without joint destruction: Assessment of serum type I collagen breakdown products. Bone 24:381-385.

Greenfield, G. 1986. Analytical approach to bone radiology. In: G. Greenfield (Ed.) Radiology of Bone Diseases 7. JB Lippincott, Philadelphia.

Group for the Respect of Ethics and Excellence in Sciences (GREES: Osteoarthritis section). 1996. Recommendations for the registration of drugs used in the treatment of osteoarthritis. Rheum. Dis. 55:552-557.

Herrmann, J.M., C. Pitris, B.E. Bouma, et al. 1999. High resolution imaging of normal and osteoarthritic cartilage with optical coherence tomography. J. Rheumatol. 26:627-635.

Hochberg, M.C., R.C. Lawrence, D.F. Everett, et al. 1989. Epidemiologic associations of pain in osteoarthritis in the knee: Data from the National Health and Nutrition Examination-I epidemiologic follow-up survey. Semin. Arthritis Rheum. (Suppl. 2) 18:4-9.

Jackson, B.F., R.K.W. Smith, and J.S. Price. 2003. A molecular marker of type I collagen metabolism reflects changes in connective tissue remodeling associated with injury to the equine superficial digital flexor tendon. Equine Vet. J. 35:211-213.

Judy, C.E., L.D. Galuppo, J.R. Snyder, and N.H. Willits. 2001. Evaluation of an in-shoe pressure measurement system in horses. Amer. J. Vet. Res. 62:23-28.

Kawcak, C.E. 2001. Current and future diagnostic means to better characterize osteoarthritis in the horse-imaging. In: Proc. Amer. Assoc. Equine Practnr. 47:164-170.

Kawcak, C.E., C.W. McIlwraith, R.W. Norrdin, R.D. Park, and S.D. James. 2001. The role of subchondral bone in joint disease: A review. Equine Vet. J. 33:120-126.

Laverty, S., M. Ionescu, M. Marcoux, L. Boure, B. Doize, and A.R. Poole. 2000. Alterations in cartilage type-2 procollagen and aggrecan contents in synovial fluid in equine osteochondrosis. J. Orthop. Res. 18:399-405.

Laverty, S., S.M. Stover, D. Belanger, T.R. O'Brien, et al. 1991. Radiographic, high-detail radiographic, microangiographic and histological findings of the distal portion of the tarsus in weanling, young and adult horses. Equine Vet. J. 23: 413-421.

Mair, T.S., J. Kinns, and R.D. Jones, et al. 2005. Magnetic resonance imaging of the

distal limb of the standing horse. Equine Vet. Educ. 17:74-78.
Marks, P.H., J.A. Goldenberg, W.C. Vezina, et al. 1992. Subchondral bone infractions in acute ligamentous knee injuries demonstrated on bone scintigraphy magnetic resonance imaging. J. Nucl. Med. 33:516-520.
Martinelli, M.J., G.J. Baker, R.B. Clarkson, et al. 1996. Magnetic resonance imaging of degenerative joint disease in a horse: A comparison to other diagnostic techniques. Equine Vet. J. 28:410-415.
McCrae, F., J. Shouls, P. Dieppe, and I. Watt. 1992. Scintigraphic assessment of osteoarthritis of the knee joint. Ann. Rheum. Dis. 51:938-942.
McIlwraith, C.W. 2005. Current state of biomarkers in equine bone and joint disease. In: Proc. Amer. Assn. Equine Practnr. (Focus on Joints). Lexington, KY.
McIlwraith, C.W. 2005. Use of synovial fluid and serum biomarkers in equine bone and joint disease. Equine Vet. J. (In press).
McIlwraith, C.W., R.C. Billinghurst, and D.D. Frisbie. 2001. Current and future diagnostic means to better characterize osteoarthritis in the horse—routine synovial fluid analysis and synovial fluid and serum markers. In: Proc. Amer. Assoc. Equine Practnr. 47:171-179.
Muller-Gerbl, M., R. Putz, N. Hodapp, et al. 1989. Computed tomography-osteoabsorptiometry for assessing the density distribution of subchondral bone as a measure of long-term mechanical adaptation in individual joints. Skeletal Radiol. 18:507-512.
Pandy, M.G., K. Sasaki, and S. Kim. 1998. A three-dimensional musculoskeletal model of the human knee joint. Part 1: Theoretical construct. Comput. Methods Biomech. Biomed. Engin. 1:87-108.
Parks, R.D., P. Steyn, and R. Wrigley. 1996. Imaging techniques in the diagnosis of equine joint disease. In: C.W. McIlwraith and G.W. Trotter (Eds). Joint Disease in the Horse. WB Saunders Co., Philadelphia. 145-164.
Price, J.S., B. Jackson, R. Eastell, et al. 1995. Age-related changes in biochemical markers of bone metabolism in horses. Equine Vet. J. 3:201-207.
Price, J.S., B. Jackson, J.A. Gray, P.A. Harris, I.M. Wright, D.U. Pfeiffer, S.P. Robbins, R. Eastell, and S.W. Ricketts. 2001. Biochemical markers of bone metabolism in growing Thoroughbreds: A longitudinal study. Res. Vet. Sci. 71:37-44.
Radin, E.L., and R.M. Rose. 1986. Role of subchondral bone in the initiation and progression of cartilage damage. Clin. Orthop. 213:34-40.
Ray, C.S., A.R. Poole, and C.W. McIlwraith. 1996. Use of synovial fluid and serum markers in articular disease. In: C.W. McIlwraith and G.W. Trotter (Eds). Joint Disease in the Horse. WB Saunders Co., Philadelphia. 203-216.
Riggs, C.M., G.H. Whitehouse, and A. Boyde. 1999a. Structural variation of the distal condyles of the third metacarpal and third metatarsal bones in the horse. Equine Vet. J. 31:130-139.
Riggs, C.M., G.H. Whitehouse, and A. Boyde. 1999b. Pathology of the distal condyles of the third metacarpal and third metatarsal bones of the horse. Equine Vet. J. 31:140-148.

Ruwe, P.A., J. Wright, R.L. Randell, J.K. Lynch, P. Jokl, and S. McCarthy. 1992. Can MR imaging effectively replace diagnostic arthroscopy? Radiology 183:335-339.

Thonar, E.J., M.E. Lenz, K. Masuda, and D.H. Manicourt. 1999. Body fluid markers of cartilage metabolism. In: Dynamics of Bone and Cartilage Metabolism. Academic Press. 453-464.

Wachter, N.J., P. Augat, M. Mentzel, et al. 2001. Predictive value of bone mineral density and morphology determined by peripheral quantitative computed tomography for cancellous bone strength of the proximal femur. Bone 28:133-139.

Widmar, W., and W. Blevins. 1994. Radiographic evaluation of degenerative joint disease in horses: Interpretive principles. Comp. Contin. Educ. 16:907-918.

Wittbjer, J., B. Nosslin, B. Palmer, and K.G. Thorngren. 1982. Bone formation of transplanted autologous bone matrix in rabbit evaluated by technetium radionuclide bone imaging. Scand. J. Plast. Reconstr. Burg. 16:23-28.

MANAGING THE SICK FOAL TO PRODUCE A SOUND ATHLETE

WILLIAM BERNARD
Equine Internal Medicine, Lexington, Kentucky

Introduction

Every breeding farm hopes for an uneventful foaling season, a high percentage of live births, and strong foals that remain healthy and grow well. Regardless of management, however, every farm has to deal with foal illness from time to time. Detecting health problems and getting the sick foal into a program of veterinary care must be done quickly to ensure the best outcome. Supporting sick foals with proper nutrition is an important factor in survival and recovery. This paper will discuss some of the more common foal diseases as well as the medical and nutritional management included in treatment.

Neonatal Foals

The ill neonate presents unique challenges as its immune system and nutritional status are not well prepared to battle disease. The neonate's immune system is slow to respond to challenges, and the foal is not nutritionally prepared for caloric interruption. Three critical factors in the therapy of the ill neonate are treatment of the underlying disease process, supportive nursing care, and nutritional support.

Nursing care of neonates (those from birth to about seven days old) includes keeping the foals clean and warm. Hydration status must be monitored; weak foals may need help in standing or lying down; and recumbent foals must be turned from side to side at regular intervals. Most importantly, the foals must receive some form of nutrition. Because these young animals have limited energy reserves, nutritional support involves providing a continuous supply of energy in a form that can be tolerated.

It is vital to avoid overfeeding. Foals that nurse enthusiastically from a bottle are in danger of overfilling their stomachs. Small frequent feedings are less likely to cause digestive upset.

Colostrum, mare's milk, or a milk replacer can be given to foals that are able to suckle. These fluids may be provided via nasogastric tube to foals that can't nurse.

Another way of delivering energy is the use of total parenteral nutrition (TPN). Although this mixture of glucose, amino acids, and lipids does not meet all requirements for normal growth and development, it does provide sufficient energy to sustain life, allowing the foal time to recover. Because of the exacting protocol, TPN must be administered in a controlled setting. An intravenous pump ensures a steady rate of delivery, avoiding sharp fluctuations in plasma glucose and insulin levels. A double-lumen catheter in the foal's neck allows the constant flow of TPN solution and the simultaneous introduction of any necessary medications through a separate tube. Blood samples are taken hourly at first to monitor glucose, with the interval lengthening as the foal's condition improves.

TPN can be used as a nutritional adjunct for any sick foal that is not able to consume adequate calories. A disease process in which TPN is particularly useful is enterocolitis (inflammation of the large intestine) characterized by severe diarrhea. This condition can be life-threatening, especially in neonatal foals. Caused by rotavirus, clostridium, salmonella, or other organisms, inflammation prevents absorption of nutrients in the gastrointestinal tract. TPN provides nourishment while allowing the gastrointestinal tract to "rest."

Foals that are too weak or uncoordinated to stand and nurse are also TPN candidates. Foals suffering from botulism, those with neurologic signs, and those in a stupor or coma may be in this category.

Several factors must be considered in planning nutritional support for the sick neonatal foal. The foal's condition dictates the starting point, and frequent changes are made as improvement is seen. In general, foals that lie on their sides and cannot achieve a sternal position (head up, weight supported on chest and trunk) without assistance are candidates for TPN. A foal in this condition is likely to develop secondary gastrointestinal problems if fed volumes of milk adequate to support nutritional requirements. Foals that can maintain sternal recumbency can usually tolerate milk, starting with small amounts during the first day.

A normal healthy foal ingests about 20% of its weight in mare's milk every day. Total intake for a foal weighing 50 kg would be about 10 liters per day. In sick foals, however, this level of intake may overwhelm digestive capability, leading to colic or other gastrointestinal problems. A guideline for an average newborn foal weighing approximately 50 kg is as follows:

$$5000 \text{ ml } (10\% \text{ bw}) \div 24 \text{ hr.} = \text{approx. } 200 \text{ ml/hr} = 7 \text{ oz/hr}$$

Intake for a sick foal that can attain a sternal position may begin at only 5 to 10% of body weight for the first 12 to 24 hours. A foal that is able to stand can usually be started at about 10% of body weight. At first, small feedings of about 10-14 ounces should be given every two hours. As the foal's condition improves, the amount of milk and the interval between feedings can be increased until the foal is getting the full 20% of body weight in milk daily. Care must be taken to make the changes gradually so as to avoid gastrointestinal complications.

Although the small amount of milk initially fed does not support rapid growth, it must be understood that sustaining life is the primary focus for extremely sick foals. Survivors are usually able to catch up in growth soon after they return to health.

Management to Prevent Illness

Colostrum, the first secretion of the mammary glands, contains antibodies that are important in the rapid response to disease. The foal loses its ability to absorb these antibodies after 24 hours, so nursing within the first few hours of life is essential. Studies have shown that foals exposed to salmonella before they ingest colostrum are at increased risk of developing an infection, a situation that can be minimized by careful attention to cleanliness. An older foal may not be affected by salmonella exposure; however, it may be quite serious in a neonate with an underdeveloped immune system and low nutritional stores. As insurance against disease, managers at some farms strip 4 to 8 ounces of colostrum from the mare and tube or suckle it into the foal immediately after birth. When bottle-feeding, care must be taken to prevent an enthusiastic foal from drinking too quickly and aspirating milk. It is also important to make sure that the hole in the bottle's nipple is not too large.

In the management of foal health, prevention of disease is far preferable to treatment, with excellent hygiene being the key. A foal may actually get its first exposure to pathogenic bacteria as it passes through the birth canal; from the time it draws its first breath, its environment is full of potentially harmful organisms.

Cleanliness is vitally important and cannot be overemphasized as a factor in preventing outbreaks of diarrhea. Some farms begin daily washing of the pregnant mare's ventral surfaces as much as a week before foaling, especially during wet weather when mares are turned out in muddy pastures. In any case, washing is important just before foaling, as the foal's early attempts to nurse may put its muzzle in contact with bacteria on the mare's legs and belly. Foaling outdoors or in a foaling barn is a choice each farm must make, and each situation has advantages and disadvantages. Foaling stalls should be thoroughly disinfected and equipment should be sterilized before use.

Overcrowding of horses should be avoided, as disease can be spread between horses by direct contact or by aerosolized bacteria carried by dust.

Common Diseases in Young Foals

One of the most common problems in young foals is enterocolitis caused by salmonella, clostridium, or rotavirus picked up from the environment or spread from other horses on workers' hands or clothing. All personnel attending a foaling should wash their hands frequently and should wear latex gloves when disinfecting the umbilicus.

It has been shown that close proximity facilitates the spread of disease, and one mare or foal shedding salmonella can lead to illness in the rest of the barn. Likewise, a cycle of diarrhea among several foals can sometimes be broken by turning the foals out on grass instead of keeping them together in the barn.

Septicemia, a generalized blood-borne infection, can follow invasion of bacteria through the mucosal membranes of the umbilicus, gastrointestinal tract, or respiratory tract. Such infection may localize in the foal's joints. Treatment varies by the organism and the number of joints involved. Antibiotics are usually effective, although organisms like salmonella that live deep in the tissues may be more difficult to eliminate. Again, prevention is achieved through excellent hygiene.

Colic is sometimes seen in very young foals, most often from meconium impaction, overfeeding, or infection. Management steps should be aimed toward prevention, as well as rapid treatment if problems occur.

HIE, or hypoxic ischemic encephalopathy, is the term given to any neurologic problem not known to be caused by infection or physical injury. The designation signifies alterations in brain function caused by a lack of oxygen and/or decreased blood flow to the brain before, during, or after birth. Terms such as neonatal maladjustment syndrome and "dummy foal" refer to the same condition. Signs including seizures, lethargy, stumbling, incoordination, and cessation of nursing may be noticed shortly after birth, but may not be noted until 24 to 72 hours later.

HIE can have a number of causes. Dystocia (difficult or delayed birth), possibly involving a compressed umbilical cord, is sometimes a factor. Placental insufficiency (placenta is not able to supply adequate oxygenated blood to the fetus) may be a cause, either because the placenta cannot keep up with rapid fetal development at the end of pregnancy or because of premature placental separation.

Mares that graze fescue pastures in late pregnancy often have abnormally thick placentas, pregnancies that are longer than average, and decreased or absent milk production. Removing mares from fescue pastures during the last months of pregnancy helps to prevent these problems. There is anecdotal evidence of a dramatic decrease in foaling problems, including HIE, on farms that have carried out pasture renovation to remove fescue and replace it with alternative forages.

Nutritional support is the key to recovery for foals suffering from HIE. Providing nursing care as well as TPN, mare's milk, or a milk replacer keeps these foals alive and hydrated until neurologic signs subside. With early care, many HIE foals recover and show normal growth and development.

Foals born prematurely or in immature condition often do not catch up to their peers in size or development, and athletic potential may be limited.

Gastrointestinal Health and Probiotics/Prebiotics

A critical factor in the health of every horse, regardless of age, is the number and type of microorganisms in the gut. In older horses, gut bacteria are essential for digestion. In young foals, the microflora are of significantly less nutritional importance; however, they are important in the host's defense against disease. Host bacteria may directly produce antibiogens (products which kill pathogens) that outcompete pathogens or prevent their adherence to the mucosal surface. The practice of coprophagy, or eating manure, is widespread among growing foals and may be a way of populating the gut with additional flora from more mature horses as the foal develops and its diet includes less milk and more forage.

The exact mechanism and the significance of bacterial function in foals are not completely understood. What is known is that any disturbance to this microbial balance—stress, travel, illness, change of diet, administration of antibiotics or other medications—has the potential to cause digestive upset. To maintain gastrointestinal health, some equine managers have turned to probiotics and prebiotics. Simply defined, probiotics are infusions of live organisms with the purpose of increasing numbers of helpful bacteria or yeast in the gastrointestinal tract. Prebiotics are designed to enhance the gut environment so as to support growth of microorganisms that are naturally present. These products have come into prominence in recent years, and many types are available to horse owners. However, their efficacy in horses of various ages is somewhat in question for several reasons.

- Especially in young foals, giving a probiotic to enhance fermentation is of little value because fermentation is not important when milk makes up the majority of the diet.

- Very few, if any, oral digestive aids have been clinically tested in foals, so their effect is not known.

- Lactobacillus strains number in the thousands; only those naturally found in the horse's gastrointestinal tract can be expected to benefit the horse. Commercial lactobacillus blends are often made up chiefly of strains found in cattle, with few or none that are specific to equines. Viability and benefits of these bovine strains are unknown.

- In older foals and mature horses, the gut contains billions of microorganisms. While digestive health products are purported to contain millions of live bacteria and/or yeast cells, studies have shown that many of the organisms die prior to use because of environmental temperature variations, elapsed time since manufacture, or other factors. Introducing too small a number of organisms may have little impact on gut function. If this is the case, many commercial probiotics are probably ineffective.

So, is there any discernable effect, good or bad, from the use of yogurt and other prebiotics and probiotics? Anecdotal evidence supports their positive effects in some cases; some managers and veterinarians don't recommend them. Horses with some conditions do seem to benefit, and therefore these products probably belong in the "can't hurt, may help" category.

Growing Foals and Weanlings

After the first few weeks, foals are stronger, more vigorous, and in better shape to survive illness because they have begun to develop at least minimal stores of energy and nutrients. Developments like diarrhea are still serious but are less often life threatening in older foals.

As in very young foals, the treatments for enterocolitis, joint infections, and severe colic include nursing care and nutritional support. Because they are more mature and have some nutritional reserves, older foals may not need the intensive fluid therapy and frequent meals that are critical to neonates. Developing specific feeds for sick foals or horses has been problematic because horses that are very ill usually cannot be coaxed to eat very much, regardless of what is offered to them.

Prevention of infectious diseases depends heavily on foal management. Vaccines are not available to protect foals against salmonella and clostridium infections. Rotavirus vaccine is available for mares but is not completely effective.

Respiratory diseases are common in foals and can range from mild to severe. Infections can develop over the course of several months with few signs, while other foals develop acute infections, sometimes including serious and debilitating pyogranulomatous lung abscesses. Causative agents include pasteurella, streptococcus and *Rhodococcus equi*. Rhodococcus lives in the soil, surviving for many years and spreading easily through airborne dust.

Many foals with respiratory infections can be treated on the farm, although extremely sick foals sometimes need to be hospitalized for intranasal oxygen therapy. Foals that are too sick to nurse may need to be fed parenterally or by nasogastric tube.

Effective antibiotic treatment depends first on identifying the organism involved and selecting specific products to combat the infective agent. With careful treatment, most foals recover well and their potential for performance is not impacted. The incidence of foal pneumonia drops as foals reach weaning age and older.

Several steps can be taken to help prevent respiratory disease. Antibody-laden plasma gathered from hyperimmunized pregnant mares can be harvested and given to newborn foals to boost immunity. Overcrowding of mares and foals should be avoided to slow the development and spread of foal pneumonia. Some farms with *Rhodococcus equi* problems have found that, during the summer months, keeping horses stalled during the day and turning them out at night prevents transmission of bacteria that are spread when foals inhale dust kicked up by mares that are troubled by flies.

Economic Considerations

While many sick foals require minor treatment that can be handled on the farm, foals that are severely ill may require care that can be given only in a clinical setting. This care can be expensive, often totaling $5,000 to $15,000 or more for treatment of the average critically ill neonate. Realistic decisions on care and management of the sick neonatal or older foal must consider this expense as compared to the foal's current and potential value.

Outlook for Athletic Performance

A study in 1991 found that a group of foals that had *Rhodococcus equi* respiratory infections earned the same amount of money in their two- and three-year-old racing years as horses that had not been sick (Bernard et al., 1991). In the same study, foals that had streptococcal respiratory infections earned less money in their three-year-old years than those with *Rhodococcus equi* infections and less money than the North American average in the two- and three-year-old years. Reasons are not clear for the parallel between streptococcus infections and decreased performance.

Conclusion

Disease prevention, early detection of illness, nursing care, antibiotic therapy, and nutritional support are important in producing healthy foals that can be expected to achieve their athletic potential. Many foals that survive illness will be fully capable of normal training and performance as mature individuals. Because of variations in farm management, genetic makeup, and response to training programs, it is impossible to predict with any certainty the probable career successes of a specific individual.

References

Bernard, W.V. 1993. Critical care in foals: Respiratory and cardiovascular support and fluid therapy. Equine Practice 1174-1185.
Bernard, W.V. 1993. Critical care in foals: Providing proper nutritional support. Equine Practice 1186-1189.
Bernard, W.V., J. Dugan, S. Pierce, and I. Gardiner. 1991. The influence of foal pneumonia on future racing performance. In: Proc. Amer. Assoc. Equine Practnr. 37:19.
Weese, J.S. 2003. Evaluation of deficiencies in labeling of commercial probiotics. Canadian Vet. J. 44:982-983.

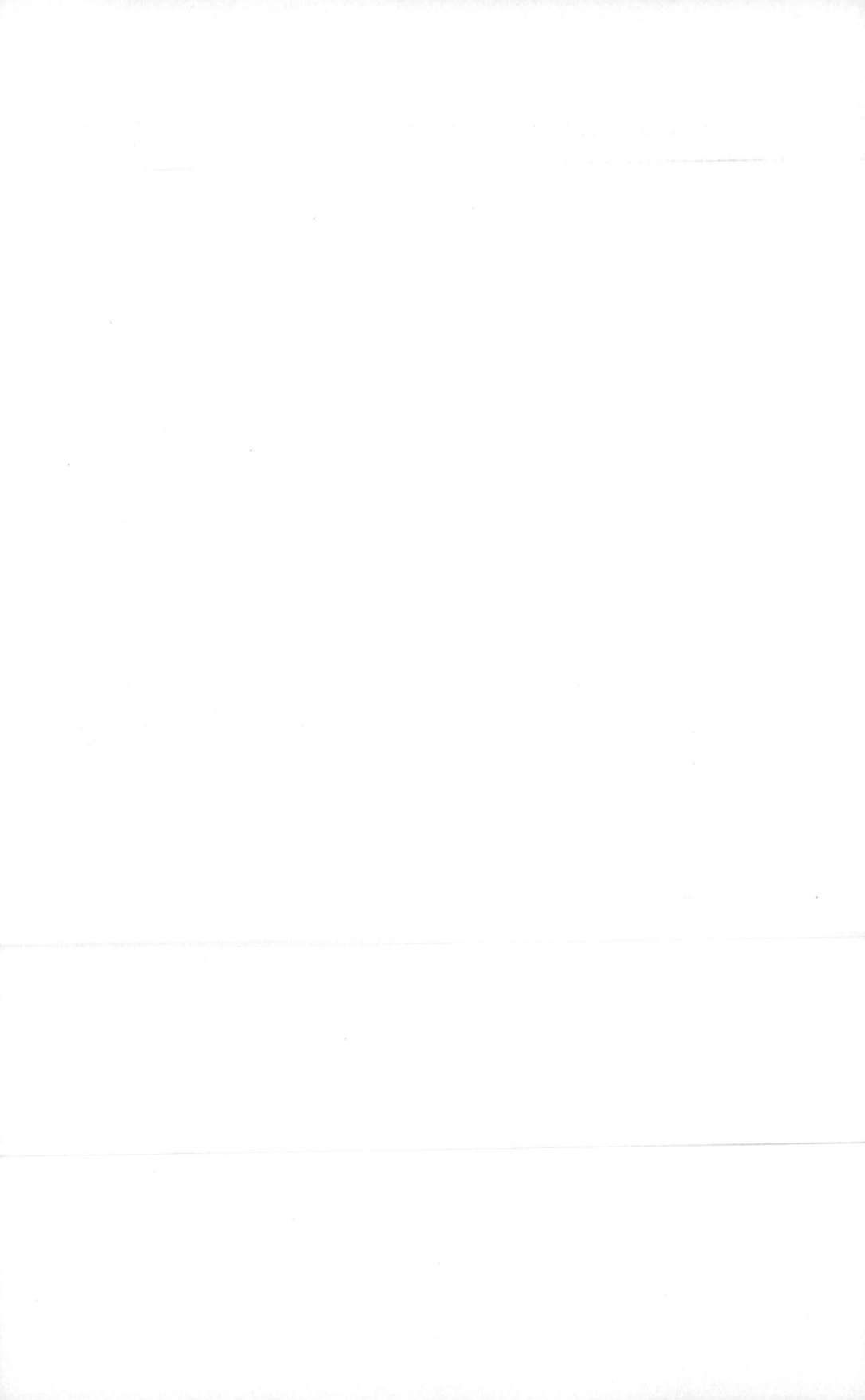

RATIONAL APPROACHES TO EQUINE PARASITE CONTROL

CRAIG R. REINEMEYER
East Tennessee Clinical Research, Inc., Knoxville, Tennessee

Introduction

Since the 1950s when phenothiazine was introduced as the first broad-spectrum anthelmintic, horse owners and veterinarians have applied dewormers in a systematic fashion to limit the transmission of equine parasites. The best-known and most widely practiced control program has been to deworm horses at bimonthly intervals throughout the year. Although this recommendation was evidence-based and highly effective when introduced in the mid-1960s (Drudge and Lyons, 1966), the reproductive behavior of target parasites has changed during the past 40 years, and resistance to certain classes of anthelmintics has further diminished the efficacy of this program.

This historical example confirms the concept that all control measures have a finite life span (Michel, 1976). Parasites are plastic organisms with the ability to adapt to, and ultimately triumph over, virtually all man-made selection pressures. Because most of these adaptations have a genetic basis, future generations of worms may not be susceptible to the same interventions that would have killed their grandparents.

Our knowledge of the biology and ecology of equine/parasite relationships has expanded greatly through research, but this information has effected few changes in control practices in the United States. Unfortunately, many horse owners and most veterinarians still expect parasite control recommendations to be packaged as a simple recipe. The intent of this presentation is not to swap recipes, but rather to examine the essential components of parasite control recommendations, and to present examples of rational programs that can be customized for specific herds in various geoclimatic regions of the United States. Recipes have finite life spans, but understanding the basic elements of parasite control gives us the power to adapt… just like the worms.

Considerations for Control Programs

TARGET ORGANISMS

Equine parasite control programs vary with the age of the host, and strongyles are the only significant parasitic pathogens of mature horses in North America. This diverse group of parasites is usually subclassified as large and small strongyles. Large strongyles were eradicated from most well-managed farms during the past decade, so small strongyles (cyathostomes) are now considered the major targets of parasite control programs for mature horses. Cyathostomes are ubiquitous, and virtually all grazing horses are infected. Horses never develop total immunity to small strongyles, and positive fecal examinations are the rule in untreated animals.

Adult cyathostomes reside in the large intestine, and the females lay eggs, which pass into the environment in the horse's feces. The eggs hatch in favorable environmental conditions, and small, worm-like larvae emerge. After two molts, a third stage larva (L3) results, which is the only phase capable of infecting another horse. Once ingested by grazing horses, infective larvae burrow into the lining of the large intestine, where they are surrounded by a fibrous capsule. After an interval ranging from a few weeks to more than two years, the capsule ruptures, larvae emerge into the lumen of the gut, and the worms mature into adults. Adult females lay eggs, and the cycle is repeated for another generation.

The current prominence of cyathostomes was achieved partially by default, but nevertheless they are valid pathogens that cause colic, weight loss, poor growth, anemia, hypoproteinemia, loss of condition, and rough hair coats (Love et al., 1999). Small strongyles also can cause larval cyathostominosis, which is a severe and potentially fatal diarrheal syndrome associated with the synchronous emergence of large numbers of immature worms from the gut wall. Even in well-managed horses, cyathostomes probably cause subclinical production losses, such as compromised feed efficiency and suboptimal performance. However, these effects remain largely uninvestigated, perhaps because Western cultures refuse to view the horse as a production animal.

Patterns of Transmission

Where? Strongyle eggs pass into the environment anywhere that a horse defecates, but translation (i.e., development into infective, third stage larvae) occurs only in pasture habitats. Stalls are usually too dry to support translation, and a large component of the moisture in wet stalls often comes from urine. The urea in urine breaks down into ammonia, which is highly toxic to developing strongyle larvae. Thus, strongyle infection is an unavoidable risk for grazing horses, but exposure for stabled animals is nil.

When? Development to the Infective Stage. Translation from eggs to infective larvae is regulated entirely by environmental conditions. Moisture and oxygen are essential, but concentrations of both within a fecal pile are usually adequate. Over a wide temperature range (45° F to 85° F), the rate of larval development is directly proportional to environmental temperature. At lower temperatures, hatching and development may require several weeks or months, whereas eggs can hatch and develop into third stage larvae in three to five days when ambient temperatures are in the high 70s (F). Beyond both temperature extremes, eggs either cannot hatch if it is too cold, or larvae develop rapidly but soon die when it is too hot.

When? Persistence of the Infective Stage. Infective L3s cannot ingest nutrients, so they survive by consuming limited, intracellular energy reserves. The duration of their survival is inversely proportional to temperature. Because very little catabolism of energy occurs at low temperatures, cyathostome larvae readily survive through northern winters (Ogbourne, 1973; Duncan, 1974). Conversely, larvae are short-lived during southern summers because energy reserves are consumed more quickly at higher temperatures (English, 1979).

The rigorous environmental limitations on the strongyle life cycle result in predictable, seasonal patterns of transmission. Given the regulatory influences of climate, it should be no surprise that the patterns of strongyle transmission differ among geographic regions. Table 1 presents the seasonal patterns of transmission in major geoclimatic divisions of the continental U.S.

Table 1. Climatic suitability for larval translation and survival, by location and season.

Season	Development/Persistence Northern Temperate Climate[A]	Development/Persistence Southern Temperate Climate[B]
Spring	++/++	++/++
Summer	++/+	--/--
Autumn	++/++	++/++
Winter	--/++	+/++

[A]Roughly above the latitude of the Ohio River
[B]Below the latitude of the Ohio River

Objectives of Parasite Control

Most owners and practitioners would agree that the ultimate goal of equine parasite control is to optimize the health and performance of horses. The responses differ, however, if one asks, "What are you trying to do when you give a dewormer?" The most frequent answer is, "Kill worms." However, killing worms per se is **not** the objective of a parasite control program. This is especially true for cyathostomes, which exert the majority of their damaging effects before they are susceptible to many dewormers.

The direct source of cyathostome infection is larvae on pasture, and those larvae developed from eggs that were deposited by grazing horses. Once strongyle eggs turn into infective larvae, the only factors that can diminish the risk of future infections are hot weather, time, and exclusion of horses from pasture. The only practical way to decrease future infection is by limiting the passage of worm eggs, and this can be accomplished by killing female worms before they reproduce. Therefore, the objective of parasite control is preventing contamination of the environment with reproductive stages (eggs) of the target parasites.

Appropriate strategies for equine parasite control must be prophylactic. A control program should not be envisioned as a regularly implemented, therapeutic procedure (like dipping a dog to remove fleas), but rather as a series of scheduled interventions that prevent parasite populations from reproducing (like preemergent herbicides). Simply reiterated, cyathostome control recommendations should attempt to limit the passage of large numbers of strongyle eggs onto pasture.

Tools of Parasite Control

Although other management techniques can be useful as adjuncts, anthelmintics (dewormers) are the mainstays of equine parasite control programs. It is essential to understand the relationships and properties of available equine anthelmintics so their characteristics can be exploited.

One finds a bewildering array of equine dewormers on the shelf at the local farmers' co-op, but the available choices for strongyles belong to only four major chemical classes (Table 2).

Table 2. Currently marketed equine dewormers by chemical class, generic name, and trade names(s).

Chemical Class	Generic Name	Trade name
Benzimidazoles	Fenbendazole	Panacur; Panacur PowerPak
	Oxfendazole	Benzelmin
	Oxibendazole	Anthelcide E.Q.
Tetrahydropyrimidines	Pyrantel pamoate	Anthelban; Exodus; Strongid Paste; Strongid-T; Pyrantel Pamoate Paste
	Pyrantel tartrate	Continuex; Strongid-C, Strongid-C 2X
Macrocyclic lactones	Ivermectin	EquiMax; Equimectrin; Equell; Eqvalan; IverCare; Ivercide; Phoenectin; Rotation 1; Zimecterin; Zimecterin Gold, etc.
	Moxidectin	Quest; Quest Plus; ComboCare
Heterocyclic compounds	Piperazine	Piperazine, various

All of the listed compounds have good efficacy against adult and immature cyathostomes in the lumen of the gut. Only two, however, are known to demonstrate activity against cyathostome larvae that are encysted within fibrous capsules in the wall of the gut. Those are moxidectin, which is effective at 0.4 mg/kg administered once, and fenbendazole (Panacur PowerPak), which is effective when given at 10 mg/kg daily for 5 consecutive days.

When cyathostomes are killed by effective anthelmintics, the fecal egg counts of treated horses should decrease by 90% or more. None of the dewormers, including the larvicides, are 100% effective, however, and strongyle egg production eventually resumes when the larvae that were encysted at the time of treatment mature and begin to reproduce. The interval between treatment and resumption of significant strongyle egg production is termed the "Egg Reappearance Period" (E.R.P.), and its duration varies with the anthelmintic used (Table 3).

Table 3. Duration of egg reappearance periods following use of therapeutic dewormers.

Class or Compound	Egg Reappearance Period (E.R.P.)
Piperazine	4 weeks
Benzimidazole	4 weeks
Tetrahydropyrimidine	4 weeks
Ivermectin	6 to 8 weeks
Moxidectin	~12 weeks

The E.R.P. is an extremely important tool to be exploited in parasite control programs. Because the primary objective is prevention of environmental contamination with worm eggs, the E.R.P. tells us how long that condition can be sustained after each treatment with a specific compound.

Anthelmintic Resistance

Resistance is defined as a measurable decrease in the efficacy of a compound against a population of worms that were previously susceptible. Resistance is not due to any change in the drug, but rather to genetic adaptations by the target parasites. How does resistance develop? Genes for resistance traits occur naturally at extremely low levels, but frequent treatments and exclusive use of one drug class provide certain advantages. Whenever resistant worms survive treatment, they are able to continue reproducing in the absence of competition from susceptible worms, and the resistant genotype becomes more frequent in the population. Continued and frequent use of the same class of drug ultimately results in a predominance of resistant genotypes in the population.

Traditionally, many horse owners "rotate" dewormers, meaning they alternate among the available chemical classes (see Table 2). Rotation was originally implemented to cover deficient spectra of the available anthelmintics, not to thwart resistance. Rotation per se is no longer as important as ensuring that all anthelmintics used are still effective.

Resistance to certain drug classes (e.g., benzimidazoles) is alarmingly prevalent, but by no means universal (Kaplan, 2002). Therefore, it behooves practitioners and/or horse owners to determine which drug classes are still effective in a herd, and which should be avoided in the future.

Monitoring Infection Status

Useful information about an animal's parasite status can be gleaned from quantitative fecal examination. This procedure counts the numbers of worm eggs per unit weight of feces, and differs from a standard fecal examination, which can only determine the presence or absence of parasite eggs (Reinemeyer and Barakat, 2004). Although the numerical results are not necessarily correlated to worm numbers or to the severity of disease, fecal egg counts are the essential tool of rational parasite control.

The most important use of quantitative egg counts is determining the spectrum of effective anthelmintics on a farm (Table 4). Subsequent follow-up can confirm the duration of the E.R.P. of various anthelmintics against resident worms (Table 4). And finally, fecal egg counts of untreated horses can determine the relative contaminative potential of individual horses within a herd (Table 4).

Quantitative fecal examination is absolutely essential if one intends to approach parasite control in a rational fashion. However, most equine practices probably don't offer this procedure for their clients at the present time. Diagnostic testing may appear to be just an additional expense, but management decisions based on the results may decrease the total cost of a farm's parasite control program due to savings on unnecessary or ineffective anthelmintic treatments.

Host Factors

Individual horses vary widely in their individual susceptibility to cyathostome infection, and those differences are reflected in the magnitude of their respective fecal egg counts (Duncan and Love, 1991). The majority of the parasites in any group of animals are concentrated in a minority of the animals. Despite this fact, all horses in a herd have been treated exactly the same when it came to parasite control. It should be obvious that rote deworming is wasted on those members of the group that apparently can handle strongyles on their own. It is also likely that the same programs could be suboptimal for the highly susceptible members of the herd.

Fortunately, it is possible to categorize the strongyle contaminative potential of each horse (Table 4). Quantitative fecal egg counts can identify the troublemakers as well as the easy keepers in a herd.

Developing Rational, Customized Control Programs

All of the factors discussed previously should be considered when designing and implementing equine parasite control programs.

Table 4. Various applications of quantitative fecal egg counting techniques.

Application	Steps
Determining anthelmintic efficacy or resistance	1. Determine egg counts in fecal samples collected from 6 or more horses prior to deworming. 2. Treat horses with label dosage of anthelmintic(s) to be evaluated. 3. Collect fecal samples from the **same** horses 10 to 14 days after deworming. 4. Perform quantitive fecal examination and calculate efficacy (fecal egg count reduction; FECR) by the formula: ([Pre-count minus post-count] / pre-count X 100). 5. Interpretation: >90% FECR = effective, <80% FECR = resistant, 80% to 90% FECR = equivocal, repeat in future.
Determining duration of Egg Reappearance Period (E.R.P.)	1. Determine egg counts in fecal samples collected from 6 or more horses prior the deworming. 2. Treat horses with label dosage of anthelmintic(s) to be evaluated. 3. Collect fecal samples from the **same** horses at 2-week intervals after deworming. 4. The E.R.P. has expired when egg counts average 50% or greater of pretreatment levels.
Determining strongyle contaminative potential	1. Collect fecal samples from all horses in a herd at least 4 weeks after the expiration of the E.R.P. for the previous anthelmintic treatment. 2. Horses with counts <100 eggs per gram (EPG) are low contaminators; those >500 EPG are high contaminators; those with 100 to 500 EPG are moderate contaminators.

The first step is to determine the spectrum of anthelmintics that are effective in a given herd. This can be accomplished by performing Fecal Egg Count Reduction (FECR) testing with all desired classes of anthelmintics (Table 4). FECR testing will identify the drugs that are viable candidates for inclusion in a program, and also reveals the classes of drugs that should never be used on the farm again.

The second step is to determine the relative strongyle contaminative potential of animals within a herd (Table 4). This procedure identifies those animals that require the greatest deworming attention, and also those that require the least.

The start of the annual strongyle transmission season will differ depending on whether the premise in question is located within the northern temperate or southern temperate region. The transmission season begins when the risk of reinfection for grazing horses changes from minimal to inevitable unless control measures are implemented. In the northern temperate U.S., this shift occurs when horses that were stabled during winter are turned out to pasture in the spring. Spring pastures still harbor residual larvae that developed during the preceding grazing season but survived on pasture through winter. Larval numbers decline during spring, thanks to the warmer weather, and ultimately will reach annual lows by about the first of June. The numbers of pasture larvae will remain low if horses are not allowed to recontaminate the environment with new worm eggs. And how does one stop egg-shedding? By killing adult parasites with anthelmintics.

In the southern temperate U.S., the shift in risk of infection occurs at the end of summer. Just prior to this time, climatic conditions are too hot and often too dry to support survival of infective larvae, even if the horses are dropping lots of worm eggs on pasture at that time. The risk of infection increases during autumn as a consequence of eggs shed recently on pasture.

Our hypothetical herds are now on pastures that are relatively clean (south) or are in the processing of being cleaned up (north), and these grazing venues will remain safe if the horses don't contaminate them with new worm eggs. A single, effective anthelmintic treatment can accomplish this, but we also know that the horses eventually will resume egg-shedding when larvae that survived treatment mature and begin to reproduce. So, the question is, "How long before we need to retreat the horses to maintain zero or at least very low egg counts?" The answer is found in the duration of the E.R.P. following the use of various drugs (Table 3).

Suppressive deworming is the practice of repeating treatment within the E.R.P. of the last compound administered. Thus, repeating treatments nose-to-tail should render fecal egg counts consistently zero or at least very low for as long as effective dewormers are used. However, we must remember that not every horse in the herd requires such an intensive program. We suggest that the low contaminators in a herd receive a single anthelmintic treatment at the beginning of the annual cycle, and another perhaps six months later. Moderate contaminators should receive two treatments administered at suppressive intervals, and the high contaminators should be treated throughout the entire transmission season (i.e., until autumn in the north or late winter in the south).

Table 5. A rational control program for horses pastured in southern temperate climates.

Contaminator Catagory	Begin Annual Program	Additional Winter Dewormings	Terminate Annual Program
Low	October	None	March
Moderate	October	One*	March
High	October	Through entire winter*	March

*Additional treatments are best administered suppressively, i.e., to coincide with expiration of the egg reappearance period of the previously used dewormer.

Table 6. A rational control program for horses pastured in northern temperate climates.*

Contaminator Catagory	Begin Annual Program	Additional Winter Dewormings	Terminate Annual Program
Low	April	None	October
Moderate	April	One**	October
High	April	Through entire summer**	October

*Northern programs are more effective if horses are stabled or held off pasture through the winter months, and first turned out in April or May.
**Additional treatments are best administered suppressively, i.e., to coincide with expiration of the egg reappearance period of the dewormer used most recently.

It is advisable to begin and end each seasonal program with a drug that is effective against migrating large strongyle larvae (ivermectin, moxidectin, or fenbendazole 10 mg/kg for 5 days) to facilitate or maintain eradication of *Strongylus* species from the premises.

Conclusion

The changing patterns of resistance among target nematodes lend an element of urgency to implementing major changes in parasite control strategies for horses in the U.S. The most critical change will be in the attitudes of horse owners and equine veterinarians because the notion of limiting treatment to certain seasons of the year seems radical, and the prospect of leaving certain animals untreated is tantamount to heresy. However, the recommendations and justifications presented in this paper will provide effective control, will decrease selection pressure for the development of anthelmintic resistance, and may accomplish both at a lower cost than current, inefficient practices.

References

Drudge, J.H., and Lyons, E.T. 1966. Control of internal parasites of the horse. J. Am. Vet. Med. Assoc. 148:378-383.
Duncan, J.L. 1974. Field studies on the epidemiology of mixed strongyle infection in the horse. Vet. Rec. 94:337-345.
Duncan, J.L., and Love, S. 1991. Preliminary observations on an alternative strategy for the control of horse strongyles. Equine Vet. J. 23:226-228.
English, A.W. 1979. The epidemiology of equine strongylosis in northern Queensland. 2. The survival and migration of infective larvae on herbage. Aust. Vet. J. 55:306-309.

Kaplan, R.M. 2002. Anthelmintic resistance in nematodes of horses. Vet. Res. 33:491-507.
Love, S., Murphy, D., and Mellor, D. 1999. Pathogenicity of cyathostome infection. Vet. Parasitol. 85:113-122.
Michel, J.F. 1976. The epidemiology and control of some nematode infections in grazing animals. Adv. Parasitol 14:399-422.
Ogbourne, C.P. 1973. Survival on herbage plots of infective larvae of strongylid nematodes of the horse. J. Helminthol. 47:9-16.
Reinemeyer, C.R., and Barakat, C. 2004. Parasite control check. Equus 319:69-78.

INDEX

A

Alfalfa 19, 22
Allergy 379
Anesthesia 321
Anthelmintics 414

B

Behavior 77
Beta-carotene 51
Biomarkers 393
Body weight 43. 137, 213, 221, 247
    feeding for change in 259
Bone development 101, 163
    disease 101
    turnover 147, 395
Bucked shins 166
Buffering 21

C

Calcium 147
Carbohydrates 29, 269
Cartilage 394
Colic, causes 318
    nutrition after episode 335
    prevalence 313
    risk factors 315
    role of grain 315
    treatment 327
Colonic ulcers 347
    treatment 351
Condition score 43
Coprophagy 406
Cortisol 97
Cribbing 77, 81, 318
Cushing's disease 272, 277

D

Developmental orthopedic disease 101, 209, 250
Dewormers 414
Diagnostic imaging 385
Digestion 17
Disease, feeding during 260
    gastrointestinal 264
    hepatic 263
    in foals 403
    renal 264
    respiratory 263, 408
    skeletal 385

E

Energy 3, 43, 89, 127, 161, 254
Enterocolitis 405
Exercise 68, 89, 97, 187, 318
Exercise-induced pulmonary
  hemorrhage 367
    diagnosis 368
    pathophysiology 369
    treatment 370

F

Fermentation 18
Fiber 2, 17, 80
Foals 137, 151
    body weight of 137
    diseases of 403
    "dummy foal" 406
Forage 3, 17, 25, 29, 303
    analysis 8
    composition 18

quality 7, 19
Fructans 20, 31, 303

G

Gastric ulcers 21, 79, 264, 347
    treatment 350
Gastrointestinal tract 173, 261
Grain analysis 9
Grass 19, 25, 29, 303
Gro-Trac 204
Growth 126, 137, 151, 155, 161, 185, 197, 203, 208, 213, 231, 247
Grazing 25, 29

H

Hay 7
    analysis 11-14
    soaking 304
Hindgut acidosis 306
Hyperlipidemia 260
Hypoxic ischemic encephalopathy 406

I

Ileus 331
Immune system 261
Impaction 333
Insulin resistance 285, 301, 355
Intracecal buffering 306

L

Lactation 148, 154
Laminitis 290, 293
    causes 290, 294, 303
    cryotherapy in treatment of 305
    genetic element 305

    pathology 295
Legumes 19

M

Malnutrition 260
Mares 141, 147, 151
Metabolic capacity 195
Metabolic syndrome 273, 284, 299
Milk 403
    replacer 403
Mineral deficiency 252
Mineral digestibility 20
Muscle development 193

N

NRC 123
Nutrient requirements 1, 7, 51, 161
    for growing horses 127, 208
    for pregnant mare 124, 151
    for sick horses 262
    values 10
Nutrition, enteral 336
    parenteral 338, 403

O

Obesity 288, 299
Osteochondrosis 101, 274

P

Parasites 318, 411
    control of 414, 416
    anthelmintic-resistant 415
    transmission of 412
Performance after illness 408
Polysaccharide storage myopathy 273

Prebiotics/probiotics 406
Pregnancy 4, 124, 133, 137, 152, 319

R

Racing performance 207, 231
    after illness 408
Recurrent exertional rhabdomyolysis 273
Reproduction 53, 68
Rhodococcus equi 408

S

Sale price 221
Sand colic 323
Senior horses 265
Skeletal development 162, 185
Skeletal disease 101, 185
Starvation 259
Stereotypies 77

T

Training 162, 198
Transport 320

V

Vitamin A 51
Vitamin E 61, 133

W

Weanlings 407
Weather 320